Promoting Student Happiness

The Guilford Practical Intervention in the Schools Series

Kenneth W. Merrell, Founding Editor
T. Chris Riley-Tillman, Series Editor

www.guilford.com/practical

This series presents the most reader-friendly resources available in key areas of evidence-based practice in school settings. Practitioners will find trustworthy guides on effective behavioral, mental health, and academic interventions, and assessment and measurement approaches. Covering all aspects of planning, implementing, and evaluating high-quality services for students, books in the series are carefully crafted for everyday utility. Features include ready-to-use reproducibles, lay-flat binding to facilitate photocopying, appealing visual elements, and an oversized format. Recent titles have Web pages where purchasers can download and print the reproducible materials.

Promoting Student Happiness

Positive Psychology Interventions in Schools

SHANNON M. SULDO

THE GUILFORD PRESS
New York   London

Library of Congress Cataloging-in-Publication Data

Names: Suldo, Shannon M., author.
Title: Promoting student happiness : positive psychology interventions in
    schools / Shannon M. Suldo.
Description: New York : Guilford Press, [2016] | Series: The Guilford
    practical intervention in the schools series | Includes bibliographical
    references and index.
Identifiers: LCCN 2015049502 | ISBN 9781462526802 (pbk.)
Subjects: LCSH: Students—Mental health. | Educational psychology. | School
    mental health services.
Classification: LCC LB3430 .S85 2016 | DDC 371.7/13—dc23
LC record available at *https://lccn.loc.gov/2015049502*

For my amazing family

*My loving parents, Joy and Dave, set the stage for a life
blessed daily by my supportive husband, Bobby,
and our entertaining children, Emma and Blake.*

About the Author

Shannon M. Suldo, PhD, is Professor in the School Psychology Program at the University of South Florida. Her research focuses on youth happiness, and she has completed numerous studies to understand factors that explain differences in students' levels of happiness. Dr. Suldo frequently presents her work at local, state, national, and international conferences, and has extensive experience implementing positive psychology interventions in elementary, middle, and high schools. She is a recipient of the Lightner Witmer Award from Division 16 (School Psychology) of the American Psychological Association and has coauthored more than 60 journal articles and 10 book chapters.

Acknowledgments

The contents of this book reflect 15 years of collaborative research conducted to better understand children's and adolescents' happiness. That journey began and grew through relationships with many remarkable individuals, primarily from two universities. Starting at the beginning—my graduate school training at the University of South Carolina—I had the great privilege of being mentored by Scott Huebner. Always ahead of the curve, Scott was interested in students' happiness well before it became popular. I thank him for introducing me to a topic that quickly became a shared passion. The extraordinary education I received at the University of South Carolina essentially paved the way for my later projects, and provided me with the skills, confidence, and desire to embrace research in all of my professional activities.

At the University of South Florida, my continued inquiry into youth happiness has been facilitated by university resources, namely, talented faculty collaborators with complementary content and methodological expertise, authentic partnerships with local schools, support for doctoral education that permits access to fantastic graduate student research assistants, seed grants for junior faculty, and true academic freedom. My research related to positive psychology has flourished over the years because of this multifaceted support; I am beyond grateful for my faculty and graduate student colleagues, as well as the children, parents, and teachers in my local schools who have participated in the research projects summarized in this book. Regarding faculty colleagues, I am especially indebted to John Ferron, Elizabeth Shaunessy-Dedrick, Robert Dedrick, and Sarah Kiefer, all of whom have made invaluable intellectual contributions to the research that formed the basis of this book. Additionally, my colleagues in the School Psychology Program have facilitated my diverse empirical pursuits since 2004 through their encouragement, appreciation, and suggestions; thank you to George Batsche, Kathy Bradley-Klug, Linda Raffaele Mendez, Julia Ogg, and Jose Castillo for being the kind of people who make coming to work a source of great personal happiness.

Most important, this book was made possible due to the ideas, enthusiasm, and hard work of many talented graduate students with whom I have had the pleasure to interact over the years. All of the studies on youth happiness that I have completed in the past decade have occurred in collaboration with the student members of my Positive Psychology Research Group, including (in roughly historical order) Emily Shaffer-Hudkins, Jessica Michalowski Savage, Allison Friedrich, Devon Minch, Troy Loker, Tiffany Stewart, Amanda March, Amanda Thalji-Raitano, Ashley Chappel Diehl, Melanie McMahan Albers, Sarah Fefer, Krystle Kuzia, Michelle Frey Hasemeyer, Brenna Hoy, Cheryl Duong Gelley, Lisa Bateman, Rachel Roth, Michael Frank, Bryan Bander, Sim Yin Tan, Brittany Hearon, Mollie McCullough, Jeff Garofano, Katie Wesley, Kayla Lawler LaRosa, Sarah Dickinson, Emily Esposito, and Gary Yu Hin Lam. These bright young women and men present more like co-investigators than students; interactions with them are often the highlights of my day, and inspire me to take new directions in my work. For instance, Jessica and Allison are responsible for guiding me to intervention research; I'm forever grateful that they expressed a desire to create and implement the first iteration of the Well-Being Promotion Program described in this book. Similarly, Amanda T.'s enthusiasm for studying the dual-factor model among high school students, followed by Melanie's and Ashley's devotion to following the sample across time, made possible an incredible dataset that we analyzed in multiple studies summarized in this book. Most recently, Brittany's and Mollie's interest in applying positive psychology interventions to elementary school children and teachers continues to broaden applications of this line of research to populations beyond my long-time focus on adolescents. In short, I am overcome with appreciation for the graduate students who volunteer their time as my research assistants, and thank them from the bottom of my heart for their contributions to inspiring, conducting, and disseminating much of the research that made this book possible. I look forward to many more years of successful collaboration with my student and faculty colleagues at the University of South Florida.

I also owe a great debt of gratitude to those friends who made possible the actual writing of this book. At The Guilford Press, thank you to Natalie Graham and T. Chris Riley-Tillman for encouraging my proposal for a contribution to the treasured Guilford Practical Intervention in the Schools Series, and then guiding me through the publication process. To my chapter coauthors, thank you for your willingness to share in this undertaking. Thank you, Julia, for providing insightful, warm, and lightning-fast feedback to each chapter. Similarly, thank you to Scott, Brittany, Jeff, Katie, Devon, and Don Kincaid for providing feedback to specific chapters most closely aligned with your expertise. Thank you to Joy Huanhuan Wang and Elizabeth Storey for your careful editorial assistance in ensuring correspondence between citations and references. Last, but so far from least, thank you to my amazing husband, Bobby Bucholtz, for offering reassurance, an endless supply of coffee and candy, and doing more than his fair share of the child care during the long periods that I became one with my laptop. Being a reasonably good scholar, teacher/mentor, clinician, wife, friend, and mother of young children is not an easy balance, and I appreciate the endless patience and support of my loved ones who have been along for the incredible ride over the years!

Contents

PART III. ECOLOGICAL STRATEGIES FOR PROMOTING YOUTH HAPPINESS

PART I

OVERVIEW OF STUDENT HAPPINESS

CHAPTER 1

Background and Rationale

INTRODUCTION TO HAPPINESS AND POSITIVE PSYCHOLOGY

What is happiness? Children's answers range from the concrete ("ice cream," "summer," "Disney World") to the expressive ("when I smile and all my teeth show!"). Adults' definitions can similarly range from reflections on pleasant but transient experiences ("a full night's sleep," "laughing with my best friend") to global reflections ("knowing my children are safe and loved," "success at work"). Helping to get us on the same page, scientists have generally settled on defining happiness with the term *subjective well-being*. This term, coined by Ed Diener at the University of Illinois at Urbana–Champaign, operationalizes happiness as composed of cognitive and emotional aspects. The cognitive component is life satisfaction—an individual's cognitive appraisal of one's quality of life. The emotional component includes the frequency with which one experiences positive feelings and negative feelings. Positive feelings include emotions like joyful, proud, excited, cheerful, and interested. Negative feelings include emotions like ashamed, mad, scared, sad, and guilty. Perhaps because it is the most stable component, people who have systematically studied subjective well-being in youth have most commonly assessed life satisfaction.

Psychologists' interest in happiness has boomed in the last 15 years, particularly since Martin Seligman's 1998 presidency of the American Psychological Association (APA), followed by the landmark special issue of the *American Psychologist* that was devoted to positive psychology. Martin Seligman and Mihaly Csikszentmihalyi served as guest editors of that special issue (Vol. 55, No. 1), which was published at the beginning of 2000. This millennial issue contained an introduction to a renewed emphasis on happiness and related constructs. The three pillars of positive psychology put forth included positive emotions and experiences (e.g., happiness), positive individual traits (e.g., character strengths), and positive institutions such as healthy schools and families (see *www.ppc.sas.upenn.edu*). Since that time, over 1,300 articles pertinent to positive psychology have been published in the professional literature (Donaldson, Dollwet, & Rao, 2015). Whereas most initial papers on positive psychology were conceptual in nature, the state of the field has progressed to the point that now a majority of papers published on positive psychology each year contain empirical tests of the early theories. A sizable minority of these studies (16%) have included children and adolescents in the research samples. This evolving literature contains abundant guidance on predictors (correlates) of happiness, benefits of happiness, and a growing number of studies testing interventions to increase happiness. In the intervention literature, initial studies with adults focused on establishing efficacy—that is, determining how well the interventions work in tightly controlled trials intended to maximize internal validity (see Sin & Lyubomirsky, 2009, for a review). Following repeated support for efficacy of these strategies, more recent attention has been directed to how the interventions work—in other words, for whom and why positive change in subjective well-being occurs (Layous & Lyubomirsky, 2014). The general public can learn about and make use of these interventions through Sonja Lyubomirsky's (2008) easy-to-read self-instructional guide that recommends evidence-based strategies for improving happiness.

The primary focus of this book is on innovations in intervention strategies developed for implementation by school-based practitioners. Full attention to happiness-increasing strategies follows sections on assessment (Chapter 2) and a review of the correlates (Chapter 3). Those bodies of knowledge are foundational to understanding the logical targets of intervention, as well as how to collect and use data to understand who may be most in need of such interventions, and how to monitor the impact of interventions on subjective well-being. As introduced in Chapter 4, positive psychology interventions first appeared in studies of adults (e.g., Seligman, Steen, Park, & Peterson, 2005), when psychologists began designing simple "cognitive or behavioral strategies to mirror the thoughts and behaviors of naturally happy people and, in turn, improve the happiness of the person performing them" (Layous & Lyubomirsky, 2014, p. 3). Soon after this initial research with adults advanced a set of promising positive psychology interventions, school and clinical psychologists working with youth tested them with adolescents, often in a group counseling modality (Marques, Lopez, & Pais-Ribeiro, 2011; Rashid & Anjum, 2008; Suldo, Savage, & Mercer, 2014), as presented in Chapter 5. More recently, applications of positive psychology research have been adapted for use in classrooms with elementary school students (Quinlan, Swain, Cameron, & Vella-Brodrick, 2015; Suldo, Hearon, Bander, et al., 2015; see Chapters 6 and 7). Evidence-based strategies for effectively involving parents in positive psychology interventions are described in Chapter 8. Considerations for adapting positive psychology interventions largely developed in Western cultures to youth from other cultural backgrounds are presented in Chapter 9. Chapter 10 situates positive psychology interventions in a multi-tiered system of supports for school-based promotion of student mental health. To set the stage, theoretical and empirical rationales for the use of positive psychology interventions are presented in Chapter 4.

Attention to happiness in schools is in line with calls to promote and protect youth mental health through providing a continuum of services with an emphasis on evidence-based primary prevention activities (Weisz, Sandler, Durlak, & Anton, 2005). Assessing a student's subjective well-being allows school mental health providers to capture psychological wellness along the complete range of functioning, from miserable to content to delighted. Identifying students with low subjective well-being is important for a number of reasons, including because of the inferior outcomes of students who have low subjective well-being even in the absence of psychopathology levels that would indicate risk (e.g., Suldo & Shaffer, 2008). Interventions that purposefully target subjective well-being are in line with a proactive, resource-building approach to mental health services, given the wealth of benefits associated with subjective well-being and the fact that high subjective well-being serves protective functions (Suldo & Huebner, 2004a). In sum, fostering subjective well-being is consistent with other universal approaches, such as Tier 1 efforts within a multi-tiered framework of mental health supports. Such efforts contrast traditional psychological services that are more reactionary in nature and focused primarily on Tier 3 efforts to remediate problems among those students with severe emotional distress.

THE DUAL-FACTOR MODEL OF MENTAL HEALTH

As established earlier, positive psychology involves the study of optimal functioning, including personal happiness as defined by "feeling good" about life (hedonic tradition) or reflected in striving for excellence and functioning well in life (eudaimonic tradition). Subjective well-being is strongly tied to the former tradition, which emphasizes emotional experiences. A student deemed to have high subjective well-being will report high life satisfaction, and experience more frequent positive affect (e.g., joy, elation) than negative affect (e.g., sadness, anger) (Diener, Scollon, & Lucas, 2009).

Subjective well-being (and life satisfaction in particular) has been the dominant indicator of well-being in most research to date on youth happiness. Other indicators of wellness merit consideration. Corey Keyes (2009) operationalizes positive mental health as including aspects of *social well-being* (e.g., positive interpersonal relationships, social contribution, community integration) and *psychological well-being* (e.g., personal growth, purpose in life, self-acceptance). Such indicators are closely aligned with the eudaimonic tradition, and are considered alongside indicators of *emotional well-being*, akin to the positive affect and life satisfaction components of subjective well-being. Keyes's model yields mental health categories that range from languishing (equivalent to mental unhealth) to flourishing (i.e., high hedonic/emotional well-being in addition to positive functioning in more than half of the social and psychological domains). Flourishing adolescents have fewer symptoms of depression and conduct problems, such as truancy and substance use, as compared with moderately mentally healthy or languishing youth (Keyes, 2006).

In 2011, Seligman revisited the original focus of positive psychology, and urged a shift in focus from what had been termed *authentic happiness* to instead *well-being theory*. Essentially, the shift de-emphasizes life satisfaction as the primary outcome to strive for, and broadens well-being to include five elements:

1. **Positive emotion.** In line with the classic emphasis on subjective well-being, this includes indicators of happiness and life satisfaction, which in abundance characterizes a *pleasant life*.
2. **Engagement.** The emphasis here is on experiences of *flow*, a term coined by Csikszentmihalyi (2014) to describe the mental zone people experience when they are fully immersed in activities that put their strengths and talents to use, which leads to an *engaged life*.
3. **Relationships.** In well-being theory, Seligman (2011) elevated the status of positive relationships to an element of well-being rather than a means by which people achieve positive emotions or meaning. This element entails desiring to be around other people and striving for strong relationships.

4. **Meaning.** The hallmark of a *meaningful life* entails a feeling of belongingness and service to something believed to be bigger than oneself.
5. **Accomplishment.** The *achieving life* is reflected in pursuing accomplishment for the pure sake of achievement (i.e., winning) regardless of the positive emotions that may or may not accompany the accomplishment, such as seen in the pursuit of wealth.

Seligman (2011) urges psychologists to consider all five elements of well-being (positive emotion, engagement, relationships, meaning, and accomplishment [PERMA]) rather than to equate well-being to positive emotions. What is unknown is the correlation between flourishing and subjective well-being; the association is likely high, given that subjective well-being reflects overall contentment (not just in-the-moment happiness), and is correlated with constructs reflected in the items that comprise measures of flourishing. One test of this multidimensional theory of well-being with more than 500 teenage boys in Australia found support for the separability of most factors, except that high levels on items tapping meaning converged with items in the relationship domain (Kern, Waters, Adler, & White, 2015). This factor-analytic study suggested a four-factor solution of well-being among youth:

1. Positive emotions (sample items: "frequently feeling cheerful, lively, joyful, etc.").
2. Engagement (sample item: "When I am reading or learning something new, I often lose track of how much time passed").
3. Relationships/Meaning (sample items: "I generally feel that what I do in my life is valuable; my relationships are supportive and rewarding").
4. Accomplishment (sample item: "Once I make a plan to get something done, I stick to it").

Those four well-being factors related differently to key youth outcomes—for instance, positive physical health co-occurred most with high positive emotions, whereas a growth mind-set was most strongly tied to high levels of accomplishment. Taken together, findings from this study provide preliminary support for a multidimensional conceptualization of well-being in line with the PERMA model. Adolescents' life satisfaction scores were strongly correlated with all dimensions of well-being ($r = .43$ with engagement, .55 with accomplishment, .63 with positive emotions, and .64 with relationships/meaning), underscoring the relevance of life satisfaction to all aspects of youth well-being.

Although well-being, and happiness in particular, has long been an ultimate goal of parents and even prioritized by our founding fathers as an unalienable right, in the 20th century psychopathology was the primary focus of most psychology research and treatment (Joseph & Wood, 2010; Seligman & Csikszentmihalyi, 2000). As chronicled by Seligman (2002), the field's focus on psychopathology stemmed from the need to treat emotionally distressed veterans who were returning from war, and the emphasis on illness tied to funding opportunities for research psychologists. Psychopathology encompasses psychological disorders and symptoms of an internalizing nature, such as depression and anxiety, as well as externalizing behavior disorders marked by hyperactivity, noncompliance, and other conduct problems. Traditionally, mental health diagnosis has been defined by the presence of symptoms of disorders and associated negative outcomes (impairment). If criteria are not met for a disorder, an individual is viewed as subclinical and is not routinely targeted for intervention.

There is an increased recognition of the distinctness of psychopathology and well-being among youth. The absence of psychopathology is correlated with but not equivalent to the presence of well-being, regardless if well-being is conceptualized in a multidimensional PERMA manner (Kern et al., 2015), as flourishing (i.e., by hedonic and eudemonic aspects of well-being; Keyes, 2006), or as high subjective well-being (Suldo & Shaffer, 2008). Rather, *complete mental health* may best be defined by few symptoms of psychopathology and intact subjective well-being. Indicators of subjective well-being easily afford examination of a more complete range of human flourishing—for instance, from problematic to satisfactory to thriving. While acknowledging the competing frameworks for defining youth well-being in a positive manner, this book focuses on the operationalization of happiness as subjective well-being in part to take advantage of the historical attention and relatively large research base on life satisfaction. Table 1.1 exemplifies how youth mental health has been defined in studies of students in middle school (Suldo & Shaffer, 2008) and high school (Suldo, Thalji-Raitano, Kiefer, & Ferron, in press) as a combination of scores on psychometrically sound measures of subjective well-being (described in Chapter 3) and psychopathology, such as the Behavior Assessment System for Children (BASC-2; Reynolds & Kamphaus, 2004) and the Achenbach System of Empirically Based Assessment (ASEBA; Achenbach, & Rescorla, 2001).

What research evidence supports the presence and utility of a dual-factor model of mental health in youth? Studies with students in elementary school (Greenspoon & Saklofske, 2001), middle school (Antaramian, Huebner, Hills, & Valois, 2010; Suldo & Shaffer, 2008), high school (Suldo, Thalji-Raitano, et al., in press), and college (Eklund, Dowdy, Jones, & Furlong, 2011; Renshaw & Cohen, 2014) indicate the importance of considering psychopathology and subjective well-being in tandem. These studies repeatedly found that most youth with minimal symptoms of psychopathology also have intact subjective well-being (a "complete mental health" profile), and many youth with elevated psychopathology experience diminished subjective well-

TABLE 1.1. Youth Mental Health Status as Defined within a Dual-Factor Model

Level of psychopathology	Level of subjective well-being	
	Low	Average to high
Low	*Vulnerable*	*Complete mental health*
	Subjective well-being below bottom 26–30th % of sample	Subjective well-being within top 70–74th % of sample
	and	and
	internalizing *T*-score < 60 and externalizing *T*-score < 60	internalizing *T*-score < 60 and externalizing *T*-score < 60
Elevated	*Troubled*	*Symptomatic but content*
	Subjective well-being below bottom 26–30th % of sample	Subjective well-being within top 70–74th % of sample
	and	and
	internalizing *T*-score ≥ 60 or externalizing *T*-score ≥ 60	internalizing *T*-score ≥ 60 or externalizing *T*-score ≥ 60

being (a "troubled" status). However, there are sizable groups of students for whom elevated psychopathology co-occurs with high subjective well-being (a status termed "symptomatic but content") or, conversely, minimal psychopathology exists simultaneously with low subjective well-being ("vulnerable" youth). Findings of differences in outcomes among the four groups, including between groups with similar levels of psychopathology but different levels of subjective well-being, illustrate how important it is to consider students' subjective well-being in assessments of their mental health.

Complete Mental Health

Within the five studies referenced above that categorized all youth into one of four groups, roughly two-thirds of students (average = 65%, range = 57–78% across samples) had a complete mental health status, defined by average to high levels of subjective well-being and low levels of psychopathology. The group of students with a complete mental health status have alternately been referred to in the literature as "well-adjusted," "positive mental health," and "mentally healthy." Students with complete mental health routinely show the best adjustment, including at the same time as the mental health assessment (Antaramian et al., 2010; Eklund et al., 2011; Greenspoon & Saklofske, 2001; Renshaw & Cohen, 2014; Suldo & Shaffer, 2008; Suldo, Thalji-Raitano, et al., in press), as well as later in the school year (Lyons, Huebner, & Hills, 2013) and even the next school year (Suldo, Thalji, & Ferron, 2011). Comparisons with classmates deemed vulnerable due to their diminished subjective well-being (despite a similar absence of mental health problems), indicated that students with complete mental health are more academically successful—they earn better grades, perform better on statewide tests of reading skills, are more behaviorally engaged in school, and have more positive attitudes about learning. These academic advantages persist, as seen in superior grades and attendance the following year. Such findings demonstrate the long-term benefits of the combination of low psychopathology and high subjective well-being. Students with complete mental health also have better physical health; superior social relationships with family, classmates, romantic partners, and teachers; stronger self-concepts; and flourish emotionally as seen in greater hope and gratitude.

Vulnerable

A small but consistently identifiable group of students (on average, 12.1% of students; range = 8–19% across samples) report diminished subjective well-being without manifesting many symptoms of psychopathology. Students with this vulnerable mental health profile have been referred to as "dissatisfied," "at risk," or "asymptomatic yet discontent." In a traditional model of mental health that focuses exclusively on psychopathology, vulnerable children would be unlikely to be targeted for intervention due to their absence of elevated scores on screening measures of internalizing or externalizing symptoms. Nevertheless, comparisons of these students' outcomes to their classmates with complete mental health indicate that their functioning is not optimal. Specifically, these students have worse physical health, lower self-concepts, poorer interpersonal and romantic relationships, and more academic risk relative to their peers who also do not have elevated psychopathology but experience high subjective well-being. For example, vulnerable middle school students experience more decline in grades over the course of the school year as compared to their peers with complete mental health.

Troubled

Approximately 12.8% of students (range = 8–17% across samples) have poor mental health on both factors: low subjective well-being and elevated psychopathology. Students with this troubled status—alternatively referred to as "distressed" or "mentally unhealthy"—routinely have the worst outcomes of any of the four groups. Research findings to date show that troubled students have the lowest self-concepts, poorest physical health, and a host of social problems including peer victimization and diminished social support. Compared to the two groups of students with low psychopathology, troubled and symptomatic but content adolescents earn similarly inferior course grades and scores on achievement tests. Research to date suggests that middle and high school students with symptoms of mental health problems are simply more likely to have academic challenges regardless of their level of subjective well-being. Nevertheless, findings from longitudinal studies suggest that the combination of elevated psychopathology and low subjective well-being places middle school students at risk for greater academic deterioration in terms of cognitive engagement and grade point averages (GPAs).

Symptomatic but Content

Roughly 10.1% of students in studies to date on the dual-factor model have reported average to high subjective well-being in spite of having elevated levels of mental health problems (range = 4–17%, with lower numbers yielded from studies that limited assessment of psychopathology to self-reports of internalizing symptoms). Students who are symptomatic but content—sometimes called "ambivalent" or "externally maladjusted"—would likely be identified on screeners of mental health problems, but in fact have some adaptive features relative to their troubled peers with low subjective well-being. These features include strong social relationships with parents, teachers, and classmates; high global self-worth; and academic engagement. Functioning in these domains is often comparable to the positive outcomes observed among students with complete mental health, suggesting that the presence of psychopathology symptoms is not always necessarily associated with poor adjustment. Findings from follow-up studies of middle school students show that youth with a symptomatic but content profile do not experience the worst academic outcomes across time; their troubled peers do.

In sum, the dual-factor model identifies two unique groups of students—those with a vulnerable or symptomatic but content mental health status—likely to be overlooked or misunderstood using only problem-focused methods of psychological assessment. Findings from a growing body of research on this dual-factor model of mental health underscore the need for a comprehensive approach that includes attention to students' subjective well-being. Viewing mental health only in terms of symptom levels is incomplete, as adjustment appears a function of students' levels of both subjective well-being and psychopathology symptoms.

BENEFITS OF SUBJECTIVE WELL-BEING

Few can argue that happiness is a valued state of being (i.e., a desirable outcome). But beyond an in-the-moment personal benefit, does happiness serve important functions that ensure well-being later down the road? Barbara Fredrickson's (2001) broaden-and-build theory answers "yes," that positive emotions cause an upward spiral. How? Whereas negative emotions are tied to avoidance and rigidity, positive emotions lead people to approach opportunities including challenges, and to think more flexibly, thus building personal knowledge and social connections. Accordingly, subjective well-being is a resource to be fostered, in that it promotes subsequent positive outcomes. Support for this theory's applicability to youth in the educational context comes from a study of high school students who were examined five times across the course of the school year (Stiglbauer, Gnambs, Gamsjäger, & Batinic, 2013). This research found that positive experiences at school—conceptualized as students' psychological needs being met through feeling connected to teachers and classmates, confident in their academic abilities, and valuing education—promoted greater positive affect. The frequent cheerful moods, in turn, facilitated more positive experiences at school. Thus, happiness was both an outcome and a cause of healthy experiences of relatedness, competence, and autonomy at school. These reciprocal relations demonstrated how students' positive affect can lead to "an upward spiral of positive school experiences and happiness over time" (Stiglbauer et al., 2013, p. 239).

While thriving at school is understandably a primary goal of school mental health providers, from a public health perspective physical health may be among the most significant outcomes. Among adults, a large body of research indicates that people with higher subjective well-being live longer, leading Diener and Chan (2011) to conclude:

> When one considers that the years lived of a happy person are more enjoyable and experienced with better health, the importance of the subjective well-being and health findings is even more compelling. It is perhaps time to add interventions to improve subjective well-being to the list of public health measures, and alert policy makers to the relevance of subjective well-being for health and longevity. (p. 32)

Physical health is one of the many outcomes that distinguished youth with different mental health statuses as indicated from a dual-factor model. As described in the prior section, students with complete mental health—defined by average to high subjective well-being along with minimal psychopathology—demonstrate superior functioning across key domains of development: academic, social, identity, and physical health. Furthermore, the adjustment advantages associated with a symptomatic but content status (in relation to their troubled peers), suggests that average to high subjective well-being may protect students with elevated psychopathology from manifesting the worst developmental outcomes.

The notion of subjective well-being as a protective factor is consistent with findings from earlier research that found a buffering effect of life satisfaction (Suldo & Huebner, 2004a). Specifically, middle and high school students who experienced more stressful life events displayed more externalizing behavior problems a year later, but only if they began the study with low life satisfaction. High life satisfaction protected students from developing increases in externalizing behaviors in the face of stress. Findings from other longitudinal research demonstrate that students' levels of subjective well-being predict their later academic adjustment, above and beyond the influence of psychopathology and initial academic performance. These studies found that subjective well-being exerted a unique influence on later student engagement (Lyons et al., 2013) and grades earned in courses (Suldo et al., 2011). The additive value of information on student subjective well-being in explaining and predicting student adjustment has implications for assessment and intervention.

INCORPORATING POSITIVE PSYCHOLOGY IN SCHOOL MENTAL HEALTH SERVICES

Whether in a schoolwide or indicated manner, assessments of youth subjective well-being are recommended as supplemental to traditional indicators of psychopathology. Chapter 2 presents multiple options for how to assess life satisfaction through self-report measures of global and domain-specific satisfaction that are free in the public domain and psychometrically sound, as developed by Scott Huebner and colleagues. The small-group positive psychology interventions presented in Chapter 5 may be particularly indicated for students with low life satisfaction. Just as school mental health providers treating students with mental illness attempt to understand the risk factors that cause and maintain a particular student's symptoms, determinants of subjective well-being include promotive factors. Tools have been advanced recently that help school mental health providers assess these external and internal assets that contribute to students' global life satisfaction. Specifically, Chapter 2 presents the Social and Emotional Health Survey as developed by Michael Furlong and colleagues (Furlong, You, Renshaw, Smith, & O'Malley, 2014). The Social and Emotional Health Survey measures 12 positive psychological "building blocks" (variables such as gratitude, zest, emotion regulation, peer support, and self-efficacy) that comprise students' level of underlying "covitality." Furlong uses the term *covitality* in reference to a latent meta-construct that reflects "the synergistic effect of positive mental health resulting from the interplay among multiple positive psychological building blocks" (Furlong, You, et al., 2014, p. 1013). Covitality, in turn, is highly predictive of subjective well-being. For instance, within high school students, the correlation between latent covitality and subjective well-being constructs is .89 (Furlong, You, et al., 2014). The measures of life satisfaction and covitality will be useful during school mental health providers' efforts to improve subjective well-being through those positive psychology interventions (Chapter 5) that target its correlates (Chapter 3), including some of the building blocks captured on the Social and Emotional Health Survey. Whereas a plethora of evidence-based interventions exist for practitioners to use with students whose mental health status indicates elevated psychopathology (see Weisz & Kazdin, 2010, for examples), the 10-session positive psychology intervention program described in Chapter 5 represents a relatively new development in the field to improve youth subjective well-being through teaching students to purposefully increase thoughts and behaviors that are consistent with theory regarding the determinants of happiness (summarized in Chapter 4).

Chapter 10 calls attention to multi-tiered systems of support (MTSS), tied to a public health approach to prevention and wellness promotion through systematic and coordinated services and practices (Doll, Cummings, & Chapla, 2014; Eber, Weist, & Barrett, 2013). Positive psychology interventions, as described throughout this book, systematically build competence and capitalize on the protective processes within students and their environments to increase subjective well-being, as well as buffer against mental health problems (Nelson, Schnorr, Powell, & Huebner, 2013; Seligman & Csikszentmihalyi, 2000). Practices to promote subjective well-being are thus essential in a prevention framework, as illustrated by research that finds diminished life satisfaction predicts the later onset of mental health problems like depression (Lewinsohn, Redner, & Seeley, 1991). This may be because the positive thoughts and activities common to happy people effectively reduce and disrupt common risk factors, such as loneliness and tendencies to ruminate on negative experiences (Layous, Chancellor, & Lyubomirsky, 2014). Empirical support for such an influence of subjective well-being on psychopathology comes from repeated assessments of youth mental health, which suggest that life satisfaction predicts later extent of psychopathology, rather than the reverse directionality. Specifically, whereas neither externalizing nor internalizing symptoms predicted later life satisfaction, middle school students with lower life satisfaction later reported higher levels of externalizing behaviors and, for boys but not girls, more internalizing symptoms (Lyons, Otis, Huebner, & Hills, 2014).

Universal strategies to promote life satisfaction may skirt issues of access and stigma associated with targeted interventions that may be indicated, as signs of problems follow diminished subjective well-being. Schoolwide efforts to promote students' subjective well-being can target the factors that correlate with life satisfaction (summarized in Chapter 3), such as the dimensions of school climate that co-occur with optimal mental health. As described in Chapter 7, universal strategies that include teacher and/or peer components may be particularly plausible in school-based applications of positive psychology given school mental health providers' proximity to these sources during the school day. Students often learn in partnership with peers, teachers, and other school support staff within an environment that can naturally reinforce a system of support and care.

APPROACHES SIMILAR TO POSITIVE PSYCHOLOGY

Researchers who identify with positive psychology are certainly not the first to focus on goals like psychopathology prevention, competence promotion and skill development, cultivation of youth strengths, or optimal functioning. Some earlier such theoretical frameworks and initiatives with compatible goals are described next.

Humanistic Therapy

Carl Rogers's person-centered approach to mental health treatment emphasizes his theory of individuals' actualizing tendency—the innate desire to maximize experience and achieve one's full potential (Joseph & Murphy, 2013). Other similarities between the person-centered approach and positive psychology include rejection of the medical model of mental health practice and an emphasis on strengths (Raskin, Rogers, & Witty, 2014). As noted by O'Grady (2013), Carl Rogers deserves credit for noting that happiness follows from purposeful efforts to live life fully and strive to reach one's potential.

Social and Emotional Learning

Developing youth into responsible, socially skilled citizens who care for one another and contribute to a strong society requires more than direct instruction in academic skills. Schoolwide curricula geared toward fostering social and emotional health fall under the umbrella of social–emotional learning (SEL). Such universal efforts to promote mental health predate positive psychology interventions, but are likewise grounded in a primary prevention framework that emphasizes positive development (Weisz et al., 2005). As described by Greenberg and colleagues (2003), in the mid-1990s, key players in educational efforts intended to prevent a host of negative outcomes, such as drug use and violence, or promote social–emotional development of good character, emotional intelligence, and civic engagement, coalesced to establish the Collaborative for Academic, Social, and Emotional Learning (CASEL). Resources disseminated on *www.casel.org* include summaries of the key features and empirical support for a growing number of schoolwide programs intended to build students' skills for managing emotions, conveying empathy and care for others, making responsible decisions, and forming positive relationships.

Positive Youth Development

Research largely from developmental psychology has identified a core set of internal factors (including social–emotional competencies), as well as external factors that shape a positive trajectory of growth into a productive adult. Core principles from the line of inquiry emphasize the powerful impact of caring relationships and communities, including informal support in a neighborhood as well as organized after-school programs, which facilitate and reinforce youth growth of internal assets. For example, purpose is one of the 20 internal assets, which complement the 20 external assets, advanced in the developmental assets framework (*www.search-institute.org*). Damon, Menon, and Bronk (2003) conceptualize the search for purpose as "key to achieving the fortuitous ends envisioned by the positive psychology movement, such as authentic happiness" (p. 120). Purpose reflects individuals' goal-directed strivings for accomplishments that are both personally meaningful and help a cause beyond oneself, such as matters important to the larger family, community, faith, or country. Asset-rich environments provide, for instance, opportunities to make a difference through helping others (e.g., adults or peers provide models of volunteerism; parents commonly discuss current events) and a safe and constructive use of time (e.g., regular participation in high-quality structured activities). Youth with such external assets have greater well-being as reflected in reduced risk-taking behavior and emotional distress (depression), and substantially higher life satisfaction (Scales et al., 2008).

Resilience Research

In general, resilience refers to "patterns of positive adaptation during or following significant adversity" (Masten, Cutuli, Herbers, & Reed, 2009, p. 118). Whereas positive youth development emphasizes contexts that engender optimal outcomes for all individuals regardless of risk level, resilience research focuses on predictors of adequate outcomes for youth who may otherwise appear on a path for developing psychopathology due to their stressors and adverse situations. Although discovered in studies of youth who experience enormous challenges, the resulting list of promotive or protective factors that distinguished those youth who did not succumb to their high risk status has substantial overlap with the assets identified within positive youth development (Masten, 2014). Commonalities include features within the child (e.g., faith and meaning/purpose; self-esteem; positive view of one's future, expressed as hope or optimism), within the family (e.g., parent involvement in schooling; authoritative parenting/support), and within the community (e.g., high levels of safety; involvement in prosocial organizations). These person-focused findings have informed the theory behind clinical applications that target the child-level correlates of superior adaptation. For example, the Penn Resiliency Program (Gillham, Jaycox, Reivich, Seligman, & Silver, 1990) referenced in Chapters 4 and 5 targets optimistic thinking and positive social relationships, protective factors implicated in the prevention of depression.

Clearly, the goals and intervention targets of positive psychology have deep roots in efforts within clinical and educational psychology, as well as in educational practices that perpetuate youth compliance with societal norms through character education approaches. Positive psychology is distinguished in part by emphasis on personal emotional growth, indexed by subjective well-being, among all youth. Even those currently satisfied students should be afforded the opportunity to become delighted, in recognition of the upward spiral caused by positive emotions that engender grander social and educational experiences (Fredrickson, 2001; Stiglbauer et al., 2013). A primary means of facilitating subjective well-being is to maximize student awareness and use of his or her character strengths, some of which are indeed synonymous with the "positive values" reflecting honesty, moral bravery, and fairness within the internal developmental assets framework. Differences include the *prescriptive* nature of many earlier character education programs that focus on building a specific set of internal assets (including those from a developmental assets or social–emotional competencies framework) within all students. This contrasts with the *descriptive* nature of many positive psychology interventions that guide students to discover their signature character strengths and nurture those strengths through intentional increased use in multiple contexts within their daily lives (Linkins, Niemiec, Gillham, & Mayerson, 2015). The latter approach is more individualized, and involves exploration of the 24 strengths captured in the Values in Action Inventory of Strengths (VIA-IS-Youth; Park & Peterson, 2006). The VIA-IS-Youth is commonly used to develop an individual profile of ranked character strengths, as described in Chapter 5.

Other interventions advanced from positive psychology to increase happiness entail strategies designed to mimic the thoughts and actions of naturally happy people (Layous & Lyubomirsky, 2014). Whereas the protective factors within resiliency research arose from a focus on people at heightened risk for adverse outcomes, the theoretical basis for targets of positive psychology interventions arose from a focus on people extreme in terms of their high subjective well-being. Of note, in contrast to the aforementioned disciplines most strongly tied to positive youth development and resilience research, advancements in positive psychology pertinent to child and adolescent populations have been led by many school psychologists who have made numerous conceptual and empirical contributions to measurement, theory, and applications in the school setting (Donaldson et al., 2015).

THE INTENDED AUDIENCE FOR THIS BOOK

Ideally, future growth in the relatively young positive psychology movement will build on key findings and lessons learned from compatible predecessor efforts. Cross-disciplinary research collaboration and dissemination efforts are also vital to preventing redundancy and fragmentation, as well as extending the reach of research developments to all those who serve youth regardless of the primary setting. In that vein, although much of the applied efforts done to date that are described in subsequent chapters have been conducted by school psychologists serving youth at school, mental health professionals from a variety of disciplines—including social work, counseling, and child clinical psychology will likely find the intervention strategies applicable to their efforts to promote children's and adolescents' happiness. Therefore, in this book the term *practitioner* is purposefully used in reference to any school mental health provider or trained clinician who is serving youth in a pediatric, outpatient, or alternative setting.

CHAPTER 2

Measuring Students' Well-Being

with E. Scott Huebner and Michael Furlong

In keeping with defining happiness through the subjective well-being construct, this chapter describes popular methods for measuring life satisfaction in practice, as well as notes how affect has been measured in research. Following is a description of the Social and Emotional Health Survey (Furlong, You, et al., 2014) developed to assess the positive psychological building blocks that provide an index of students' covitality, which predicts the subjective well-being outcome. Reproducible copies of these life satisfaction and covitality measures are provided in the Appendix.

MEASURING SUBJECTIVE WELL-BEING

How can well-being best be assessed in children? You might think you can readily "see" a child's level of subjective well-being, or more specifically, his or her life satisfaction. Some personal characteristics are relatively easy to observe, whereas others are not. You might believe that a child's typical observable feelings, such as sadness or joy, would reflect his or her life satisfaction. Nevertheless, although children's judgments of their quality of life are positively correlated with their positive emotions, they are not interchangeable. A child can report high life satisfaction yet also demonstrate relatively few positive emotions and/or frequent negative emotions (Huebner, 1991b). When asked to estimate their children's life satisfaction, parents' reports are

E. Scott Huebner, PhD, is Professor in the School Psychology Program in the Department of Psychology at the University of South Carolina.

Michael Furlong, PhD, is Professor in the Department of Counseling, Clinical, and School Psychology at the University of California, Santa Barbara.

moderately correlated with their children's reports, leaving room for error (Huebner, Brantley, Nagle, & Valois, 2002). To most accurately measure children's subjective well-being, school professionals use the standardized self-report instruments described below, in which students serve as the "experts" regarding their levels of life satisfaction. The self-report format is the primary assessment vehicle because children's perceptions of the quality of their lives are not only relatively inaccessible through other methods (e.g., direct observation), but also because children's reports are increasingly considered important in their own right (Ben-Arieh, 2008).

Before we focus on the multiple measures practitioners can use to measure youth life satisfaction, it should be noted that several of the studies of youth subjective well-being referenced in other chapters examined both the cognitive and affective dimensions. The latter emotional dimension has been assessed most commonly with the 27-item Positive and Negative Affect Scale for Children (PANAS-C; Laurent et al., 1999). Individuals who administer the PANAS-C can select the time frame that children should consider when reporting their emotional experiences. Are you interested in how someone is feeling *right now*? Or in what emotions he or she has experienced in the *past 24 hours*? Or in the *past few weeks*? Logically, more accurate recall, as well as transience in moods, is associated with shorter durations. In research that attempts to capture students' subjective well-being in order to understand their happiness in relation to other factors, we have asked students to reflect on the extent to which they have felt various feelings and emotions *during the past few weeks*. In other studies that have collected affect ratings quite frequently as part of a progress monitoring system—for instance, to look for change in emotions over the course of different activities—we have changed the directions to ask students to rate how often they have experienced the various feelings and emotions *within the past day*.

Three major approaches have been employed in the assessment of life satisfaction: global, general, and multidimensional life satisfaction. The global approach assumes that life satisfaction reports are best obtained using domain-free questions (e.g., "My life is going well") versus domain-based questions (e.g., "My life *at school* is going well"). In this approach, children formulate their responses to the questions based on their own unique criteria. In contrast, general life satisfaction reports are based on the sum of questions covering a variety of specific domains (e.g., questions addressing satisfaction with school life, family life, and friends). Thus, the total score is based on the sum of the particular domain-based questions that have been included by the test developer. Thus, if one measure includes items measuring satisfaction with domains that differ from another measure, the "general" or total scores should be different because the total scores reflect varying combinations of domains. For example, Cummins and Lau's (2005) measure for youth is based on the total of scores on seven domains including material well-being, health, productivity, intimacy, safety, place in community, and emotional well-being, whereas Huebner's (1994) measure is based on the domains of family, friends, school, self, and living environment. In contrast to a focus on total scores reflecting "overall" well-being, multidimensional measures of life satisfaction have been designed to assess multiple domains of importance to children, yielding a profile of separate scores for each domain. The selection of which measure or measures that a professional wishes to use should thus be based on which particular domains of life satisfaction he or she wants to measure.

Regardless of the particular measure, all life satisfaction measures represent a positive psychology approach to youth well-being. In contrast to conceptual models (and associated measures) that infer positive well-being from the absence of psychopathological symptoms, life satisfaction measures are consistent with the World Health Organization's (1948) early definition of health as a state of complete physical, mental, and social well-being. Life satisfaction measures are all designed to differentiate levels of life satisfaction above (as well as below) a neutral point of satisfaction. In this fashion, a "high" level of life satisfaction is not defined simply as the absence of dissatisfaction. Children who are "mildly satisfied" can be differentiated from children who are "moderately" and "highly" satisfied with their lives as a whole or with specific domains.

Extensive reviews of the psychometric properties of life satisfaction measures are available in Proctor, Linley, and Maltby (2009a). If a global assessment of youth life satisfaction is desired, the Students' Life Satisfaction Scale (SLSS; Huebner, 1991a, 1991b) has been recommended (Proctor et al., 2009a). If a multidimensional measure is desired, the Multidimensional Students' Life Satisfaction Scale (MSLSS; Huebner, 1994) has been recommended (Proctor et al., 2009a). In addition to the MSLSS, a much shorter measure, the Brief Multidimensional Students' Life Satisfaction Scale (BMSLSS; Seligson, Huebner, & Valois, 2003, 2005) has been developed for large-scale monitoring and research studies, as well as clinical screening and intervention studies.

Students' Life Satisfaction Scale

The SLSS is a brief, seven-item self-report measure that was designed for use with children ages 8–18. The items require children to judge their satisfaction with life as a whole, thus the items are written to be context free (see above). Supplemental positive and negative affect items were developed and used along with the SLSS items during its development in order to clarify the distinctiveness of the life satisfaction construct tapped by the SLSS in relation to related subjective well-being variables (Huebner, 1991a, 1991b).

Administration and Scoring

The SLSS can be administered to individuals or groups. The initial version of the SLSS used a 4-point frequency response option scale (e.g., Huebner, 1991b). However, subsequent research suggested that a 6-point extent format was more appropriate (Gilman & Huebner, 1997). This revised format consists of response options of 1 = *strongly disagree*, 2 = *moderately disagree*, 3 = *mildly disagree*, 4 = *mildly agree*, 5 = *moderately agree*, and 6 = *strongly agree*. Higher scores thus indicate higher degrees of life satisfaction. The complete measure and instructions can be found in the Appendix.

The SLSS has been used with nonclinical samples of students ranging in age from 8 to 18 years. Studies of nonclinical samples began in the 1990s (e.g., Dew & Huebner, 1994; Huebner, 1991b) and have continued to the present. Additional samples from clinical and other special populations have included at-risk students (Huebner & Alderman, 1993); adjudicated adolescents (Crenshaw, 1998); gifted students (Ash & Huebner, 1998); and students with learning disabilities (McCullough & Huebner, 2003), emotional disturbance (Huebner & Alderman, 1993), hearing impairments (Gilman, Easterbrooks, & Frey, 2004), and chronic health conditions (Hexdall & Huebner, 2007). The SLSS has also been used in international studies as well (e.g., Marques, Pais-Ribeiro, & Lopez, 2007; Park & Huebner, 2005).

Psychometric Properties

Studies have supported the unidimensional nature of the scale. Estimates of internal consistency typically fall in the .80s. Research on stability coefficients and changes related to interventions suggests that children's responses are relatively stable yet sensitive to systematic intervention programs. SLSS scores show meaningful patterns of convergent and discriminant validity correlations. For example, SLSS scores are positively related to the occurrence of positive life events, negatively related to negative life events, and unrelated to intelligence test scores (see Huebner & Hills, 2013, for a review of the psychometric properties of the SLSS).

Multidimensional Students' Life Satisfaction Scale

The original version of the MSLSS consisted of 40 items, however, an abbreviated version has been developed with 30 items (Huebner, Zullig, & Saha, 2012). The shorter version eliminated 10 negatively keyed items included in the original version, increasing its brevity, yet maintaining adequate reliability. The remaining number of items for each subscale range from five (school domain) to seven (family and self domains). In contrast with children's judgment of their life satisfaction with their lives as a whole, the MSLSS was designed to assess children's judgments of their life satisfaction in major, specific life domains. The MSLSS thus provides a multidimensional profile of children's life satisfaction judgments, in an effort to ensure more focused assessment and intervention information. For example, students reporting relatively high degrees of satisfaction with their schooling experiences along with relatively low degrees of satisfaction with their family experiences may necessitate differing intervention programs from students who indicate dissatisfaction with school and family circumstances.

Specifically, the MSLSS was designed to (1) provide a profile of children's satisfaction with five important, specific life domains (i.e., school, family, friends, self, living environment); (2) show relevance across the wide age range of 8–18 years; and (3) be applicable across varying ability levels (i.e., children with mild developmental disabilities through gifted children). The particular domains were selected following focus groups, essays, and ratings from pilot studies of elementary school- through secondary school-age students.

Administration and Scoring

The 30- or 40-item versions of the MSLSS may be administered to individuals or groups. Similar to the SLSS, the current version of the MSLSS employs a 6-point response options scale, in which 1 = *strongly disagree* to 6 = *strongly agree*. Higher scores thus indicate higher degrees of satisfaction in each domain. Because the subscales consist of unequal numbers of items, the domain scores can be made comparable by summing the item responses and dividing by the number of items in the domain. The complete 40-item measure and instructions can be found in the Appendix. The reverse-keyed items that were eliminated from the abbreviated version (Huebner et al., 2012) are indicated by an asterisk for users who would like to consider using the shorter version.

Like the SLSS, the MSLSS has been used in a variety of studies with samples of clinical and nonclinical groups of children and adolescents. The MSLSS has also been utilized with youth in other nations (cf. Gilman et al., 2008).

Psychometric Properties

Internal consistency (alpha) coefficients for the 40-item MSLSS range from .70 to .90, and test–retest coefficients for 2- and 4-week time periods fall mostly in the .70–.90 range, providing further support for the reliability of the scale. The results of exploratory and confirmatory factor analyses have supported the dimensionality of the MSLSS. Convergent and discriminant validity have also been demonstrated through predicted correlations with other self-report subjective well-being measures, parent reports, teacher reports of school behavior, and social desirability scales. Unique aspects of the applicability and validity of the MSLSS in the assessment of the well-being of several specific groups of children with exceptionalities, such as students with intellectual disabilities and behavior disorders, have been reported on in various publications (see Huebner & Hills, 2013, for a review of the psychometric properties of the MSLSS).

Brief Multidimensional Students' Life Satisfaction Scale

The BMSLSS (Seligson et al., 2003) was designed to fill the need for a reliable and valid measure of life satisfaction that was relevant, developmentally appropriate, and sufficiently brief to be useful in screening contexts or in large-scale surveys of children and adolescents, such as national and cross-national surveys. Specifically, it was designed to reflect the conceptual model underlying the MSLSS. The BMSLSS is thus a five-item self-report measure that assesses satisfaction with respect to each of the five domains included on the MSLSS, as described above—that is, students rate their satisfaction on a single item for each of the five domains of family life, friendships, school experiences, self, and living environment. A single item covering satisfaction with life overall can also be included.

Administration and Scoring

The BMSLSS can be administered to groups or individuals. Response options are on a 7-point scale (Andrews & Withey, 1976) that ranges from 1 = *terrible* to 7 = *delighted*. Evidence for the usefulness of a 5-point response option scale, in which 1 = *very dissatisfied* to 5 = *very satisfied*, has also been provided for the BMSLSS by Athey, Kelly, and Dew-Reeve (2012). The measure and instructions can be found in the Appendix.

Consistent with studies of the SLSS and MSLSS, the BMSLSS has been employed in research with children from ages 8 to 18. It has been used in two large-scale studies in the United States in particular. The BMSLSS was included in the 1997 South Carolina Youth Risk Behavior Survey of the Centers for Disease Control and administered to over 5,500 high school students in South Carolina (Huebner, Drane, & Valois, 2000) and in a study of 2,502 middle school students in South Carolina (Huebner, Valois, Paxton, & Drane, 2005).

Psychometric Properties

Reliability (alpha) coefficients for the BMSLSS generally fall within the .70–.80 range. Evidence for stability across short- and longer-term time periods has also been provided. The BMSLSS items show a unidimensional factor structure and a meaningful pattern of convergent and discriminant validity correlations with scores on the lengthier MSLSS (for reviews of the psychometric properties of the BMSLSS, see Huebner & Hills, 2013; Huebner, Seligson, Valois, & Suldo, 2006) and with other measures (e.g., positive affect, negative affect, social desirability responding).

Summary of Hedonic Subjective Well-Being Measurement

Although psychometrically sound measures of global and domain-based life satisfaction for children and adolescents were relatively slow to be developed, a variety of developmentally appropriate measures for youth are now available. Recent developments should help facilitate the determination of the effectiveness and efficacy of intervention efforts, such as those described in this book. As these measures are refined and better normative samples become available, school professionals should be able to confidently monitor students' well-being, perhaps providing "routine well-being check-ups" (Frisch, 1998, p. 36), as well as to study the effects of individual and group intervention programs.

Based on suggestions by Harter (1985) for self-concept assessments, Huebner, Nagle, and Suldo (2003) suggested that the clinical utility of such life satisfaction measures may be increased by a kind of "testing of the limits" procedure. Such a procedure would aim to elucidate some of the processes used by individuals or small groups of children to determine their responses to the various items. For example, following students' completion of the measures, open-ended questions could be asked, such as "What makes you agree/disagree that your life is going well?" or "What are the major things you think about when you say you like/dislike school?" Such procedures may be especially useful in some cases to inform interpretations derived from the responses of youth with disabilities (Brantley, Huebner, & Nagle, 2002; Griffin & Huebner, 2000).

The readers should note that the SLSS, MSLSS, and BMSLSS are available at no cost and can be used without additional permission from the author(s). Therefore, practitioners and researchers may use them or modify them as necessary to suit their purposes.

MEASURING PSYCHOLOGICAL DISPOSITIONS THAT UNDERLIE SUBJECTIVE WELL-BEING

When implementing positive psychology interventions in school contexts, there are three core considerations when selecting measures to use to evaluate students' needs at intake as well as program effectiveness. First, and foremost, is the selection of a general measure of subjective well-being, as described in the first section of this chapter. Using the BMSLSS or the SLSS scales alone or in combination with the PANAS-C provides an efficient and well-documented index of subjective well-being.

Unitary Strength Measures

A second consideration is deciding whether it makes sense to focus on one or more unitary positive psychology constructs that are associated with thriving subjective well-being. In this vein, companion measures of hope (Snyder, 2005) and gratitude (Froh et al., 2011), for example, provide information about constructs that are related to positive youth development but which themselves are not direct measures of subjective well-being. These latter assessments are measures of psychological dispositions or skills. Fortunately, there are a range of pertinent measures from which to select, with the strongest evidence base for the unitary constructs of optimism, forgiveness, mindfulness, and grit, in addition to the aforementioned hope and gratitude. The use of now well-developed measures of those constructs is based on a theory of change in which well-being cannot be "taught" directly, but it is possible to be fostered via the enhancement of internal psychological dispositions that have direct and indirect effects on subjective well-being.

Multidimensional Strength Measures

A third consideration, and the one discussed in more detail in the remaining sections of this chapter, is deciding whether any of the recently developed multidimensional measures might provide an appropriate, comprehensive understanding of how a positive psychology intervention has impacted students. Olenik, Zdrojewski, and Bhattacharya (2013) provide a review of measures that assess multiple indicators associated with positive developmental trajectories leading toward higher levels of subjective well-being. These measures are designed to evaluate integrated constructs that are thought to complement one another and when present together promote more robust psychological development.

Positive Youth Development—Short Form

One measure (two versions) with a solid research foundation based on national longitudinal studies of the 4-H program is the Positive Youth Development—Short Form (PYD-SF; 34 items) and the Positive Youth Development—Very Short Form (17 items; Geldhof et al., 2014). The PYD-SF measures the core components of Learner's five C's of positive youth development: competence, confidence, connection, character, and caring/compassion, which when fostered during adolescence increases the odds that a youth will "be on a life trajectory marked by mutually influential person–context relations that contribute to self, family, community, and civil society" (Geldhoff et al., 2014, p. 164).

PERMA Model

Seligman's (2011) PERMA model (positive emotions, engagement, relationships, meaning, and accomplishment; described in Chapter 1) provides another multidimensional framework of youth strengths considered to foster "flourishing." In the short time since its development, schools, particularly in Australia (e.g., White & Waters, 2015), have infused PERMA's constructs into their educational structure. Recently, the preliminary development of a strengths assessment based on the PERMA model has been reported (Kern et al., 2014). This instrument has 34 items that assess positive emotions (alpha = .92), engagement (alpha = .68), relationships (alpha = .85), and accomplishment (alpha = .84). More research is needed to refine the "meaning" component of this PERMA measure. This instrument also has companion internalizing distress scales (depression and anxiety), which could be used within a dual-factor evaluation framework, as described in Chapter 1.

Child Trends Flourishing Children Project

Another comprehensively developed multicomponent assessment was created by the Child Trends Flourishing Children Project (FCP; Lippman et al., 2014; see also *www.childtrends.org/ our-research/positive-indicators/positive-indicators-project/#box*). The FCP assessment is a set of 19 brief measures designed to measure the following components associated with flourishing subjective well-being (each of the 19 FCP components are described in individual pages on the Child Trends website): (1) *personal flourishing* (gratitude, forgiveness, hope, life satisfaction, goal orientation, purpose, spirituality); (2) *flourishing in school and work* (diligence and reliability, educational engagement, initiative taking, trustworthiness and integrity, thrift); (3) *flourishing in relationships* (positive friendships with peers, positive relationships with parents); (4) *relationship skills* (empathy, social competence); (5) *helping others to flourish* (altruism, helping family and friends); and (6) *environmental stewardship* (environmental stewardship).

Social Emotional Health Survey—Secondary

The Social Emotional Health Survey—Secondary (SEHS-S) is a multidimensional assessment of adolescents' psychological strengths. The SEHS-S conceptual foundation is based on the supposition that as all youth develop they address fundamental developmental tasks that have implications for their subjective well-being. As this developmental process unfolds, a youth builds basic self–other attitudes or cognitive dispositions. These dispositions help a youth organize his or her world and his or her place in it to foster positive development and protect against psychological distress. In addition, the SEHS-S model suggests that these dispositions work together to foster higher levels of subjective well-being (Jones, You, & Furlong, 2013). The combined and interactive effect of positive psychological dispositions has been called *covitality* (Renshaw et al., 2014). See Renshaw and colleagues (2014) for a description of the conceptual and research groundings of SEHS-S components.

The SEHS-S assesses core psychosocial strengths based on a higher-order model that consists of four latent traits (each comprised of three measured subscales): *belief-in-self* (with subscales of self-efficacy, self-awareness, and persistence), *belief-in-others* (with subscales of school support, peer support, and family coherence), *emotional competence* (with subscales of emotional regulation, behavioral self-control, and empathy), and *engaged living* (with subscales of gratitude, zest, and optimism) (Furlong, You, Renshaw, Smith, & O'Malley, 2014). Figure 2.1 shows the SEHS-S conceptual model.

ADMINISTRATION AND SCORING

This 36-item instrument is used with youth ages 13–18 years. For 10 of the 12 subscales, the students' self-reports are completed using a 4-point scale (1 = *not at all true of me*, 2 = *a little true of me*, 3 = *pretty much true of me*, and 4 = *very much true of me*). The gratitude and zest

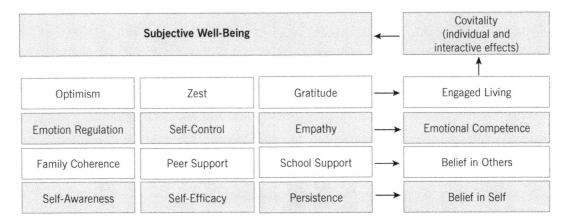

FIGURE 2.1. SEHS-S measurement components and their relation to subjective well-being.

measured subscales use a 5-point response scale: (1 = *not at all*, 2 = *very little*, 3 = *somewhat*, 4 = *quite a lot*, 5 = *extremely*). The SEHS-S items are listed in the Appendix.

PSYCHOMETRIC PROPERTIES

To date, six studies have examined the psychometric properties of the SEHS-S. Confirmatory factor analyses provided construct validity support for the SEHS-S higher-order measurement model, as shown in Figure 2.1 (Furlong, You, et al., 2014; Ito, Smith, You, Shimoda, & Furlong, 2105; Lee, You, & Furlong 2015; You et al., 2014). Each analysis reproduced the same higher-order structure with high factor loadings (all in the .50–.91 range) and no double-loading items. Evidence supporting measurement invariance has been found for gender (Furlong, You, et al., 2014; Ito et al., 2015; Lee et al., 2015), younger and older adolescents (You et al., 2014), and for five ethnic groups (Latino, white, Asian, black, and multiethnic) of California students (You, Furlong, Felix, & O'Malley, 2015). Reported internal consistency reliabilities have been consistent and favorable across previous studies: belief-in-self (.75–.84), belief-in-others (.81–.87), emotional competence (.78–.82), engaged living (.87–.88), and covitality (total score across the 36 items = .91–.95).

Prior research has found that the SEHS-S covitality index is positively associated with subjective well-being. Lee and colleagues (2015; $r = .56$) and Kim, Dowdy, and Furlong (2014; $r = .57$) reported strong correlations between covitality and subjective well-being, as measured by the SLSS and the PANAS-C. Using a more complex structural equation model, Furlong and colleagues (2013), Lee and colleagues (2015), and Ito and colleagues (2015) found that an increase of 1 standard deviation in the covitality index was associated with a nearly 1 standard deviation increase in subjective well-being (betas = .89–.94). You and colleagues (2014) reported that each 1 standard deviation increase of covitality was associated with about a two-thirds decrease of psychological distress as measured by the Behavioral Emotional Screening Survey (BESS; Kamphaus & Reynolds, 2007).

To convey in a more practical way the strength of the relation between covitality and subjective well-being, Figure 2.2 presents data from the Furlong and colleagues (2013) sample.

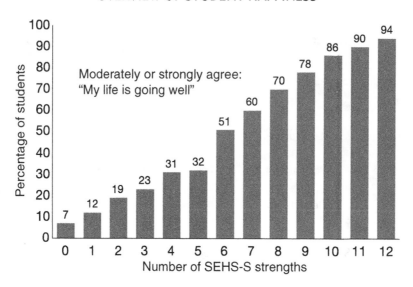

FIGURE 2.2. Percentage of students responding moderately or strongly agree with the SLSS item "My life is going well" by number of SEHS-S strengths.

Here, if students' average response to the three items in each of the 12 subscales was in the positive direction (3 on a 4-point response scale and 4 on a 5-point response scale), then they were considered to have the strength—students could therefore have from 0 to 12 SEHS-S strengths. Figure 2.2 shows the comparison between the number of students' strengths and percentage of students who responded either "moderately" or "strongly" agreeing with the SLSS item "My life is going well." As shown, for each additional individual SEHS-S positive psychological disposition, there was an increase in the proportion of students who responded affirmatively to this prototypic life satisfaction item.

Furthermore, students' SEHS-S responses have shown positive links to other quality-of-life indicators of importance to school psychologists and all educators: *feeling safe at school* (Furlong et al., 2013), *academic course grades* (Furlong et al., 2013; Lee et al., 2015), *prosocial behaviors at school* (Ito et al., 2015), and *personal adjustment* (Jones et al., 2013). In addition, studies reported negative relations between covitality and substance abuse, depression (Furlong, You, et al., 2014; Lee et al., 2015), attention-deficit/hyperactivity disorder, school problems, and internalizing symptoms (Jones et al., 2013; You et al., 2015).

Social Emotional Health Survey—Primary

The Social Emotional Health Survey—Primary (SEHS-P) is based on the general SEHS-S covitality model, but given less cognitive complexity among children ages 8–12, it includes fewer psychological disposition components. Survey length and readability were key considerations when developing the SEHS for this age group. During the preliminary phase of SEHS-P development, items were drafted to represent four subscales: gratitude, zest, optimism, and persistence. These four strengths were selected because of the positive relations between the former three and children's happiness, and because of the importance of task persistence to overall school success. The development of the SEHS-P included exploratory analysis using a pilot study sample and a separate analysis of readability and comprehension of all words included in the items. See Furlong and colleagues (2013) for a complete description of scale development.

ADMINISTRATION AND SCORING

The SEHS-P is a 16-item student-report measure designed to measure four latent, positive psychological dispositions with four items per scale. These four dispositions have all been shown to be linked with various aspects of positive student development and combine to measure one overarching trait, called covitality. In addition to the 16 items measuring psychological dispositions, the SEHS-P also has four supplemental items that measure students' self-perceptions of their prosocial behavior at school. The SEHS-P items are listed in the Appendix.

PSYCHOMETRIC PROPERTIES

Using a sample of more than 2,600 students in grades 4–6 from 26 schools, Furlong and colleagues (2013) carried out a series of exploratory and confirmatory factor analyses. The results indicated support for a model in which gratitude, zest, optimism, and persistence all loaded well onto a second-order covitality factor. Additional analyses found that the SEHS-P factor structure was equivalent for both boys and girls; this was also found for the prosocial behavior subscale. Adequate internal consistency reliability was found for all subscales: gratitude (.70), zest (.75), optimism (.66), persistence (.76), covitality (.88), and prosocial behavior (.80). Concurrent validity was evidenced by positive correlations among the covitality index, prosocial behavior, and school connectedness. High SEHS-P covitality scores were also associated with higher feelings of being safe at school and reduced bullying victimization.

SCHOOLWIDE APPLICATIONS OF THE SEHS

Within the context of this book's model describing how positive psychology interventions can be infused within a schoolwide continuum of mental health supports (see Chapter 10), a complementary approach is suggested when integrating strengths and quality-of-life assessments into practice. The first step recognizes the importance of monitoring the well-being of all students when considered from a positive psychology perspective because the health and well-being of all students is important, in fact, it is a fundamental student right (Kosher, Ben-Arieh, Jiang, & Huebner, 2014). Schools, for example, have implemented universal assessment of students' well-being using one of the life satisfaction measures described earlier in this chapter (the SLSS or the BMSLSS). These brief assessments are easily administered and scored using paper-and-pencil formats, or adapted into online formats (e.g., via SurveyMonkey), which facilitates using data to monitor students' well-being over time. When used at the whole-school level, the percentage of students with positive mental health (e.g., SLSS *T*-scores of 40 and higher, or mean scores of 4.0 or higher) has been used as an index of positive student development and school climate.

The next step involves assessment with those students with relatively low or below-threshold life satisfaction. For example, using universal well-being screening results schools have used SLSS *T*-scores (≤ 40) and BMSLSS *T*-scores (≤ 40) to identify those students who reported less than optimal well-being. Following this approach, the SEHS-S, which provides a profile of positive student strengths, is used in combination with a measure of personal distress (implementing the dual-factor complete mental health model) to provide data with which to make decisions about targeted service delivery. For example, high schools have administered the SEHS-S with the BESS (Kamphaus & Reynolds, 2007) as part of the social–emotional health screening process. As in traditional school-based mental health screening, those students with elevated or higher BESS self-reports are identified, but, in addition, the BESS scores are compared with the SEHS-S strength ratings. Elevated BESS (T-score > 60) scores and low SEHS-S scores (raw scores < 85 out of 150—maximum covitality score [lowest 1 standard deviation]; Furlong 2015) have been used to identify the subgroup of students most in need of Tier 2 services. As shown in Table 2.1, the balanced assessment of student distress and psychological assets provides data for more nuanced decision making—most notably, this procedure identifies a group of students who do not report high levels of distress on the BESS, but who nonetheless report very low social–emotional strengths. When these students also report low SLSS or BMSLSS scores, they are a primary group of students who could most directly benefit from the positive psychology interventions described in later chapters of this book. Dowdy and colleagues (2015); Furlong, Dowdy, Carnazzo, Bovery, and Kim (2014); and Moore and colleagues (2015) provide additional information about how the SEHS-S has been used by schools to monitor the social–emotional health of students.

Substantial research evidence shows that increases in students' SEHS-S profiles are strongly associated with thriving subjective well-being (Furlong, You, et al., 2014; You et al., 2015), a primary outcome examined in applications of positive psychology interventions. Therefore, assessments such as the SEHS-S are of great potential use in efforts to monitor the effects of positive psychology interventions.

TABLE 2.1. Percentage of Students at One High School in Priority Groups Derived from Screening Using the SEHS-S and the BESS

SEHS-S strength groups	BESS distress groups		
	Normal risk ($T < 60$)	Elevated risk ($T = 60–69$)	Extremely elevated risk ($T \geq 70$)
Low strengths (≤ 85)	4. Languishing 2%	2. Moderate risk 3%	1. Highest risk 3%
Low average strengths (86–106)	5. Getting by 23%	3. Lower risk 5%	
High average strengths (107–127)	6. Moderate thriving 41%	9. Inconsistent 4%	8. Inconsistent 1%
High strengths (≥ 128)	7. High thriving 18%		

Note. Shading indicates highest-priority students for follow-up. The percentages of students shown are actual values from one high school; however, these percentages will vary by school. The same dual-factor approach can be used with the SEHS-P. For more information, see Furlong (2015).

SUMMARY

A primary goal of many positive psychology interventions is to foster higher levels of well-being, which, in turn, fuels positive developmental trajectories. Although subjective well-being cannot be directly "taught," it can be fostered via other internal psychological dispositions that have direct and indirect effects on subjective well-being via comprehensive positive psychology interventions. What these approaches have in common is that they propose core strengths that when developed form the foundation for broad positive development in family, school, and community contexts. As positive psychology interventions are now including multiple components, likewise comprehensive measurement approaches are needed to assess student needs and to evaluate effectiveness. The measures described in this chapter offer resources for progress monitoring and data-informed implementation of positive psychology interventions.

CHAPTER 3

Factors Associated with Youth Subjective Well-Being

Early research on student happiness involved observational studies to determine what happy youth looked like in terms of common environments, personalities, activities, and/or demographic features. The development of a thorough understanding of what factors are and are not associated with indicators of subjective well-being, including positive affect and life satisfaction both globally and within domains, was necessary in part to enable psychologists to recommend intervention targets that were likely to deliver the biggest bang for the buck in efforts to promote happiness. For example, if happy kids were distinguished by extensive involvement in organized after-school activities and minimal time playing video games, then it may make sense to recommend parents do what they could to structure their children's use of free time accordingly (although stronger recommendations would be based in evidence that experiments that *changed* after-school behaviors were actually tied to changes in the child's happiness). Researchers have identified the factors correlated with subjective well-being (hereon referred to as "correlates" in this book, but also referred to as determinants and predictors in other works) through three primary methods. In the first method (qualitative studies), youth are asked to share the factors that they believe most determine their life satisfaction appraisals. Perceived correlates are the themes that emerge across student reports. In the second method (cross-sectional studies), youth subjective well-being ratings are gathered at the same time as data on other factors such as quality of relationships or youth activities and attitudes. Correlates are the factors that vary along with subjective well-being levels (e.g., youth with higher levels of extraversion and lower levels of neuroticism tend to be the same youth who report greater life satisfaction). In the third method (longitudinal studies), data on possible correlates are collected prior to the final wave of student subjective well-being ratings. Here, correlates are the factors that ultimately predict which students have higher or lower subjective well-being (e.g., children who perceive greater parent support go on to report higher life satisfaction months and years down the road).

The first time I systematically reviewed the research literature in search of those types of studies was the year 2000 and I was working on my master's thesis at the University of South Carolina. At the time, there were so few published studies on youth life satisfaction that I had to synthesize the research findings pertinent to adults' subjective well-being in order to suggest plausible hypotheses about the likely influence of parenting practices on adolescent life satisfaction. In the intervening 15 years, we have thankfully learned a great deal about the determinants of happiness specific to children and adolescents. In fact, the number of empirical studies has grown so exponentially that researchers have published numerous journal articles and book chapters to synthesize the findings across categories of correlates (e.g., family, peers, school, internal assets) into literature reviews; quite recent examples include *Assessment and Promotion of Life Satisfaction in Youth* (Huebner, Hills, & Jiang, 2013) and *Life Satisfaction and Schooling* (Huebner, Hills, Siddall, & Gilman, 2014). Even a review published 5 years prior to those (*Youth Life Satisfaction: A Review of the Literature*; Proctor et al., 2009b) located 141 empirical studies of life satisfaction in children and adolescents. Clearly, a review of all the studies pertinent to correlates of students' life satisfaction is outside the scope of this book. Instead, this chapter contains summaries of the robust correlates of subjective well-being as identified in the aforementioned secondary sources. The interested reader is encouraged to access those lengthier pieces for further detail or to identify the primary sources that informed the conclusions in the reviews (as summarized within this chapter). This chapter also contains findings from selected empirical studies published since the aforementioned works, as well as a few studies that were not cited in the three reviews. These primary sources were selected for particular attention because they illustrate, refine, or expand upon conclusions from previously published reviews of correlates.

WHAT ARE THE MAIN CATEGORIES OF CORRELATES?

In casting a broad net, those studies that defined subjective well-being and then asked children questions like "What are you considering when you judge how satisfied you are with your life?" (Suldo, Frank, Chappel, Albers, & Bateman, 2014) or "What things facilitate well-being?" (Navarro et al., 2015), suggested a similar set of categories that matter, at least in the eyes of youth. The broad categories are remarkably similar across samples, robust to age (elementary to high school age), country (e.g., Spain, Norway, Thailand, Canada), and cultures within a country (e.g., in the United States, a Mexican American sample as well as a cross-section of students in diverse high schools). In all studies, many youth described their happiness as influenced by relationships as well as internal qualities, specifically:

- Family support, including parents who provide love and affection as well as open communication marked by trust; harmonious (vs. conflict-ridden) interactions and expressed positive affect in the home; and spending sufficient time together.
- Friendships, which provide companionship, acceptance, and assistance, as well as access to enjoyable activities.
- Personal attitudes, such as a positive outlook on life, confidence in one's self.

In over half of the qualitative studies, additional influences cited include:

- Schooling experiences, including access to formal education, personal academic performance, and relationships in the classroom.
- Physical health, including feeling well, having minimal illnesses or health conditions that limit activities.

Themes that may be considered minor since they emerged in some but not most samples include:

- Personal abilities and behaviors, including primary strategies for coping with stress, self-advocacy skills.
- Use of free time, including involvement in extracurricular activities and access to friends.
- Financial resources, including having enough money to meet basic needs, personal employment demands.
- Living environment and community, including safety, security, and comfort.
- Physical appearance.
- Goal-directed activity and aspirations.
- Stressful life events, including death of a loved one, parent separation.
- Chronic stressors, including arguments with friends or family members, and a heavy academic workload.

The youth who participated in interviews and focus groups that yielded the above list of likely correlates have proven pretty insightful. Specifically, cross-sectional and longitudinal studies with different, larger samples have generally confirmed that the factors above, although identified in an atheoretical manner, indeed covary with differences between youths' levels of subjective well-being. The few additional correlates likely involve a perspective that is beyond a given student's present-oriented snapshot. For instance, empirical studies have repeatedly found an inverse relationship between age and life satisfaction among youth, such that life satisfaction declines across the adolescent years. The next pages summarize what empirical studies have indicated are the primary correlates within each category.

STUDENT-LEVEL CORRELATES

Demographic Factors

Most studies find that average levels of life satisfaction are comparable across different demographic groups within a given country. Whereas other ratings of self such as self-esteem tend to favor boys, research has not yet found consistent main effects of gender or racial group in subjective well-being. When exceptions emerge, effects are of small magnitude and not easily understood. Taken together, research supports the notion that boys and girls from majority and minority ethnic groups are equally likely to be happy. In contrast, cross-sectional and longitudinal studies with samples from all over the globe (e.g., Israel, Hong Kong, Germany, United Kingdom, United States) have found declining trends in life satisfaction across the adolescent years (e.g., Helliwell, Layward, & Sachs, 2015). The effect of socioeconomic status is not as linear. Although the size of the effect is often small in magnitude, children living in poverty routinely report lower well-being relative to youth from families who do not qualify for government aid, such as free or reduced-price meals at school. However, once basic needs are met, there is little if any relationship between family income and quality of life.

Personality

Early research focused on extraversion and neuroticism found that both were robust correlates of subjective well-being, exerting positive and negative influences, respectively. Thanks to advances in measurement tools, researchers can now reliably assess adolescents' levels on all of the "Big Five" personality traits. When examined in relation to indicators of happiness, my graduate students and I recently found that the Big Five personality factors account for about 47% of the variance in high school students' life satisfaction levels (Suldo, Minch, & Hearon, 2015). Neuroticism emerged as the strongest predictor. Openness, conscientiousness, and extraversion were also significant and unique predictors of greater life satisfaction, as was a higher level of agreeableness for girls, but not for boys.

Attitudes

The self-oriented beliefs that have had positive correlations with children's and adolescents' subjective well-being include general self-esteem, self-efficacy in multiple areas (such as with regard to social, academic, and emotional situations), and an internal locus of control. In a related line of research, greater hope and optimism (often rooted in attributions pertinent to personal control and ability) have emerged as strong correlates of life satisfaction. Greater life satisfaction has also been reported by youth who have higher levels of other character strengths, including gratitude, love, and zest.

Activities

Preliminary mixed-methods research suggests that some of the distinguishing features of vulnerable teenagers—those students with low subjective well-being but an absence of mental health problems—involve how they spend their free time. In particular, our research suggests that their subjective well-being may be suppressed because challenges balancing employment with social, family, and academic demands contribute to feeling overwhelmed and overcommitted (Suldo, Frank, et al., 2014). Furthermore, when they had downtime, students in this subgroup seemed more inclined to select unstructured, solitary activities that were aligned with their personal interests. In general, large-scale studies have found a positive correlation between participation in extracurricular activities that are more structured by design, such as school-based clubs and team sports, and youth life satisfaction. Indeed, none of the troubled students in the aforementioned qualitative study mentioned anything about extracurricular activity participation when discussing factors that determine happiness, suggesting sports, musical pursuits, clubs, and the like were off their radar. Recent research in Israel found that high school students who participated in additional sports and arts classes at school had higher subjective well-being than peers who only took required classes (Orkibi, Ronen, & Assoulin, 2014). Thus, taking part in organized athletic and artistic pursuits either during the school day or after school appears correlated with elevated subjective well-being.

Health

As discussed in Chapter 1, happier children tend to have fewer symptoms of mental health problems as well as better physical health. No surprise given the relationship between healthy habits and those ultimate outcomes, recent research has found that one healthy behavior—getting more hours of sleep in a typical night—predicted greater subjective well-being 6 months later (Kalak, Lemola, Brand, Holsboer-Trachsler, & Grob, 2014). This trend held for all three age groups examined (ages 10–11, 12–13, and 14–15), and was not better explained by a reverse effect (i.e., subjective well-being did not predict later sleep trends). Such findings underscore the importance of ensuring adequate sleep among high school-age youth who tend to sacrifice it to accommodate competing demands. Other healthy behaviors that predict greater life satisfaction during adolescence include good eating habits (eating breakfast every school day, infrequent consumption of soft drinks), near-daily rigorous physical activity, and infrequent or no smoking (Moor et al., 2014).

Left unchecked, stress exerts a negative effect on life satisfaction, in part through causing increases in internalizing forms of mental health problems. Global life satisfaction declines as stress in multiple contexts increases, including stressors pertinent to schoolwork, parent–child relations, social struggles, and financial problems (Suldo, Dedrick, Shaunessy-Dedrick, Roth, & Ferron, 2015). As such, developing effective stress management strategies may also be considered a health-facilitating behavior. Saha, Huebner, Hills, Malone, and Valois's (2014) longitudinal study of middle school students found that students' later global life satisfaction was most tied to their tendency to cope with stressors like arguments with friends by seeking social support. Similarly, the high school students with elevated life satisfaction tend to respond to school-related stressors by turning to family members, among using other adaptive strategies involving time and task management efforts, cognitive reappraisal, and athletic diversions (Suldo, Dedrick, Shaunessy-Dedrick, Fefer, & Ferron, 2015). In contrast, students with the lowest life satisfaction more frequently respond to academic stressors through keeping problems to themselves, giving up, or deteriorating emotionally.

FAMILY-LEVEL CORRELATES

The family context is a central determinant of subjective well-being throughout the lifespan. The highest levels of life satisfaction are seen among youth who feel securely attached to and accepted by their parents, and perceive close relationships with parents that feature open communication and self-disclosure. In addition to such strong parent–child relationships, parenting practices consistent with an authoritative parenting style are robust correlates of youth subjective well-being. These authoritative parenting practices include promotion of youth's psychological autonomy (e.g., encouragement of age-appropriate decision making), behavioral supervision and monitoring, and high levels of responsiveness as indicated by expressions of warmth, care, and emotional support (see Suldo & Fefer, 2013, for a review). Case in point, Tolan and Larsen (2014) followed nearly 4,000 adolescents from 25 middle schools and found three trajectories of life satisfaction: stable high, improving, and declining. The ecological predictors that distinguished these groups the most at the beginning and end of middle school were parenting practices. Students whose life satisfaction stayed high from sixth to eighth grade repeatedly reported the most parental involvement (e.g., children and parents work together in household activities) and communication (e.g., frequent discussions about daily events).

Stability and predictability at home also contributes to life satisfaction. Although some studies found diminished life satisfaction among children from divorced parents, subsequent research found mean differences among students from different family structures (e.g., divorced vs. intact two-parent) were better explained by the economic disadvantage more common to single-parent families (Shek & Liu, 2014). The level of harmony between parents seems to matter even more. Chappel, Suldo, and Ogg (2014) examined the combined and unique influence of four categories of family stressors (low socioeconomic status, disrupted family structure, cumulative major life events, and perceived interparental conflict) on adolescents' life satisfaction, and found interparental conflict exerted the strongest influence. Specifically, those middle school students who reported their parents' arguments were more frequent, long lasting, and intense (e.g., involved yelling) had significantly lower life satisfaction as compared with their peers who reported less conflict between their parents. Chapter 4 contains a discussion of how happiness levels of a child's mother and father, and others within the home, affect the child.

FRIEND-LEVEL CORRELATES

Healthy relationships at home set the stage for positive friendships that feature feelings of attachment to one's peers, which co-occur with greater life satisfaction. Feeling accepted by one's peers is related to greater life satisfaction, particularly among early adolescents in cultures with relatively less emphasis on family values (Schwarz et al., 2012). Beyond the cross-sectional studies that find perceptions of support and popularity co-occur with greater life satisfaction, longitudinal studies find that friendship experiences during adolescence cast a long shadow. Case in point, the negative effects of peer rejection and the protective nature of having at least one friend—at age 15—were apparent in the life satisfaction of adults in their 40s (Marion, Laursen, Zettergren, & Bergman, 2013). For individuals who had reported at least one same-age friend at age 15, level of rejection from classmates (also when 15 years old) was not related to life satisfaction in middle adulthood; whereas for individuals without a friend during adolescence, greater classmate rejection was a significant predictor of lower life satisfaction nearly 30 years later. Such significant effects of interpersonal relationships at school are revisited in the next section.

SCHOOL-LEVEL CORRELATES

The primary school-based correlates of students' happiness involve school climate (including relationships with people at school) and students' personal academic success. Student success is most often thought of in terms of skills—that is, demonstrated knowledge in specific areas. Indicators of engagement that predict skill attainment are also important to consider given their role as academic enablers. Thus, a comprehensive view of academic success involves attention to student skill as well as school-related behavior (behavioral engagement) and attitudes (affective engagement; Suldo, Gormley, DuPaul, & Anderson-Butcher, 2014).

Climate

School climate is a multidimensional construct that often reflects perceptions of interpersonal relationship quality (including student–teacher and student–student interactions), parent involvement, safety and order, fairness in discipline and resource allocation, and physical appearance of the school building. Across samples of secondary students, the interpersonal dimensions and parent involvement emerge as the strongest correlates of life satisfaction.

Student–Teacher Relationships

For middle school students, the aspects of teacher support that seem most salient to children's subjective well-being include emotional support that causes students to feel cared for and treated fairly, and tangible assistance during the learning process; boys and girls differ some in perceptions of how teachers show such support (Suldo et al., 2009). Research that has compared the influence of school-related support from multiple sources (parents, peers, teachers) on life satisfaction finds that although parent support for learning exerts the strongest effects on *global* life satisfaction later in the school year, student–teacher relationships are the strongest predictor of subsequent *school* satisfaction (Jiang, Huebner, & Sidall, 2013). Positive student–teacher relationships may spur children's interest and engagement in classroom and after-school activities, which in turn may contribute to global life satisfaction. Empirical tests of path models have supported school satisfaction as a mediator of the relationship between student engagement and global life satisfaction. Such findings have implications for school climate initiatives that address the facets of school climate that are tied to students' subjective well-being.

Classmate Relationships

Social relationships with classmates can lead to distress or wellness depending on the nature of the interactions. For instance, negative experiences with peers (e.g., rejection, lack of popularity) can adversely impact the development of friendships, leading to loneliness and low subjective well-being. Using an experience sampling method in which youth reported their momentary happiness while engaged in different daily activities, Csikszentmihalyi and Hunter (2003) found students in middle and high school experienced the lowest levels when they were by themselves, whereas happiness was highest when they were with friends. In addition to proximity to friends, more recent survey research with high school students has underscored the influence of kind interactions with classmates. Specifically, students who received more positive social acts (ranging from compliments to assistance in times of need) from peers at one's school reported greater levels of life satisfaction and positive affect (Suldo, Gelley, Roth, & Bateman, 2015). These effects were significant above and beyond the negative influence of peer victimization; relational forms of victimization exerted a particularly strong effect on life satisfaction. In sum, students who feel excluded, talked about negatively, unpopular, lonely, or otherwise treated poorly by classmates are likely to experience diminished subjective well-being, whereas students who feel their classmates provide companionship, care, and support are likely to experience elevated subjective well-being.

Academic Skills

Across studies that have examined associations between students' life satisfaction and objective indicators of skills, such as course grades and achievement test scores ascertained from school records, the bivariate correlation has generally been around .20 (e.g., Lyons & Huebner,

2015; Suldo et al., 2011). The small but reliable (statistically significant) association suggests that middle and high school students who perform well in their studies tend to be a bit happier. Some exceptions have been found in students with a particular background. For example, among high school students in Germany who are in the most selective academic track (akin to college preparatory programs), the relationship between life satisfaction and students' GPA was more pronounced for students whose mothers had a high level of educational attainment (Crede, Wirthwein, McElvany, & Steinmayr, 2015). In contrast, life satisfaction was unrelated to GPA for children whose mothers had a less rigorous academic history (i.e., had not been in the most selective track themselves). Crede and colleagues (2015) speculated that students from high-achieving families may experience greater pressure to excel, which fuels life satisfaction when grades are good; in contrast, perhaps children who have gained entry to an academic track higher than their mothers are already considered academically successful, contributing to reduced pressure such that lower grades would not necessarily co-occur with lower life satisfaction.

Academic Enablers

Global life satisfaction is generally more strongly linked to engagement in the classroom, in terms of on-task and compliant behavior, as well as valuing schooling. Among middle school students, Lyons and Huebner (2015) identified moderate correlations between students' life satisfaction and indicators of behavioral and cognitive engagement. Another academic enabler that is a robust correlate of life satisfaction is academic self-efficacy beliefs. Students who believe they can learn and achieve tend to be happier. Coupled with the aforementioned small relationship between actual academic performance and life satisfaction, it seems plausible that experiencing academic challenges in the classroom does not doom a student to low happiness. Instead, a struggling student's teacher may help keep subjective well-being intact by supporting the student's academic efficacy beliefs. Some strategies for facilitating efficacy beliefs in the classroom include arranging opportunities for mastery experiences that are well matched to the child's skill level, and verbal persuasion to convey the teacher's belief in the child's ability to succeed (Bandura, 1997).

SUMMARY

This chapter has described methods of establishing factors associated with youth subjective well-being and summarized the most prevalent correlates that have been identified in the literature. Although not all student-, family-, friend-, and school-level correlates of well-being are malleable, those that may be enhanced within the school environment are particularly promising targets for happiness-increasing interventions. This research sets the stage for another important question addressed in Chapter 4: To what extent do efforts to improve these correlates lead to changes to students' subjective well-being?

PART II

STUDENT-FOCUSED STRATEGIES FOR PROMOTING YOUTH HAPPINESS

Theoretical Framework Underpinning Design and Development of Positive Psychology Interventions

Guidance for practitioners interested in promoting student subjective well-being can be gleaned from two bodies of literature. The first pertains to studies that have identified potentially malleable factors within the environment (e.g., peers, family, and school) as well as within individuals (e.g., cognitions and activities) that are correlated with increased life satisfaction among children and adolescents. Although the bulk of these studies have been cross-sectional and thus the directionality of associations is unknown, efforts to increase the correlates of subjective well-being summarized in Chapter 3 may logically contribute to elevations in subjective well-being. The second route, which has been made possible by advances in the first route, is to apply one of a growing number of positive psychology interventions that have been shown to improve subjective well-being, primarily through manipulating one's purposeful thoughts and behaviors. While implementing interventions that have support for efficacy may appear the most appealing route for those interested in increasing subjective well-being, several caveats about the literature on empirical interventions for subjective well-being are warranted. First, this research is relatively recent (i.e., only began in the past 15 years) and has not yet been subjected to replication by independent research teams. Second, the majority of published studies have been limited to samples of adult participants; studies with youth participants have only emerged in the past 5–10 years (although such studies are increasing in prevalence). As such, applying some interventions requires a leap of faith that what works with adults will also work with youth. This chapter presents the positive psychology interventions that have been evaluated with a focus on subjective well-being as an outcome. To set the stage, the chapter begins with a larger question: Is it even possible to make enduring change in one's level of happiness, or are some people just born to be happy like others are born to be tall?

STABILITY OF HAPPINESS

A growing body of research has focused on if, why, and how people's happiness levels change, and why some people simply seem happier than others regardless of their circumstances. In a landmark paper, Sonja Lyubomirsky, Ken Sheldon, and David Schkade (2005) summarized the scientific arguments against and for people's potential to make lasting changes in happiness. The research synthesized in that paper is based largely on studies of adults, but the implications are applicable across the lifespan. Prior to presenting a framework that directs attention to the most plausible opportunities for sustaining increasing happiness, Lyubomirksy and colleagues first acknowledge three robust sources of pessimism.

Genetically Determined Set Point

There is considerable evidence of a biological component to happiness. The substantially higher correspondence of subjective well-being levels among identical twins (even those reared apart) as compared to fraternal twins demonstrates the genetic nature of subjective well-being (Lykken, 1999). The heritability of happiness accounts for about 50% of the variance between individuals. This biological set point is commonly conceptualized as a range of typical happiness expression. For example, some people tend to naturally demonstrate higher levels of happiness and seem a lot happier than most. Other people have a lower set point in happiness, and may not often seem happy. On a scale of 1 (*lowest*) to 7 (*highest*), some people's level of happiness is naturally high and their range could be 5–7. On the other hand, some people may demonstrate a much lower range such as 0–2. Evidence of this set point in youth is provided later.

Relationship between Personality and Happiness

By definition, the traits that make up one's personality are consistent across situations and are stable. Personality traits—especially neuroticism but also extraversion—are among the most consistent correlates of subjective well-being in adults (Steel, Schmidt, & Shultz, 2008) as well as in youth as described in Chapter 3. This serves as a source of pessimism for the potential to effect lasting change in happiness given that aspects of personality (e.g., temperament) may be present from birth and are thus closely related to the genetic set point. In short, having a personality profile that is linked to diminished happiness is not generally something people can do much to "fix." Evidence of the stable relationships between personality and subjective well-being in youth is provided later.

Hedonic Adaptation

The phenomenon of the *hedonic treadmill* is that while happiness may spike following some good fortune or plummet after a major life stressor, people adapt relatively quickly to their circumstances and/or increase their aspirations for positive events, which drives a return of one's happiness level back to baseline. For instance, Brickman, Coates, and Janoff-Bulman's (1978) classic study compared the happiness levels of adults in three extreme groups of adults: winners of the state lottery, people who had become paralyzed as the result of an accident, and controls from the same geographic region. The happiness of lottery winners was similar to that of the ordinary adults in the control group, and the happiness of the paralyzed adults was not as low as might be expected based on the extent of their injuries. These counterintuitive similarities suggest that the effect of life-changing circumstances is short-lived due to humans' tendency to adapt to any positive or negative change. Such adaption is beneficial for individuals who experience an extremely negative situation, such as a loss or trauma. But it is the bane of clinicians who work to improve people's lives only to see them return to baseline. Gains in happiness through behavior change efforts are only temporary; such activities must be continued in order for higher levels of happiness to be maintained. One's happiness levels quickly adapt and shift back to the lower bound of our genetic set point if intentional positive activities are not maintained over time. This is similar to weight loss—people can work hard to get to their goal weight, but if they then stop the eating or exercise habits that got them there, the weight creeps back on. In order to continue the upward spiral of happiness that flows from positive interventions, those efforts must be sustained.

In spite of these realities that illustrate the durability of one's predetermined happiness range, for better or for worse, research with adults indicates that the frequency with which they engage in strategies to increase or maintain happiness, such as through pursuing career goals, partying, exercising, helping others, or praying, indeed predicts a significant and substantial amount of variance—16%—in people's happiness after accounting for the enormous influence of personality (Tkach & Lyubomirsky, 2006). A more recent study of 900-plus college students examined their personality traits in addition to their natural use of happiness-inducing behaviors, such as nurturing relationships, savoring, acts of kindness, goal-directed activities, optimism, flow, spirituality, gratitude, forgiveness, meditation, and positive health actions (frequent healthy eating, daily exercise; Warner & Vroman, 2011). These young adults' personality traits (the Big Five taken together) explained 35% of the variance in their happiness levels (as measured by a four-item subjective happiness rating scale, not complete subjective well-being). The set of 14 happiness-inducing behaviors predicted an additional 10% of variance in happiness, above and beyond the influence of the Big Five traits. Ones that were particularly salient included cultivating optimism, nurturing relationships, savoring, and avoiding worry.

Taken together, such findings support the notion that genetics is not the only piece of the happiness equation. It is possible to avoid hedonic adaptation and increase one's level of subjective well-being into the upper range of one's set point through purposeful activities and ways of thinking (Sheldon & Lyubomirsky, 2006a). Although positive circumstantial changes also predict increases in subjective well-being, gains may be more enduring if paired with actions that train attention to or keep fresh positive changes in life circumstances. Such efforts to savor (continued appreciation) and derive pleasure from a change in different and unexpected ways (continued variety) are key to preventing hedonic adaptation (Sheldon & Lyubomirsky, 2012). Notably, people who experience rapid growth in positive emotions soon after adapting a happiness-increasing behavior, such as loving-kindness meditation, are more likely to stick with that behavior change (Cohn & Fredrickson, 2010). Schueller's (2010) research evaluated six positive exercises, and found that only the savoring exercise caused significant increases in happiness and decreases in depression among the entire sample of adults (i.e., regardless of personal preference for the savoring activity). For the other five happiness-increasing behaviors, the extent to which well-being benefits were reaped was in part a function of how much the particular happiness-inducing exercise resonated with the participant (e.g., is viewed as enjoyable and easily completed), which in turn related to who stuck with the practice of positive change (Schueller, 2010). Thus, lasting gains in subjective well-being may vary as a function of preference, variety, and appreciation, as well as be moderated by other features that contribute to optimal person–activity fit when intentional positive activities are undertaken (Lyubomirsky & Layous, 2013).

ARCHITECTURE OF SUSTAINABLE HAPPINESS MODEL

This body of research, largely with samples of adults, led Lyubomirsky and colleagues (2005) to conclude that happiness is influenced by three distinct components.

Genetic Set Point

For each person, the largest determinant of happiness is the genetic set point, which is constant, stable, and controlled by biological factors. This means that our baseline level of happiness is controlled by what we're born with and can look different for each individual. As described above, this genetic set point of happiness as determined by biological factors makes up approximately 50% of our personal happiness. Keeping in mind the genetic basis to happiness and the set point, Seligman (2002) comments that "happiness is not a competition. Authentic happiness derives from raising the bar for yourself, not rating yourself against others" (p. 14). Accordingly, indicators of happiness are often interpreted in an ipsative manner, rather than compared against norms that reflect happiness of other same-age youth or a criterion that would reflect a socially imposed standard for sufficient happiness. In asserting how genetic factors contribute more to a happiness set *range* as opposed to a set *point*, Sheldon, Boehm, and Lyubomirsky (2013) explain:

> Although a particular person may have limited potential for joy and ebullience and more of a tendency towards gloom and pessimism compared to others, that person might still at least achieve a chronic state of guarded contentment, which is better than chronic dejection and fear. Everyone has a characteristic range of possible subjective well-being states, and thus the goal becomes to find ways to stay in the top end of one's own possible range (vs. regress back to one's own mean). (p. 904)

Life Circumstances

Circumstances are incidental but relatively stable facts of an individual's life. This category includes demographic variables such as gender, ethnicity, age, socioeconomic status, and physical appearance. Other static circumstances that are arguably more within personal control include the geographic region in which one lives, occupational status, and specific possessions. Children and adults alike often envision changes in circumstance as a means to happiness. We anticipate that greater happiness would flow from living in a sunnier climate, driving the newest car, carrying the latest iPhone, or having an easier job. While there are some incremental happiness advantages to some circumstances, and positive changes in life circumstances can contribute to moving one's level of happiness within his or her set range, taken together life circumstances account for only about 10% of an individual's happiness. Accordingly, a widely discussed study of nearly half a million Americans found that the incremental benefits of a higher income on happiness maxed out at $75,000 annually (Kahneman & Deaton, 2010). Adults whose income exceeds that threshold do not appear to experience greater positive affect, as indicated by happiness, enjoyment, and smiling/laughter within a day.

Intentional Activity

Intentional activity includes varied actions and thoughts in one's daily life, such as amount of exercise, looking at things in a positive light, and setting goals (Lyubomirsky et al., 2005). This category of contributors to happiness is much more flexible to change and includes ways of thinking and behaving that are selected to be part of one's attitudinal and behavioral repertoire or not. These intentional activities are undertaken in daily life (for good or bad) and met with various degrees of pleasure and success. Purposeful efforts to cultivate personal attitudes and goal-directed behavior known to co-occur with happiness—for example, making an active choice to cultivate one's strengths—offer the best and most lasting potential to maximize one's happiness level. Taken together, intentional activities determine about 40% of the variance in happiness, thus reflecting a sizable target for interventionists.

Lyubomirsky and colleagues' (2005) ideas behind the "architecture of sustainable change" remains the prevailing model of salient issues involved in efforts to improve happiness levels. Empirical tests of this theory in its totality among samples of children and youth are lacking. However, a growing body of research has examined aspects of the model, including some of the sources of pessimism and optimism for lasting change in youth happiness. Highlights from this body of work are summarized below. In general, findings demonstrate the applicability of the model to practitioners who desire to promote students' happiness.

EVIDENCE FOR THE GENETIC SET POINT IN YOUTH

Twin Studies

Findings in support of the genetic set point largely come from studies of twins. Most observable traits, like physical features (e.g., weight) and abilities (e.g., intelligence), are influenced by a combination of genetics and environment. Monozygotic twins are genetically identical, whereas dizygotic (often called fraternal) twins share roughly 50% of each other's genes. When monozygotic twins resemble each other more on a given variable, like weight or score on an intelligence test, than dizygotic twins on the same variable, a genetic effect on that factor is indicated. Furthermore, a higher correlation between dizygotic twins as compared to correlations between a twin and a nontwin sibling suggests an effect of a specific environment shared by the twins (but not the nontwin sibling). Correlations of less than 1.0 between monozygotic twins on a given factor also indicate that the factor is influenced by environmental features.

Are these genetic influences as evident in youth as they are in adults' happiness? Bartels and Boomsma (2009) set out to determine if people are indeed born to be happy by examining subjective well-being among participants in the Netherlands Twins Registry. This study examined data from a sample of over 4,000 youth who were twins, and almost 1,000 of their nontwin siblings. The sample included 770 identical twin pairs and 590 fraternal twin pairs of the same gender, as well as 503 fraternal twin pairs that included one boy and one girl in the set. When they were between the ages of 12 and 23 (most twins were 14–16), the twins and some nontwin siblings reported their subjective well-being on two indicators of life satisfaction and two indicators of positive affect (general happy mood). Findings from this study supported the notion that up to half of the variance in youth subjective well-being levels is attributable to genetic effects. Within monozygotic twins, the average correlation between two identical twins in a set was strong—about .42 (r ranged from .31 to .53 depending on the indicator of subjective well-being examined and the gender of the twins). Within dizygotic twins and nontwin siblings, the average correlation was small—about .14 (r ranged from .08 to .26 depending on the indicator of subjective well-being used and gender). The findings supported a genetic influence on subjective well-being regardless of the specific component (cognitive vs. affective) examined, because the correlation among monozygotic twins exceeded the correlation among the dizygotic twins and twin–sibling pairs on each of the four indicators. Bartels and Boomsma explained, "The implication of this finding is that distinct measures of subjective well-being are not distinct at the genetic level. All four measures, used in this study, load on similar sets of genes" (p. 619).

Further analyses of this dataset indicated that genetic factors accounted for close to 50% of the variance in subjective well-being scores, consistent with Lyubomirsky and colleagues' (2005) model. For both indicators of life satisfaction, heritability explained 47% of the variance, with the remaining 53% of individual differences in life satisfaction attributable to nonshared environmental factors. Heritability estimates were somewhat smaller for emotional indicators of subjective well-being, specifically accounting for 36–38% of the variance in positive affect. Importantly, the genetic architecture of subjective well-being was the same across youth gender and age. Although older youth reported lower levels of subjective well-being, the strong genetic basis for an individual's rating of life satisfaction or happiness held across adolescents and young adults in the sample. This well-designed study supports the notion that roughly 50% of the variability in a youth's subjective well-being level will be inherited, regardless of the youth's age or gender.

Evidence Beyond Twin Studies

In the absence of access to an identical twin to study, how can researchers test the happiness set-point theory? Sheldon and Lyubomirsky (2006a) offer three ideas: (1) examine an individual's personality as a proxy for what is inherited, (2) examine the well-being of an individual's biological family members, or (3) examine an individual's average well-being score as compiled across multiple ratings over many years. By definition, youth spans a restricted number of years. Therefore, findings from studies pertinent to the first two methods are summarized in the next sections. But first, it's important to establish the extent of change in subjective well-being that may be expected during youth.

As described in Chapter 1, defining youth mental health as the combination of subjective well-being and psychopathology can yield four mental health groups: complete mental health (average to high subjective well-being, low psychopathology), vulnerable (low subjective well-being, low psychopathology), symptomatic but content (average to high subjective well-being, elevated psychopathology), and troubled (low subjective well-being, elevated psychopathology). In a longitudinal study of change and stability in adolescents' mental health, McMahan (2013) found that 61% of students had the same mental health status 1 year later. Nearly one-quarter (23%) of students changed their relative subjective well-being level (from low to average/high or vice versa) across the 1-year interval; the remaining 16% of students changed only in psycho-pathology level (from not elevated on symptoms of internalizing or externalizing to within the elevated range, or vice versa). Table 4.1 summarizes the stability and change with each group.

As previously reported, the bulk of typical secondary students are likely to have complete mental health (Suldo, Thalji-Raitano, et al., in press). McMahan (2013) followed the sample of high school students from that study and found that the greatest stability occurs within the complete mental health group; students who begin with worse levels of subjective well-being, psychopathology, or both are more like to change (in either direction) from year to year. Of the total sample of 425 high school students who took part in both years of the study, about 12.5% of youth moved into a higher subjective well-being group (e.g., vulnerable to complete mental health or troubled to symptomatic but content), 11% moved into a lower subjective well-being group (e.g., complete mental health to vulnerable or symptomatic but content to troubled), 11.5% moved into a higher psychopathology group (e.g., complete mental health to symptomatic but content or vulnerable to troubled), and 13% moved into a lower psychopathology group (e.g., symptomatic but content to complete mental health or troubled to vulnerable).

The Critical Influence of Personality on Subjective Well-Being

What factors predicted which youth would stay happy or troubled, and which students would experience change in their mental health status? McMahan (2013) examined students' status on a number of correlates of youth subjective well-being, including (1) circumstantial variables that are demographic in nature (gender, socioeconomic status, ethnicity) as well as the cumulative number of major life stressors that the student experienced in the prior 6 months, (2) attitudinal variables such as self-esteem and self-concept, and (3) personality characteristics (extraversion, neuroticism, conscientiousness, openness to new experiences, agreeableness). McMahan also examined students' baseline quality of interpersonal relationships (with parents, teachers, and

TABLE 4.1. Mental Health Groups as Indicated by the Dual-Factor Model across Two Time Points Separated by 1 Year among 425 High School Students

	Initial mental health group			
	Complete mental health ($n = 270$; 63.5% of sample)	Troubled ($n = 61$; 14.4% of sample)	Vulnerable ($n = 47$; 11.1% of sample)	Symptomatic but content ($n = 47$; 11.1% of sample)
Proportion of group that had this same status 1 year later	80%	36%	30%	17%
For students with a different mental health status next year, what group did they move to?	SBC (10%) Vulnerable (7%) Troubled (4%)	CMH (25%) SBC (20%) Vulnerable (20%)	CMH (45%) Troubled (15%) SBC (11%)	CMH (47%) Troubled (19%) Vulnerable (17%)

Note. CMH, complete mental health; SBC, symptomatic but content.

peers) and schooling experiences (i.e., school connectedness, school achievement) in order to determine which demographic, intrapersonal, and environmental characteristics predict students' later mental health status. In line with the genetic set-point theory in which stability of mental health is largely predicted by stable factors like personality, McMahan found that neuroticism was the strongest predictor of consistent complete mental health. Results of logistic regression analyses indicated that students with lower neuroticism scores had more than five times the odds than those with higher levels of remaining in the complete mental health group. A life circumstance factor also mattered, although less strongly. Specifically, students of higher socioeconomic status had twice the odds of retaining a complete mental health status than students of lower socioeconomic status. There was also a trend for better academic achievement to predict stability in this optimal mental health status, which may reflect a circumstantial variable (i.e., consistently successful student) or behavioral patterns (i.e., persistence with academic assignments) depending on a given student's personal focus on achieving a high GPA. Of students who began the study with worse mental health, improving to complete mental health was largely predicted by personality features. Specifically, students with lower levels of neuroticism had 10 times the odds of moving to the complete mental health group than their more neurotic peers, and students with higher levels of agreeableness had twice the odds of becoming complete mental health.

These personality factors also predicted which students worsened in their mental health status; students with higher levels of neuroticism had nearly eight times the odds of becoming troubled than students with lower levels, whereas students with higher levels of extraversion had only half the odds of becoming troubled as students with lower levels of extraversion. In addition to extraversion serving as a protective factor, students with higher self-esteem at baseline were less likely to become troubled than students with lower levels of self-esteem. Personality (specifically, low levels of extraversion, high levels of neuroticism) was the largest determinant of which students stayed troubled across time. Research with other samples of youth has supported the critical influence of personality on individual differences in subjective well-being, as described in Chapter 3 (Suldo, Minch, et al., 2015).

Interestingly, stressful life events as reported at the first time point did not predict change or stability in mental health, suggesting that the presence or absence of adverse life circumstances did not cast a lasting shadow among teenagers. Why did frequent experiences of negative (stressful) life events not predict which students remained troubled at both time points? At the initial time point, students reported the number of stressful life events they experienced in the 6 months prior. The yearlong interval was likely sufficient time to permit adaptation to these circumstances; students had considerable time to adjust to the stressful experiences they incurred 12–18 months prior to reporting their mental health at Time 2.

Well-Being of Family Members

To learn more about the determinants of happiness among those students who had a particularly stable mental health, individual interviews were conducted with six to 10 students from each of the four aforementioned groups (Suldo, Frank, et al., 2014). The interview included questions about the happiness levels of family members. Students were asked, "How happy are the people in your immediate family, such as a parent or a sibling? On a scale of 1 to 5, how would you rate the well-being (overall happiness, satisfaction with life) of each person living in your home?" (1

= *very slightly or not at all happy*; 3 = *moderately happy*; and 5 = *extremely happy*). As results of analyses for that series of items have not been published previously, they are presented in detail below:

Of the 30 students, 21 lived with both biological parents (in three cases, the parents were no longer together but the children had residences in both homes). The students' ratings suggested that those with happier fathers also tended to be those with happier mothers ($r = .44$, $p < .05$). Therefore, for the students who rated both biological parents, ratings for mothers and fathers were combined to create an average parent happiness level. For the other students, only the rating provided for the biological parent living in the home was examined (three mothers, four fathers; two students did not live with either parent and were excluded from the analyses presented next).

Parents' happiness levels differed significantly as a function of their child's mental health status, $F(3,34) = 7.78$, $p < .001$. Parent happiness levels were rather high in the groups of students with average/high subjective well-being ($M = 4.63$, $SD = 0.35$, among the group of youth with complete mental health; $M = 4.33$, $SD = 0.75$, among symptomatic but content students). In contrast, students in the two mental health statuses defined by low subjective well-being were more likely to rate their parents as only moderately happy ($M = 2.95$, $SD = 0.84$, among the group of troubled students; $M = 3.28$, $SD = 0.94$, among vulnerable students). As shown in Figure 4.1, parents' global happiness levels (as perceived by their teenage children) paralleled the children's own levels of life satisfaction. The children's life satisfaction scores reflect their average score on the SLSS, as completed at two time points (a few months earlier in the year, and 1 year prior to that). We also examined children's composite score on the SLSS and PANAS

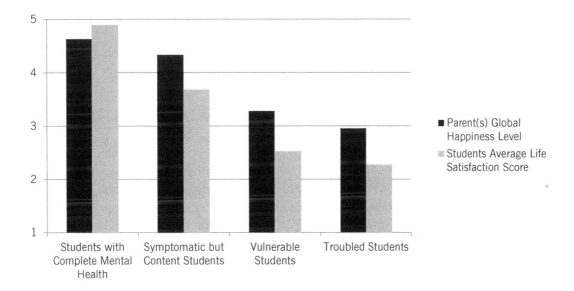

FIGURE 4.1. Correspondence between parents' and children's happiness levels among students with stable mental health. The SLSS is on a 1–6 scale. Average SLSS scores were converted to a 1–5 scale to permit direct comparison with the ratings of parent happiness from the 1–5 scale used in the global questions.

(life satisfaction + positive affect – negative affect) averaged across the same two time points, referred to as average subjective well-being.

Regression analyses indicated that children's ratings of their biological parents' happiness explained 57% of the variance in their own average subjective well-being score, $F(1, 26) = 34.84$, $p < .001$, $R^2 = 57.26$. When life satisfaction scores were predicted, parents' happiness explained 42% of the variance in students' average life satisfaction score, $F(1, 26) = 18.81$, $p < .001$, $R^2 = 41.98$. Interestingly, adding the average rating of the happiness levels of one's brother(s) and/or sister(s) in subsequent regression models did not explain a statistically significant amount of additional variance in either children's subjective well-being or life satisfaction scores; instead, it was the parents' happiness that drove the effect of family members' happiness on students' happiness. Although based on a small sample, these preliminary analyses provide support for the notion that even among high school students, the happiness levels of a child's parents shows up in children's happiness levels.

Significant associations between parents' and children's happiness are also present when each party rates his or her own life satisfaction. In a sample of 148 fourth- and fifth-grade students and their biological parents (137 mothers, 109 fathers), statistically significant correlations indicated that happier children came from happier mothers ($r = .26$, $p < .01$) and fathers ($r = .29$, $p < .01$; Hoy, Suldo, & Raffaele Mendez, 2013). Similar to the study above with high school students in which parents' happiness was indexed by child perception, Hoy and colleagues found a moderate, significant relationship between fathers' and mothers' life satisfaction levels ($r = .38$, $p < .001$), in this case after matching parents' independent reports of their subjective well-being. These findings are consistent with other research suggesting that (1) adults tend to pair up with partners of similar levels of subjective well-being and experience changes in happiness as a couple (Bookwala & Schulz, 1996; Hoppmann, Gerstorf, Willis, & Schaie, 2011); and (2) children born into households with happier parents are likely to inherit a similar disposition favoring high subjective well-being, in part due to shared values and behavioral choices modeled at home (Headey, Muffels, & Wagner, 2014). Are those children of parents with low subjective well-being simply out of luck?

EVIDENCE FOR OPTIMISM FOR CHANGE IN HAPPINESS

A growing body of research supports that one's happiness can be improved, for lasting periods, after participating in activities intended to increase positive emotions. Originally, these activities were created and tested in adults. The activities are not complex; instead, they are brief, scripted, often self-administered activities that were developed to mimic the thoughts and behaviors of already happy people (Layous & Lyubomirsky, 2014). Researchers like Sonja Lyubomirsky, Ken Sheldon, Robert Emmons, Laura King, Martin Seligman, and others recruited samples of adults to participate in brief activities and compared changes in their happiness with that of adults randomly assigned to control conditions. They found that adults who made behavior changes that involved increasing their displays of kindness (Lyubomirsky et al., 2005), grateful thinking (Emmons & McCullough, 2003), hopeful thinking (Layous, Nelson, & Lyubomirsky, 2013; Sheldon & Lyubomirsky, 2006b), identifying and using their signature character strengths in new ways (Seligman et al., 2005), and/or savoring their positive experiences

(Kurtz, 2008; Schueller, 2010) sustained lasting gains in aspects of subjective well-being, often indicators of life satisfaction, positive emotions, and happiness.

POSITIVE PSYCHOLOGY INTERVENTIONS

Such evidence of the potential of positive change in well-being has fueled public interest in positive psychology, in part to help people become happier. Beyond the experimental attempts referenced above to purposefully promote happiness, there is abundant historical research on constructs that predated positive psychology but are now considered under the positive psychology umbrella due to empirical associations with well-being. With increased respect for subjective well-being as an important outcome, other studies of traditional clinical interventions that target remediation of the etiological basis of problems (e.g., cognitive errors, behavioral withdrawal) now may be evaluated with an eye toward impact on indicators of well-being or quality of life. Thus, one might wonder which strategies should be considered a positive psychology intervention. Is it anything with the word *positive* in the activity name or outcome assessment battery? Parks and Biswas-Diener (2013) suggest that an activity that can be defensibly conceptualized as a positive psychology intervention meets the following criteria:

- *Content.* The intervention focuses on positive topics, namely, the positive aspects of one's life such as environmental assets and personal strengths, rather than problems (stressors, personal deficits).
- *Target variable.* The primary goal of the intervention is to build a positive variable, such as subjective well-being (hedonic well-being) or meaning (eudemonic well-being), either as an outcome variable or a target, mediator, or mechanism of further positive change.
- *Research.* The intervention has been scientifically evaluated and findings from research studies provide empirical support that the intervention affects the positive variable, which in turn leads to positive outcomes for the intended population.
- *Population.* The intervention intends to promote wellness among people who are not distressed. Among clinical populations, targeting a theoretically appropriate positive variable with the goal of ameliorating pathology counts, whereas focusing on fixing weaknesses or targeting positive variables without theoretical rationale would not.

In a growing body of research, positive psychology interventions have also been tested in samples of youth, including children and adolescents through school-based services. The targets and activities that have been examined most often in intervention studies with students include:

- *Gratitude,* including such activities as "counting blessings" and recording positive events in a journal, and performing a gratitude visit (write and deliver a letter of thanks).
- *Kindness,* enhanced through performing three to five acts of kindness in a designated day.
- *Personal identification of strengths,* often through a "you at your best" writing about a time the student excelled followed by reflection on personal strengths shown at that time.

- *Use of character strengths* (i.e., 24 positive traits valued across cultures that are identified in the VIA classification system) in new ways.
- *Hope and goal-directed thinking,* involving activities such as visualizing desired future (goals) and creating pathways (steps to pursue) toward that vision.
- *Optimistic thinking style,* featuring a permanent, personal, and pervasive view toward positive events in the future based on the explanation of life events in the past.
- *Serenity,* often fostered through mindfulness mediation to train awareness to the present moment.

Some of the first published studies provided support for brief positive psychology interventions with middle school students, specifically interventions that targeted hope (Marques et al., 2011) and gratitude (Froh, Sefick, & Emmons, 2008). Other researchers have focused on cultivating strengths in youth through school-based programs. In the United Kingdom, such programs developed by Carmel Proctor, Jennifer Fox Eades, and colleagues include Celebrating Strengths (Fox Eades, 2008) and Strengths Gym (Proctor et al., 2011). In New Zealand, the Awesome Us program developed by Denise Quinlan, Nicola Swain, Dianne Vella-Brodrick, and colleagues at the University of Otago is a relatively brief classwide intervention that teaches children in grades 5 and 6 how to spot and use character strengths (Quinlan, Swain, et al., 2015). In the United States, Martin Seligman, Jane Gillham, Karen Reivich, and colleagues at the University of Pennsylvania developed a positive psychology curriculum for high school students (Positive Psychology for Youth Project) that emphasizes exploring and applying signature strengths (Gillham et al., 2013; Seligman, Ernst, Gillham, Reivich, & Linkins, 2009). In addition to those programs that focus on strengths, other universal interventions with theoretical underpinnings in positive psychology have appeared in countries around the world. For example, in Australia, Toni Noble and Helen McGrath developed Bounce Back!, a schoolwide program that teaches students (kindergarten–grade 8) how to cope effectively with stressors; the curriculum integrates principles from positive psychology (e.g., cultivating positive emotions, optimistic thinking, positive relationships) into a school's English language arts curriculum (McGrath & Noble, 2011). In Canada, Kimberly Schonert-Reichl and colleagues (Schonert-Reichl & Lawlor, 2010; Schonert-Reichl et al., 2015) have examined MindUP, a universal social and emotional learning program that uses classroom-based lessons and daily breathing activities to teach elementary and middle school students how to become mindful as well as to increase positive emotions through gratitude, optimism, and kindness. In Israel, Anat Shoshani and Sarit Steinmetz (2014) pioneered a schoolwide application of positive psychology (e.g., gratitude, goal fulfillment, character strengths, and positive relationships) in a universal approach to promote the well-being of all children in a middle school.

In collaboration with numerous talented graduate students at the University of South Florida, I developed a school-based intervention that incorporates many of these activities from the positive psychology literature into a comprehensive, multitarget intervention. We refer to this intervention as a Well-Being Promotion Program during our conversations with youth and families. The intervention was originally developed for implementation with small groups of middle school students, as described in Chapter 5. Following empirical support for a positive impact of the intervention on students' life satisfaction (Suldo, Savage, et al., 2014), we augmented it to include components for parents (Roth, Suldo, & Ferron, 2016), as well as teachers and classmates

(Suldo, Hearon, Bander, et al., 2015). The program modifications for younger and older students, classwide application, and parent inclusion are described in Chapters 6, 7, and 8, respectively.

HOW WELL DO POSITIVE PSYCHOLOGY INTERVENTIONS IMPROVE YOUTH SUBJECTIVE WELL-BEING?

The process of developing any educational intervention generally starts with foundational research to inform the design and developmental of a theory-driven intervention. Fully developed interventions or strategies are then assessed for impact on the intended outcome, beginning with tightly designed efficacy trials (Institute of Education Sciences & the National Science Foundation, 2013). Table 4.2 indicates how each stage in the sequence of development of basic knowledge to the intervention development and evaluation process is relevant to the process of evaluating interventions intended to promote youth happiness.

As recently as 10 years ago, I could not direct interested practitioners to any evidence-based strategies for increasing student happiness, as such research simply did not yet exist. Fortunately, in the past decade, rapid advances in basic knowledge of measurement and correlates of youth subjective well-being have enabled researchers to apply findings from exploratory research, especially studies within the area of positive psychology on the internal and environmental factors implicated in children's subjective well-being, to the design and development of interventions intended to promote subjective well-being. Table 4.3 contains a summary of the design features and findings from this growing number of published outcome studies of positive psychology interventions with youth samples. Most efforts can best be described as pilot studies in nature. Although often tested with relatively small samples of students, such studies provide important information needed to determine if attempting to integrate a given positive psychology intervention in school mental health efforts is feasible and worthwhile. Some of the experimental studies included in Table 4.3 have examined the impact of a fully developed theory-driven intervention via random assignment of students to intervention or control conditions. Given the heavy involvement of the intervention developers in these studies, the next logical step in the evaluation of the impact of school-based positive psychology interventions involves attempts at independent replication of positive effects. In the absence of effectiveness and scale-up research, the knowledge base on school-based positive psychology interventions may best be described as preliminary but promising.

A review of the key findings included in Table 4.3 makes clear that a growing body of research demonstrates positive change in at least some aspects of subjective well-being following youth participation in time-limited, school-based interventions that targets correlates of subjective well-being. Further research is needed to determine if the promise of an intervention varies as a function of age or other student features, such as academic skill level or behavior challenges. Additionally, further application and evaluation of these positive psychology interventions with larger and diverse youth samples is justified by the initial outcomes that suggest many school-based positive psychology interventions are associated with lasting gains in multiple indicators in subjective well-being, particularly positive affect. The preliminary findings provide considerable optimism for the potential of educational interventions to cause sustainable positive changes in youth happiness.

TABLE 4.2 Types of Research in the Development and Evaluation of School-Based Interventions

Type	Purpose	Sample research questions
Foundational	Inform theory and methodological issues about a specific phenomenon or desired outcome, such as optimal mental health	• What are the key elements of happiness? • How can youth happiness be measured in reliable and efficient ways?
Early-stage or exploratory	Identify correlates of the desired outcome, particularly those potentially malleable factors associated with the outcome	• Are changes in happiness possible? • What internal and environmental factors are correlated with youth happiness?
Design and development	Apply findings from observational studies to create interventions to achieve the outcome; carry out initial small-scale tests of the intervention to determine feasibility in the intended setting by the intended end user, and promise the intervention may achieve the intended outcome	• What are the critical factors to target in an intervention to increase youth happiness? • Which interventions seem to work, in that children are happier after taking part in the strategies? • Can these strategies be carried out in classrooms, by teachers and school mental health providers?

Studies of impact: How well does a *fully developed* intervention achieve its intended outcomes?

Efficacy	Determine the impact of an intervention under *ideal* conditions, such as with extensive implementation support often from the intervention developer	• Does the mental health of children who take part in the intervention improve relative to same-age peers who do not receive an intervention? • If yes, which mental health indicators (aspects of subjective well-being or psychopathology) show an effect? • Do these gains last after the intervention period is over?
Effectiveness	Determine the impact of an intervention in *routine* practice, such as in a school with no support from the intervention developer	• How effective is a targeted positive psychology intervention when delivered by a school psychologist to students with room for growth in happiness (Tier 2) as part of a school's multi-tiered system of mental health supports?
Scale-up	Determine the impact of an intervention in *routine* practice and *across settings and populations* in order to examine generalizability of positive impact across diverse groups	• How effective is a classwide positive psychology curriculum when delivered by health teachers to all high school freshmen (Tier 1) as part of a district's plan for universal mental health services?

TABLE 4.3. Empirical Evaluations of Positive Psychology Interventions with Samples of Youth

Author(s)	Description of PPI	Measures	Sample	Duration	Key findings
			Target: Gratitude		
Froh, Sefick, & Emmons (2008)	Counting one's blessings—daily listing of up to five things that one was grateful for since yesterday.	BMSLSS, PANAS-C, GAC, one-item indicator of global life satisfaction	$N = 221$ middle school students (grades 6 and 7), in 11 classes assigned to gratitude ($n = 76$), hassles (daily journaling about hassles in your life in past day; $n = 80$), or no-intervention control ($n = 65$)	Daily for 2 weeks.	Relative to hassles condition, significant ($p < .05$) effect on gratitude and negative affect at postintervention and 3-week follow-up. Relative to both comparison conditions, significantly higher school satisfaction at postintervention and 3-week follow-up. At postintervention (but not follow-up), marginally ($p < .10$) greater life satisfaction relative to hassles condition. No changes in positive affect.
Froh, Kashdan, Ozimkowski, & Miller (2009)	Gratitude visit—write and deliver a letter to one person for whom you are grateful. Then, one individual meeting with interventionist focused on sharing and reflecting on the visit.	PANAS-C, GAC	$N = 89$ youth (grades 3, 8, and 12), randomly assigned to gratitude ($n = 44$) or control in which students journaled about daily events ($n = 45$)	Over 2 weeks, five 10- to 15-minute writing sessions (either gratitude letter or daily events journal). Gratitude condition also delivered letter by end of second week.	Only for youth who began with low positive affect: compared to control, significantly ($p < .05$) greater gratitude and positive affect postintervention. At 2-month follow-up, elevated positive affect maintained and marginal ($p < .10$) maintenance of gratitude. No significant effect on negative affect.
McCabe, Bray, Kehle, Theodore, & Gelbar (2011); McCabe-Fitch (2009)	Three good things—nightly listing of three positive things that one experienced that day. Gratitude letter—after gratitude was defined, students were instructed to independently write and deliver (preferably in person, but mail or e-mail acceptable) a letter of thanks to someone who had done something kind for them but whom they had never thanked.	SHS, PANAS-C, SLSS	$N = 50$ middle school students (grades 7 and 8), randomly assigned to gratitude ($n = 26$; gratitude letter + gratitude journaling) or control in which students journaled about life details (daily events; $n = 24$)	In one meeting, students were instructed to journal each night for 1 week. Gratitude condition also instructed (in same meeting) to write and deliver a gratitude letter by end of the same week.	Relative to students in control condition, a small, positive affect on happiness became apparent at 2-month follow-up. Small, positive effect size for positive affect at postintervention and 2-month follow-up (interpreted with caution due to baseline differences in positive affect that favored experimental group). No effect on life satisfaction or negative affect.

(continued)

53

TABLE 4.3. *(continued)*

Author(s)	Description of PPI	Measures	Sample	Duration	Key findings
Froh et al. (2014)	Grateful thinking—classroom curriculum intended to teach students about the social–cognitive appraisals involved in receiving benefits from others (understanding a benefactor's intention, cost incurred, and benefits bestowed).	GAC, grateful thinking (benefits–appraisal vignettes); also in Study 1: behavioral gratitude (wrote a thank-you note); also in Study 2: PANAS-C, BMSLSS	Two samples of elementary school students. Study 1: $N = 122$ in six classes (all grade 4), randomly assigned to intervention ($n = 62$) or attention control (discussion of mundane social activities; $n = 60$). Study 2: $N = 82$ in four classes (grades 4 and 5), randomly assigned to intervention ($n = 44$) or attention control ($n = 38$)	Five 30-minute classwide lessons from the benefits–appraisal or control curriculum, either daily for 1 week (Study 1) or 1 day per week for 5 weeks (Study 2).	Study 1: Compared to control, significant ($p < .05$) increases in grateful thinking, grateful behavior, and grateful mood at postintervention. No follow-up data reported. Study 2: Compared to control condition, significant ($p < .05$) growth in grateful thinking, grateful mood, and positive affect, with significant between-group differences evident by 7- and 15-week follow-up. No significant effects of intervention on negative affect or life satisfaction.
Owens & Patterson (2013)	Draw a picture of something for which they were grateful that happened that day.	PANAS-C, BMSLSS, GSE	$N = 62$ elementary students (ages 5–11), assigned to a condition: gratitude ($n = 22$), alternate PPI—best possible selves ($n = 23$), or active control (draw about anything they did that day; $n = 17$)	One session per week for 4–6 weeks.	Relative to other two conditions, no significant effects on affect, life satisfaction, or self-esteem. No follow-up data reported.
Layous, Nelson, Oberle, Schonert-Reichl, & Lyubomirsky (2012)	Acts of kindness—students instructed to perform three acts of kindness in a week and report these acts via an in-class survey.	PANAS-C, SWLS, SHS, sociometric ratings of peer acceptance	**Target: Kindness** $N = 415$ elementary school students (ages 9–11) in 19 classrooms randomly assigned to acts of kindness ($n = 211$) or active control intended to be mildly pleasant (visit three places; $n = 204$)	Weekly, for 4 weeks.	Students in both conditions had significant ($p < .05$) increases in positive affect, and marginal ($p < .10$) increases in life satisfaction and happiness; no advantage of intervention condition on these outcomes. In both groups, significant increases in peer acceptance, but kindness group

increased significantly more than controls on peer acceptance.

Target: You at your best—no studies with school-age youth[a]

Target: Character strengths

Study	Measures	Sample	Duration	Intervention	Results
Proctor et al. (2011)	SLSS, PANAS, RSE	$N = 319$ middle school students (ages 12–14), in strengths gym ($n = 218$) or no-intervention control ($n = 101$)	Over 6 months, weekly classwide lessons focused on a specific strength. Teachers completed three to 12 lessons ($M = 5.6$).	Strengths gym program—delivered classwide by teachers, lessons correspond to the 24 VIA strengths, intended to build a student's personal strengths and the recognition of strengths in others.	Compared to control, significant ($p < .05$) increases in life satisfaction and marginal ($p < .10$) gains in positive affect. No significant effects on negative affect or self-esteem. No follow-up data reported.
Rashid et al. (2013)	PPTI, SLSS, SSIS	$N = 59$ middle school students (grade 6), in two schools, one assigned to strengths classroom ($n = 33$) and the other to no-intervention control ($n = 26$)	Throughout entire academic year, weekly teacher integration of strengths in classroom curriculum; discussion of strengths with parents over winter break.	Teacher training in the VIA classification system, ways to build strengths at school, and links between strengths and the curriculum. Student identification and use of signature strengths in problem solving and in a self-improvement project, recognizing strengths of characters in curriculum. Also, two parent psychoeducation sessions focused on their child's signature strengths.	Within intervention condition, improvements in teacher-rated social skills and parent-reported problem behavior (composite of externalizing, internalizing, and hyperactivity symptoms). Compared to control, no significant effects on life satisfaction or well-being assessed by the PPTI (positive emotions, engagement, meaning). No follow-up data reported.
Quinlan, Swain, Cameron, & Vella-Brodrick (2015)	SLSS, I-PANAS-SF, EVDL, MCI, CINSS, SUS	$N = 196$ elementary school students (grades 5 and 6; most ages 9–10), in nine classrooms assigned to the strengths condition ($n = 140$; six classrooms) or no-intervention control ($n = 56$; three classrooms)	Six weekly 90-minute group sessions; one review session 1 month later	Student identification and use of strengths in problem solving, goal pursuit, and relationship building; recognizing strengths in self (e.g., via reflection of activity strengths, as shown in "you at your best") and in other people like classmates (i.e., strengths spotting). Classroom teacher co-facilitated sessions.	Compared to control condition, significant growth in positive affect, emotional and behavioral classroom engagement, classroom emotional climate (cohesion, less friction, satisfaction of intrinsic needs for autonomy and relatedness), and strengths use evident by 3-month follow-up. No significant effects of intervention on negative affect or life satisfaction.

(continued)

TABLE 4.3. *(continued)*

Author(s)	Description of PPI	Measures	Sample	Duration	Key findings
			Target: Positive emotions like serenity via mindfulness		
Schonert-Reichl & Lawlor (2010)	Mindfulness education program (adapted from Kehoe & Fischer, 2002)—delivered classwide by teachers, lessons target self-awareness, focused attention, positive emotions, self-regulation, management of negative emotions and negative thinking, and goal setting; also, daily mindfulness attention exercises with affirmations and visualizations.	PANAS, RI, SDQ, TRSC	$N = 246$ students (grades 4–7) in 12 schools; six intervention classrooms ($n = 139$) and six classrooms ($n = 107$) in a wait-list control condition	Over 4 months, 10 weekly 40- to 50-minute classwide lessons. Also, students completed mindfulness exercises three times per day (3 minutes per practice) for at least 9 weeks.	Compared to control, significant ($p < .05$) increases in optimism, teacher-rated improvements in attention/concentration, and social–emotional competence, as well as decreases in externalizing behavior problems; marginal ($p < .10$) gains in positive affect; for preadolescents only (grades 4 and 5), significant increases in self-concept. No significant effects on negative affect or self-concept (for students in grades 6 and 7). No follow-up data reported.
Schonert-Reichl et al. (2015)	MindUP program (Hawn Foundation, 2008)—delivered classwide by teachers, lessons target self-regulation (e.g., mindful smelling, mindful tasting), prosocial behavior, positive emotions (via gratitude, optimistic thinking), and a caring classroom environment (e.g., via acts of kindness); also, daily mindfulness exercises (deep breathing, attentive listening).	IRI, RI, SDQ, SGQ, MAAS-C, SPQC; executive functions tasks; sociometric ratings of peer acceptance, prosocial and aggressive behavior; math grades	$N = 99$ students (grades 4–5) in 4 schools; two intervention classrooms ($n = 48$) and two classrooms in a business-as-usual control condition (i.e., a social responsibility program; $n = 51$)	Over 4 months, 12 weekly 40- to 50-minute classwide lessons. Also, students completed mindfulness exercises three times per day (3 minutes per practice) for 12 weeks.	Compared to control, significant ($p < .05$) increases in executive functions (speed on tasks), optimism, mindfulness, school self-concept, and social–emotional competence (perspective taking, empathy, peer-nominated prosocial behavior and acceptance), as well as decreases in depressive symptoms and aggression; marginal ($p < .10$) higher year-end math grades. In both groups, significant increases in social responsibility. No follow-up data reported.
			Target: Positive emotions via savoring—no studies with school-age youth[a]		
			Target: Hope		
Marques, Lopez, & Pais-Ribeiro (2011)	Building hope for the future program—teaches students	SLSS, CHS, SWS, MHI-5	$N = 62$ middle school students (grade 6);	Five weekly 1-hour group sessions and 1 1-hour group	Compared to control, significant ($p < .05$) increases in hope,

Study	Intervention	Measures	Sample	Dosage	Findings
	to create clear goals, identify pathways to achieve goals, harness mental energy to pursue goals, and reframe barriers as challenges to be overcome. Also, one psychoeducational session on hope for parents and teachers.		intervention (n = 31) and matched comparison group (n = 31)	meeting with parents and teachers.	life satisfaction, and self-worth. All gains maintained at 6- and 18-month follow-up. No changes in mental health problems or grades earned in courses.
Owens & Patterson (2013)	Best possible selves—draw a future version of yourself as happy and interested.	PANAS-C, BMSLSS, GSE	N = 62 elementary school students (ages 5–11), assigned to best possible selves (n = 23), alternate PPI—gratitude (n = 22), or active control (n = 17)	One session per week for 4–6 weeks.	Relative to other two conditions, significant increases in self-esteem. No significant effects on affect or life satisfaction. No follow-up data reported.
Green, Grant, & Rynsaardt (2007)	Delivered by teachers trained as life coaches, meetings focused on setting goals, identifying resources to achieve goals, developing action steps and solutions, and evaluating progress.	THS, CogHS, DASS-21	N = 56 female high school students (ages 16–17) randomly assigned to life coach (n = 28) or a wait-list control (n = 28).	Ten 45-minute individual coaching sessions over the period of two semesters (28 weeks).	Relative to control, significant increases in hope (total; also agency and pathways) and cognitive hardiness, and decreases in depression. No changes in stress or anxiety. No follow-up data reported.

Target: Optimism

Study	Intervention	Measures	Sample	Dosage	Findings
Brunwasser, Gillham, & Kim (2009); Gillham, Hamilton, Freres, Patton, & Gallop (2006)	Penn resiliency program—depression prevention curriculum focused on helping children cope with daily stressors by developing a realistic, optimistic explanatory style (e.g., challenge pessimistic beliefs by considering alternative explanations and examining evidence), as well as social and problem-solving skills.	CASQ, CDI	Meta-analysis of 17 evaluations of PRP in relation to a control group, with a combined sample of 2,498 youth ages 8–18	Twelve weekly 90-minute group sessions.	Meta-analysis found that students in intervention condition had immediate reduction in depressive symptoms, a significant but small effect that was more robust at 6- and 12-month follow-up, as compared to youth receiving no intervention. Some studies (e.g., Gillham et al., 2006) report positive effects of intervention condition on an optimistic explanatory style for positive events, for up to 2 years.

(continued)

TABLE 4.3. (continued)

Author(s)	Description of PPI	Measures	Sample	Duration	Key findings
Rooney, Hassan, Kane, Roberts, & Nesa (2013); Johnstone, Rooney, Hassan, & Kane (2014)	Aussie optimism program—positive thinking skills program. Delivered classwide by teachers, lessons aimed to prevent depression and anxiety among children by improving optimistic thinking via cognitive–behavioral strategies aligned with Seligman's (1990) theory of optimism.	CASQ, CDI, SCAS	N = 910 students (grades 4 and 5) from 22 schools, randomly assigned to intervention (n = 467) or control group (n = 443, regular health education curriculum)	Ten 1-hour weekly sessions led by teachers.	Students in both conditions had significant (p < .05) increases in optimism and decreases in anxiety symptoms at postintervention, as well as 6- and 18-month follow-up; no advantage of intervention condition on optimism or anxiety. Intervention condition improved significantly more on immediate reduction in depressive symptoms. Positive intervention effects on depression not evident at follow-up points (42 and 54 months later); symptoms in both groups declined at a similar rate.
			Multitarget		
Rashid & Anjum (2008); Rashid et al. (2013)	Positive psychotherapy, with multiple PPIs: you at your best, gratitude journaling, identification and use of signature strengths in a self-improvement project, recognizing signature strengths of family members, and savoring. Parents invited to final session (student presentation of signature strengths project).	SLSS, PPTI, SSRS, CDI	N = 22 middle school students (grade 6), randomly assigned to intervention (n = 11) or no-intervention control (n = 11)	Eight weekly 90-minute group sessions.	Compared to control, significant increase in well-being and parent-rated social skills. At 6-month follow-up, gains in well-being (but not social skills) were maintained. Gains in positive affect maintained at 2-month follow-up. No changes in life satisfaction, depressive symptoms, or teacher-rated social skills.
Suldo, Savage, & Mercer (2014)	Multiple PPIs: you at your best, gratitude journaling, gratitude visit, acts of kindness, identification and new uses of signature strengths, savoring,	SLSS, PANAS-C, YSR	N = 55 middle school students (grade 6), randomly assigned to intervention (n = 28) or wait-list control (n = 27)	Ten weekly 1-hour group sessions.	Compared to control, significant (p < .05) increase in life satisfaction. Gains maintained at 6-month follow-up (although the control group caught up by

Author	Intervention	Measures	Sample	Dosage	Results
	optimistic thinking, hope (best-possible future self).				follow-up). No significant effects on affect or psychopathology.
Roth, Suldo, & Ferron (2016)	Same as Suldo et al. (2014) above, plus two follow-up sessions (PPIs were reviewed). Also, one parent psychoeducational session and weekly notes for parents.	SLSS, PANAS-C, BPM-Y	N = 42 middle school students (grade 7), randomly assigned to intervention (n = 21) or wait-list control (n = 21)	Twelve weekly 50-minute group sessions, and one 1-hour parent group meeting.	Compared to control, significant (p < .05) increases in life satisfaction and positive affect, and reductions in negative affect. Gains in positive affect maintained at 2-month follow-up. Marginal (p < .10) reductions in internalizing and externalizing psychopathology at postintervention, maintained (p < .10) at follow-up for internalizing.
Suldo, Hearon, Bander, et al. (2015)	Multiple PPIs: you at your best, gratitude journaling, gratitude visit, acts of kindness, identification and new uses of signature strengths, and cultivating student–teacher and student–student relationships. Also, one teacher psychoeducational session and teacher co-facilitated sessions.	MSLSS, SLSS, PANAS-C	N = 12 elementary school students (grade 4). No control group.	Ten weekly 50-minute classwide lessons and one 50-minute teacher meeting.	Significant (p < .05) increases in positive affect and satisfaction with self. Marginal (p < .10) increases in global life satisfaction and satisfaction with friends and living environment. All gains maintained at 2-month follow-up. No changes in students' attendance or discipline referrals.
Gillham et al. (2013); Seligman, Ernst, Gillham, Reivich, & Linkins (2009)	Multiple PPIs within a positive psychology curriculum delivered classwide by teachers. Primary focus is on identification and new uses of signature strengths. Also targets positive emotions, purpose, and resilience via gratitude journaling, gratitude visits, savoring, optimism, and talks about the meaning of life (e.g., social relationships, connections to institutions and values).	SSRS, others unspecified	N = 347 high school students (grade 9), randomly assigned to language arts classes with a positive psychology curriculum or language arts as usual (n per group unspecified)	Throughout entire academic year, 20–25, 80-minute small-group or classwide sessions with follow-up homework to apply skills, and reflections on these experiences through journaling.	Preliminary findings (students followed through grade 11): improvements in social skills (as rated by teachers and parents), teacher-rated learning strengths, and student-rated school enjoyment and engagement. No effects on depressive symptoms, anxiety symptoms, overall achievement, or participation in extracurricular activities. Only for students who began with regular classes (not honors classes): improved achievement in language arts.

(continued)

TABLE 4.3. *(continued)*

Author(s)	Description of PPI	Measures	Sample	Duration	Key findings
Shoshani & Steinmetz (2014)	Multiple PPIs within a positive psychology curriculum delivered schoolwide by extensively trained teachers. Primarily targets positive emotions, gratitude (e.g., gratitude journaling, gratitude visits), goal fulfillment, optimism, character strengths, and strong relationships at home and school (and positive school climate).	SWLS, BSI symptom subscales, RSE, GSES, LOT-R	$N = 1,038$ middle school students (grades 7–9) in Israel, in two schools: intervention school ($n = 537$ students and 80 teachers) and a matched school serving as a wait-list control, with social sciences as usual ($n = 501$)	Throughout 1 school year, 15 classwide sessions, each with theory, experiential activities, and multimedia material. Class sessions ran in parallel with 15, 2-hour workshops for all educators in the school.	Compared to control, from baseline to 1-year follow-up, significant ($p < .05$) increases in self-esteem, self-efficacy, and optimism, and decreases in anxiety and depression. No significant effect of intervention condition (school) on life satisfaction.

Note. BMSLSS, Brief Multidimensional Students' Life Satisfaction Scale (Seligson, Huebner, & Valois, 2003); BPM-Y, Brief Problem Monitor—Youth (Achenbach, McConaughy, Ivanovo, & Rescorla, 2011); BSI, Brief Symptom Inventory (Derogatis & Spencer, 1982); CASQ, Children's Attributional Style Questionnaire (Seligman et al., 1984); CDI, Children's Depression Inventory (Kovacs, 1992); CHS, Children's Hope Scale (Snyder et al., 1997); CINSS, Children's Intrinsic Needs Satisfaction Scale (Koestner & Veronneau, 2001); CogHS, Cognitive Hardiness Scale (Nowack, 1990); DASS-21, Depression Anxiety and Stress Scale (Lovibond & Lovibond, 1995); EVDL, Engagement versus Disaffection with Learning (Skinner, Kindermann, & Furrer, 2009); GAC, Grateful Adjectives Checklist (McCullough, Emmons, & Tsang, 2002); GSE, Global Self-Esteem subscale of the Perceived Competence Scale for Children (Harter, 1982); GSES, General Self-Efficacy Scale (Schwarzer & Jerusalem, 1995); I-PANAS-SF, International Positive and Negative Affect Schedule—Short Form (Thompson, 2007); IRI, Interpersonal Reactivity Index (Davis, 1983); LOT-R, Life Orientation Test—Revised (Scheier, Carver, & Bridges, 1994); MAAS-C, Mindful Attention Awareness Scale for Children (Lawlor, Schonert-Reichl, Gadermann, & Zumbo, 2014); MCI, My Class Inventory (Fisher & Fraser, 1981); MHI-5, Mental Health Inventory with five items (primarily anxiety and depression symptoms) of the Short Form—36 Health Survey (Ware, Snow, Kosinski, & Gandek, 1993); PANAS, Positive and Negative Affect Schedule (Watson, Clark, & Tellegen, 1988); PANAS-C, Positive and Negative Affect Schedule for Children (Laurent et al., 1999); PPI, positive psychology intervention; PPTI, Positive Psychotherapy Inventory—Children's Version (Rashid & Anjum, 2008); RI, Resiliency Inventory (Song, 2003); RSE, Rosenberg Self-Esteem Scale (Rosenberg, 1965); SCAS, Spence Children's Anxiety Scale (Spence, 1998); SDQ, Self-Description Questionnaire (Marsh, Barnes, Cairns, & Tidman, 1984); SGQ, Social Goals Questionnaire (Wentzel, 1993); SHS, Subjective Happiness Scale (Lyubomirsky & Lepper, 1999); SLSS, Students' Life Satisfaction Scale (Huebner, 1991b); SPQC, Seattle Personality Questionnaire for Children (Kusche, Greenberg, & Beilke, 1988); SSIS, Social Skills Improvement System (Gresham & Elliott, 2008); SSRS, Social Skills Rating System (Gresham & Elliot, 1990); SUS, Strengths Use Scale (Govindji & Linley, 2007); SWLS, Satisfaction with Life Scale (Diener, Emmons, Larsen, & Griffin, 1985); SWS, Self-Worth subscale of the Self-Perception Profile for Children (Harter, 1985); THS, Trait Hope Scale (Snyder et al., 1991); TRSC, Teachers' Rating Scale of Social Competence (Kam & Greenberg, 1998); VIA, Values in Action; YSR, Youth Self-Report form of the Achenbach System of Empirically Based Assessment (ASEBA; Achenbach & Rescorla, 2001).

[a]To date, there are no published evaluations of "you at your best" or savoring in a study in which it was isolated as an intervention activity or target (e.g., to prolong positive emotions). Positive effects have been observed in multitarget positive psychology interventions that begin with a positive introduction that includes the "you at your best" activity, and later include instruction and rehearsal of savoring (Rashid & Anjum, 2008; Roth, Suldo, & Ferron, 2016; Suldo, Savage, & Mercer, 2014).

HOW DO POSITIVE PSYCHOLOGY INTERVENTIONS WORK TO INCREASE SUBJECTIVE WELL-BEING?

Barbara Fredrickson's (2001) broaden-and-build theory provides perhaps the most logical, evidence-based, and pervasive explanation of how the positive emotions that emit from positive psychology interventions propel the lasting gains in subjective well-being. Thinking gratefully, performing acts of kindness, and envisioning a best-possible self create and direct focus to positive feelings about one's past, present, and future, respectively. In brief, such positive emotions create an upward spiral, marked by increased cognitive capacity and behavioral flexibility that, over time, permits individuals to *build* personal social, psychological, and physical resources. The linchpins of this theory are expanded below, followed by highlights of the vast empirical support for this theory.

Positive Emotions

"Feeling good" at a particular moment comes in different forms, sparked by different activities, attended to uniquely by different people. Table 4.4 lists the most common positive emotions.

Broaden

Positive emotions open up our minds, broaden the scope of our attentional field, and create new opportunities for additional (positive) experiences. Such expanded thinking and vision paves the way for enhanced creativity, and enhances speed and effectiveness of problem solving. Fredrickson's (2009) impressive collection of scientific studies of the functions of positive emotions demonstrates that they "broaden your outlook, bringing more possibilities into view. With positivity, your thoughts and actions surface more spontaneously; you're better able to envision future prospects and win–win solutions" (p. 61).

This increased flexibility in thought is beneficial in daily task completion and effort allocation, and perhaps even more noticeably helpful when major stressors trigger coping responses. People with greater positive emotion tend to handle stress better, with superior and deliberate problem-solving strategies. They see more solutions in the face of adversity. Whereas negative emotions fuel narrowing in on a restricted coping repertoire with impulsive selection of often ineffective behavioral responses, positive emotions and open-mindedness go hand in hand.

Build

Increases in positive emotions are followed by growth in resources across four areas:

1. *Mental resources:* better habits of mind, such as being mindful (present) of our surroundings, savoring pleasant events, and generating multiple pathways to reach goals.
2. *Psychological resources:* more self-acceptance and enhanced character strengths, such as purpose in life and optimism.
3. *Social resources:* become more attractive to others, forge more trusting and satisfying

relationships, strengthen connections to others, and perceive more support from close others.

4. *Physical resources:* better health, in part through reduced stress-related hormones and increased hormones responsible for emotional bonding and growth; enhanced immune systems; and better sleep.

Gains in these areas are referred to as resources purposefully. When stressors are encountered in the future, regardless of whether these stressors are positive (e.g., opportunities) or negative (e.g., a setback), one can draw on these resources to navigate the stressor more successfully.

TABLE 4.4. Common Positive Emotions

Emotion	Synonyms and key features	Leads to
Joy	Feel great pleasure, delight, and happiness; light and glowing	Energy and involvement
Gratitude	Appreciate some positive event or gift that came our way in life; recognize the good in humanity	Urge to give back or give forward
Serenity	Feel content and appreciative for safe circumstances; such peace often follows other positive emotions like joy and amusement	Savoring of the circumstance and reflection on how to build it in our life more often
Interest	Feel fascinated, pulled to further discovery; feel alive and open to further exploration of new ideas	Acquisition of new knowledge and skills
Hope	Feel like a dire situation might improve, that possibilities for betterment exist	Persistence, ingenuity, and planning for a better future
Pride	Feel pleased with self following an achievement; recognition of one's value; confidence	Grit and seeking more opportunities for achievement
Amusement	Urge to laugh following something unexpected and humorous, most often in a social context	Sharing of laughter with another person, which builds connections
Inspiration	Witness human excellence, of character or talent; rapt attention on another's divine qualities	Pursuit of personal betterment and strive for excellence
Awe	Witness goodness on a grand scale; feel overwhelmed by greatness, full of amazement, and temporarily transfixed	Recognition of connectedness to something larger
Love	Positive emotions above occur in the context of a safe, close relationship; a momentary state when a positive emotion is shared with another person	Production of hormones that strengthen bonds and intimacy

Note. Derived from Fredrickson (2009).

Empirical Support

Research indicates that a ratio around 3:1 positive to negative emotions experienced over time is the likely tipping point for experiencing flourishing mental health (Fredrickson, 2013). Notice that the goal is not an unrealistic 3:0 or even 1:0; negative emotions such as anger, guilt, fear, and disgust are acknowledged to be unavoidable in life. Striving to eliminate negative emotions would be futile. Instead, striving to increase positive emotions until they are three times more prevalent appears sufficient to overcome the strength of negative emotions. Experimental research confirms that positive emotions can be induced and cause positive effects on well-being, for instance through loving-kindness meditation, which involves training warm and caring feelings toward oneself and others (see Garland et al., 2010, for a review) or many of the activities named in Table 4.3.

Increasing Positive Emotions

Based on a plethora of studies of evidence-based strategies for increasing positive emotions, Fredrickson (2009) advanced a "toolkit" of a dozen strategies from which people can select in attempts to improve their personal ratio closer to the 3:1 goal. Youth adaptations of most strategies are described in detail in Chapters 5–8, and target gratitude, kindness, identification and use of character strengths, disputing negative thinking (via developing an optimistic explanatory style), savoring positive emotions, visualizing a positive future, and creating strong social connections. Other strategies that are outside the scope of this book but are nonetheless plausible routes include developing distractions that can be used to divert one's attention when rumination and negativity surface, and increasing time in nature. Fredrickson also emphasizes the value of mindfulness in daily activities (cultivate curiosity about, and acceptance of, whatever your current experience entails) as well as during meditation (with or without thoughts of loving-kindness). Practitioners interested in learning more about developing mindfulness in youth are encouraged to look into mindfulness-based stress reduction (MBSR) for adolescents (Biegel, Brown, Shapiro, & Schubert, 2009) or the MindUP program referenced in Table 4.3 (*http://thehawnfoundation.org/mindup*).

CHAPTER 5

The Well-Being Promotion Program
A Selective Intervention for Adolescents

with Jessica Savage

This chapter presents a comprehensive, multitarget positive psychology intervention developed to improve adolescents' subjective well-being. The "Well-Being Promotion Program" was originally designed for implementation with small groups of youth via 10 weekly meetings during a single class period (approximately 45 minutes). When implemented as intended, the intervention was associated with improvements in sixth-grade students' life satisfaction over the course of the 10-week program (Suldo, Savage, & Mercer, 2014). This chapter contains a description of Seligman's (2002) theoretical framework that guided development of intervention targets (i.e., positive feelings about students' past, present, and future) and specific activities focused on gratitude, kindness, character strengths, optimistic thinking, and hope. We also describe the features of the intervention that align with current thinking in best practices in positive psychology interventions. Then, we overview the goals and activities within each of the 10 sessions; the complete manual for the practitioner who intends to lead a group is presented in the Appendix. The session-by-session protocols in the manual detail procedures for each activity, along with reference to the research-based underpinnings. This chapter also includes a summary of the design and development process, including existing empirical support for the multitarget positive psychology intervention when implemented as intended with small groups of adolescents during regular school hours. Finally, we provide a detailed example of a recent implementation of the Well-Being Promotion Program, to help make concrete how the procedures described in this chapter and the Appendix have been enacted with success in our work with middle school students.

Jessica Savage, PhD, is a school psychologist in Hillsborough County Public Schools and a 2011 graduate of the School Psychology Program at the University of South Florida.

THEORETICAL FOUNDATIONS OF THE INTERVENTION

Early in the history of positive psychology, Seligman (2002) asserted that people are capable of increasing their happiness levels into the upper range of their set points through intentional activities. He proposed a multidimensional view of increasing happiness, including attention to past, present, and future aspects of emotional life. In this theory of authentic happiness, developing feelings of satisfaction with one's past entails activities to strengthen gratitude for positive events and forgiveness associated with negative events. In terms of the present, Seligman discussed happiness levels as dependent on both pleasures—immediate, fading sensations—and gratifications that come from full absorption in a task. Positive feelings in the present involve enhancing momentary pleasures through savoring and mindfulness, as well as increasing gratifications via use of one's talents and character strengths in new and meaningful ways. Positive emotions about the future were theorized to stem from hopeful and optimistic thinking. An optimistic explanatory style increases the ability to cope with trauma as well as generates positive emotions (Seligman, 1990).

We developed the Well-Being Promotion Program described in this chapter based on Seligman's (2002) framework for increasing happiness and recommendations for improving optimal well-being throughout the lifespan. Our student-focused program includes developmentally appropriate modifications, including gratitude interventions and application of character strengths identified with the VIA classification system. Our selection of specific activities was also informed by knowledge of other researchers' positive psychology interventions that had worked to increase adults' happiness; we modified such activities targeting kindness, savoring, and goal-directed thinking (hope) to be suitable for use with secondary school students. Aside from the introduction and termination sessions, each session is categorized into one of three phases, differentiated by a focus on the past, present, and future aspects of emotional well-being. Specifically, Sessions 2–9 contain activities intended to increase happiness into the upper levels of one's range through (1) expressions of gratitude for past events, (2) gratifications through novel use of character strengths, and (3) positive future-oriented emotions through development of an optimistic explanatory style and hopeful, goal-directed thinking. The activities ultimately contained in the 10 sessions of the core program are in line with theory and studies on effective positive psychology interventions, many of which provided the basis for Fredrickson's (2009) "toolkit" of 12 evidence-based strategies recommended for use to increase frequency of positive emotions.

OVERVIEW OF THE WELL-BEING PROMOTION PROGRAM

We intend the manualized intervention found in the Appendix to provide extensive guidance to practitioners who seek to implement positive psychology interventions within school-based practice. The practitioner will still need to provide examples from personal experience and make modifications as necessary to accommodate student needs. In addition to becoming familiar with the background information presented in the preceding chapters of this book, practitioners should read all session protocols carefully prior to initiating the intervention. Such familiarity with the intervention in its entirety will help the practitioner to orient him- or herself to the nature of each of the three phases and key ideas that resurface across sessions.

As can be seen in the Appendix, each session protocol begins with an overview of the goals, procedures, and materials needed for a successful meeting. Detailed descriptions of intervention activities follow, sometimes with brief rationales for how activities relate to the topic of the session. These brief rationales recap information provided in further depth in the text chapters of this book. Directions for practitioners to complete in-session activities are presented in bulleted lists. Within particular activities, wording of instructions and explanations of concepts is important for clarity. Thus, recommended verbatim instructions for practitioners (i.e., group leaders) to share with students are denoted in *italics*.

Table 5.1 contains a summary of the targets and primary activity within each session. All sessions contain practitioner-facilitated discussions of concepts relevant to happiness, directions for how to complete specific positive psychology interventions (alternately referred to as exercises, activities, and strategies), and homework assignments that involve completion or rehearsal of the activity taught during the group session.

POSITIVE INTRODUCTION—SESSION 1

The first session contains an introduction to the intervention purpose and meeting logistics, in addition to completion and discussion of the you at your best activity. Specifically, students

TABLE 5.1. Overview of Core Sessions in the Well-Being Promotion Program for Small Groups of Adolescents

Session	Target	Strategies
1	Positive introduction	You at your best
Positive emotions about the past		
2	Gratitude	Gratitude journals
3	Gratitude	Gratitude visit
Positive emotions about the present		
4	Kindness	Acts of kindness
5	Character strengths	Introduction to strengths (VIA classification system)
6	Character strengths	Survey assessment of signature character strengths
7	Character strengths; savoring	Use of signature strengths in new ways; savoring methods
Positive emotions about the future		
8	Optimistic thinking	Optimistic explanatory style
9	Hope	Best-possible self in the future
10	All	Termination; review of strategies and plan for future use

write about a time when they were at their best, then share and reflect on the personal strengths displayed in the story. This activity was intended to create an initial well-being increase that would help engage students in the intervention process. In a large community sample, adults who self-administered that activity incurred an immediate boost in happiness as well as reduction in symptoms of depression, relative to adults in an active placebo condition (Seligman et al., 2005). However, these positive effects did not maintain past the postintervention data collection. Because the differences between conditions were not evident at 1-week or 1- to 6-month follow-up assessments, Seligman and colleagues concluded the exercise

> is not an effective intervention, at least not in isolation. We add "in isolation" because in our multiexercise programs (which have not yet been subjected to a randomized controlled trial), we use this exercise to introduce the signature strengths interventions, and it is possible that telling an introductory story about one's highest strengths, followed by the effective signature strength exercise, may amplify the benefits on happiness and depression. It seems plausible— given that three of the interventions were effective when delivered alone—to suppose that a package of positive interventions, perhaps including ones that were ineffective in isolation, might well exceed the beneficial effects of any single exercise. Such packages—likely containing some moves that are truly inert, some moves that are inert in isolation but effective in a package, and some moves that are always active—are what any therapy consists of. (pp. 419–420)

In this first session, students are also introduced to Lyubomirsky, Sheldon, and Schkade's (2005) model of sustainable happiness. This provides a rationale for the group's focus on learning, rehearsing, and purposefully enacting thoughts and behaviors intended to increase positive feelings about the past, present, and future. An initial homework activity is assigned (reread and expand the you at your best story). Students learn that they can earn small treats, such as candy and school supplies, contingent on homework completion. We also routinely provide the same treats at the end of each session to reinforce participation in group discussions and activities.

PHASE 1:
PAST-FOCUSED POSITIVE EMOTIONS—SESSIONS 2 AND 3

Positive emotions about the past include pride, fulfillment, contentment, and satisfaction (Seligman, 2002). Emotional valences about the past are driven by thoughts and interpretations of historical events, actions, and relationships. When one dwells on past events that he or she has interpreted negatively, negative emotion is perseverated. In contrast, focusing thoughts on positive interpretations of past events can hold emotion in the upper range of one's set point. Gratitude amplifies the intensity and frequency of positive memories.

Gratitude

Gratitude is often referred to as an emotional response to the reception of a personal positive outcome from another individual that was neither deserved nor earned (Emmons &

McCullough, 2003). One may experience a grateful emotion for a number of reasons, including receipt of gifts, favors, emotional support, or a collective effort such as reflected in a donation (Bono, Froh, & Forrett, 2014). Research supports long-term mental health benefits of gratitude among adolescents; as described in Bono and colleagues (2014), higher and increasing levels of gratitude predicted fewer negative emotions and depression, as well as greater positive emotions, life satisfaction, and happiness.

Intervention activities targeting gratitude that have shown positive effects on one or more aspects of subjective well-being among adolescents include "counting blessings," sometimes called "gratitude journaling" (Froh et al., 2008), and expressing gratitude to another through writing and delivering a letter of thanks, termed a *gratitude visit* (Froh, Kashdan, Ozimkowski, & Miller, 2009). Among adults who self-administered a randomly assigned intervention online, individuals who completed a gratitude visit incurred the largest gains in happiness immediately afterward and up to 1 month later; however, effects were gone by 3-month follow-up (Seligman et al., 2005). In the same study, individuals who carried out a "three good things" activity (write down three things that went well each day and their causes, nightly for 1 week) experienced gains in happiness that became evident at 1 month after the intervention conclusion, and maintained through 6-month follow-up. College students asked to keep a gratitude journal daily for 10 weeks experienced increased global life satisfaction but no changes in positive or negative affect (Emmons & McCullough, 2003). Other studies with adults who wrote down three good things daily for shorter durations—1 week (Odou & Vella-Brodrick, 2013) or 4 weeks (Sheldon & Lyubomirsky, 2006b)—found decreased negative affect but still no change in positive affect.

Completing multiple activities targeting gratitude may be particularly mood boosting. Relative to control conditions that receive no intervention, higher levels of happiness have been found among samples of college students (Senf & Liau, 2013) and middle school students (McCabe, Bray, Kehle, Theodore, & Gelbar, 2011; McCabe-Fitch, 2009) who were assigned to both count their blessings nightly *and* perform a gratitude visit.

Session 2 introduces gratitude and gratitude journaling. Gratitude journals are used as a means of focusing student thoughts on things, people, and events for which they are thankful. In separate journal entries, students are asked to write down five small-to-large things (events, people, talents, etc.) for which they are grateful. The intensity is high for the first week, in that students are asked to journal daily. This is in line with Emmons and McCullough's (2003) finding that higher intensity led to greater increases in happiness. In later sessions, journaling for homework is assigned on a once-per-week basis due to the introduction of other activities.

Session 3 opens discussion of the content of those journals, introduces enactment of gratitude through visits, and makes the connection among thoughts, feelings, and actions. The gratitude visit starts with the development of an expression of gratitude through a written letter, followed by an in-person delivery of the letter to the targeted individual. The practitioner should help students generate a short list of people in their lives who had been especially kind to them, and choose a person from the list to whom they could enact a face-to-face visit. The practitioner should help the student write the one-page letter, which details reasons why the student is grateful to that person. Students report the outcome of the planned gratitude visit at the next session.

PHASE 2:
PRESENT-FOCUSED POSITIVE EMOTIONS—SESSIONS 4–7

Positive emotions within the present include joy, zest, ecstasy, calm, and excitement, and in general are associated with a state of flow (Seligman, 2002). These are often the emotions that people have in mind when they discuss happiness. There are two distinct types of present positive emotions: pleasures (raw sensory feelings) and gratifications (full engagement or absorption in activities that are enjoyed through thinking, interpreting, and tapping into strengths). Since pleasures are fleeting, momentary, and of short duration, the focus in this intervention is on increasing gratifications, which are more highly related to long-term happiness. Gratifications are not as easy to come by as are pleasures. They require identification and development of character strengths, challenging those strengths, and absorbing oneself into strength-related activities. Sessions 4–7 facilitate engagement in activities intended to be enjoyable and produce gratifications through tapping into strengths. In Session 4, we begin by focusing on the character strength of kindness due to its relationship with increases in subjective well-being in prior research. Within Sessions 5–7, students are taught about their signature character strengths and how they can be utilized in new and unique ways to achieve increased gratifications. In Session 7, students learn how to savor positive emotions, such as those that result from using one's strengths (Bryant & Veroff, 2007).

Kindness

"Acts of kindness" are actions that benefit others or make others happy, at the cost of personal time or effort. Adults who carried out five acts of kindness per week (Lyubomirsky et al., 2005) and children who carried out three kind acts in a week (Layous, Nelson, Oberle, Schonert-Reichl, & Lyubomirsky, 2012) have experienced gains in subjective well-being. Simple remembrance of kind acts and associated positive emotions increased subjective well-being among adults who counted their acts of kindness (Otake, Shimai, Tanaka-Matsumi, Otsui, & Fredrickson, 2006).

In Session 4, students are introduced to kindness as a strength, and are asked to perform five acts of kindness during one designated day per week. The dosage (kind acts concentrated in a single day) is purposeful, as prior research found increases in well-being for adults who perform the acts in 1 day as compared with spreading them out over the course of 1 week (Lyubomirsky et al., 2005). Some examples of acts of kindness include doing household chores typically assigned to parents (e.g., walking the dog, washing dishes), helping sibling(s) or classmates with school assignments, and helping the teacher clean up the classroom. In Session 5, students recount and share some of the kind acts they completed. Such retelling provides a method of active savoring of these experiences.

Character Strengths

Although building good character in youth has long been the goal of many character education programs in schools, positive psychology has further fueled this focus through a theoretically driven perspective. Peterson and Seligman (2004) conceptualized character strengths as a set of

24 individual positive traits (e.g., creativity, persistence, bravery, leadership) that are classified into a set of six virtues that are cross-culturally valued and grounded in moral principles. (For more information on this VIA classification system, see *www.viacharacter.org*.) Every person possesses a unique profile of "signature" strengths (i.e., "top five" character traits) that are frequently exhibited, highly regarded, and individually celebrated (Peterson & Seligman, 2004). In research with adults, a brief (1-week) intervention that involved identifying one's signature strengths through completion of an online survey of VIA strengths, followed by use of signature strengths in novel ways daily, caused positive effects on happiness and reduced depressive symptoms; these improvements in mental health were maintained throughout a 6-month follow-up period (Seligman et al., 2005). Seligman (2011) reiterated the centrality of character strengths to all aspects of well-being: "In well-being theory, these twenty four strengths underpin all five elements, not just engagement: deploying your highest strengths leads to more positive emotion, to more meaning, to more accomplishment, and to better relationships" (p. 24).

Park and Peterson (2006) adapted the original adult-focused VIA survey to be appropriate for use with youth (ages 10–17) through a lengthy self-report instrument: the Values in Action Inventory of Strengths for Youth (VIA-Youth). The VIA-Youth yields individual profiles of ranked character strengths that correspond to self-identified behaviors. School-based interventions with youth that use the VIA classification system in efforts to cultivate individual's strengths and to encourage the recognition of strengths in others have yielded positive effects on middle school students' life satisfaction (Proctor et al., 2011) and elementary school students' positive affect and classroom engagement (Quinlan, Swain, et al., 2015).

Session 5 introduces the concept of character strengths, using the VIA classification system as a framework. Students learn to define and recognize each of the 24 character strengths. They revisit their you at your best activity to identify personal strengths demonstrated in their stories. Based on their preliminary understanding of the meanings of the VIA strengths, their current self-awareness, and their peers' input, they guess what their signature strengths may be.

In Session 6, students complete the 198-item VIA-Youth (for ages 10–17) online (see *www. authentichappiness.org*). A 96-item version of the VIA Youth Survey recently became available at *www.viacharacter.org*; this version retained the four items that load most strongly on each strength. The psychometric properties of the short form are strong and it is easier to administer (i.e., has fewer reverse-scored items). As students complete the VIA Youth Survey, the practitioner helps each student (1) review the computer-generated report that lists and describes their character strengths, (2) identify their signature strengths, and (3) select one signature strength to use in a new way each day for the next week. Due to the complexity of some strengths, such as appreciation of beauty and art, perspective, and prudence, planning multiple feasible activities may be challenging for youth. Practitioners assist students to brainstorm as many unique ways to enact a given strength as possible. Students are encouraged to add in new ways that occur to them throughout the week.

Session 7 introduces students to the value of using strengths across all key domains of life. For adults, these domains include work, love, and raising children (Seligman, 2002). For adolescents, we focus on school, friendships, and family. Students select a second signature strength to apply in new ways across these domains. Students are asked to record their feelings after each use of their chosen signature strength in order to enhance the connection between thoughts, actions, and feelings of well-being. Students are also introduced to methods of savoring positive feelings, such as those that stem from use of signature strengths.

Savoring

Savoring refers to efforts to attend to, appreciate, intensify, and elongate the positive qualities in one's life through sharing, celebrating, grateful thinking, focusing, and reflecting on the positive event and associated feelings (Bryant & Veroff, 2007). Reacting to positive events through savoring strategies causes a greater boost in happy mood. Research with young adults indicates that habitual savorers (i.e., people who consistently savor positive daily events) are more likely to maintain that happy mood even between positive events (Jose, Lim, & Bryant, 2012). Savoring may be particularly beneficial when the frequency of positive events in one's life is relatively low; among young adults with fewer daily positive events, those who savored more were happier than those who savored less (Jose et al., 2012). Savoring appears to provide a way to extract the most possible from the present, prior to directing attention to the future. Based on their extensive research, Sheldon and Lyubomirsky (2012) suggest "there may be an ideal balance between present-oriented and forward-looking modes of living, a balance that, if achieved, produces the highest level of well-being" (p. 679).

Savoring responses appear similarly adaptive for youth. In one study, early adolescents (ages 10–14) were tracked for 4 days and asked to report the best thing that happened to them each day, and their initial emotional reaction when the event first occurred—specifically, to what extent they felt happy, excited, and proud (Gentzler, Morey, Palmer, & Yi, 2013). When later interviewed about the best event during that daily tracking period (the event rated as most intensely positive), adolescents reported their current level of positive affect about the event, and also their behavioral responses to the event in the intervening week. The youth most prone to savoring or *maximizing* the event through sharing it with someone, celebrating, or reflecting on how good they felt were more likely to maintain highly positive emotions about the event. In contrast, youth who *minimized* the event through a maladaptive style of attributions featuring downplaying the significance of the event, thinking it was unlikely to happen again, or viewing the positive feelings as transient, had more parent-rated symptoms of internalizing and externalizing forms of mental health problems.

Research with young adults in which college students were instructed in savoring for brief periods (2 weeks) found significant increases in happiness (Kurtz, 2008) and decreases in negative affect and depressive symptoms (Hurley & Kwon, 2012). Findings from preliminary studies in youth suggest that some features of the situation and the person may make a given student more inclined to savor, while other situations may require more guidance to do so (Gentzler, Ramsey, Yi, Palmer, & Morey, 2014). Among middle school students, the more positive affect (feelings of happiness, excitement, and pride) that immediately follows a positive event, the more likely the youth is to savor the positive event and feelings over the next week. Gentzler and colleagues (2014) also found students with some temperament tendencies were more inclined to savor, including a temperament high in effortful control (high capacity to control one's behavior and maintain attention), which may engender better regulatory abilities in general.

Session 7 introduces a rationale for savoring, and offers two ways to savor. The first method involves sharing the experience with someone else, akin to how students have celebrated their progress with positive psychology activities to date in the group. The second method involves purposefully absorbing oneself in the positive experience by focusing on the event and the related positive feelings. For homework, students record which method(s) they used to savor uses of their signature strengths.

PHASE 3:
FUTURE-FOCUSED POSITIVE EMOTIONS—SESSIONS 8 AND 9

Positive emotions about the future include faith, trust, confidence, hope, and optimism (Seligman, 2002). This phase of the intervention targets (1) optimism, in terms of an optimistic explanatory style for current events that leads to positive expectations for future events; and (2) hope, in terms of an expectation of and motivation for goal accomplishment. Session 8 is devoted to optimistic thinking. We focus on several dimensions of one's explanatory style, namely, attributions of permanence, pervasiveness, and personalization. Students practice an optimistic explanatory style that is associated with resilience in that negative life events come to be viewed as temporary, isolated, and externally caused. In contrast, positive events are viewed in terms of traits and abilities, which engenders optimism for continued success. Activities in Session 9 are based on Snyder, Rand, and Sigmon's (2005) hope theory, which is focused on the "belief that one can find pathways to desired goals and become motivated to use those pathways" (p. 257). Students learn a method for increasing a hopeful perspective through visualizing their "best-possible self in the future" and planning ways to achieve those goals.

Optimistic Thinking

Optimism has been described as both (1) a general disposition related to expectations for the future (Scheier & Carver, 1985), and (2) a cognitive explanatory style encompassing the belief that future events are closely tied to the explanation of past events (Abramson, Seligman, & Teasdale, 1978). Seligman (1990) described a method of developing optimistic thinking called learned optimism. It is a cognitive-behavioral method for changing one's explanatory style in making attributions about events. In learned optimism, young people are taught to view positive life events as permanent, pervasive, and due to personal effort and traits, while negative life events are interpreted as temporary, limited to the immediate incident, and resulting from external forces (Seligman, Reivich, Jaycox, & Gillham, 1995).

School-based initiatives to promote optimism in part to prevent depression include the Penn Resiliency Program (Gillham et al., 1990), a 12-session curriculum designed to train children (ages 10–13) to develop an optimistic explanatory style and positive social skills, and the Aussie Optimism Program—Positive Thinking Skills (Rooney, Hassan, Kane, Roberts, & Nesa, 2013), a 10-module program for students in grades 4 and 5 that also involves cognitive-behavioral strategies to cultivate learned optimism. Among middle school students, the Penn Resiliency Program has yielded positive effects on an optimistic explanatory style for positive events and, among high-symptom students, reduced occurrence of clinical disorders (Gillham, Hamilton, Freres, Patton, & Gallop, 2006), as well as reduced depressive symptoms in students at two of three schools (Gillham et al., 2007). Children who participated in the Aussie Optimism Program also experienced positive changes in optimism as well as reduced symptoms of anxiety and depression (Rooney et al., 2013).

Session 8 introduces optimistic thinking in terms of explanatory style. Most applications of learned optimism entail lengthy curricula like the Penn Resiliency Program and the Aussie Optimism Program to fully teach and rehearse this complex skill. Because optimistic thinking was intended to be one of many targets within our comprehensive positive psychology intervention, we developed a scaled-down version of learned optimism that focuses on the key dimensions of the explanatory style advanced by Seligman (1990). In Session 8, students are helped to consider ways they think about why various good and bad events happened in their lives. An optimistic explanatory style includes attributions of *permanency* to positive life events. Good events are viewed in terms of traits and abilities, for example, "I made the goal because I'm talented in sports." In contrast, negative life events are conceptualized as temporary; students consider the transient mood, effort, or situational features that contributed to a negative event, for example, "I didn't study enough to get an A, so I'll have to try harder for the next test" or "Even Beckham would have missed that ball—I'll probably make the next goal I try for." Optimists see the positive as *pervasive,* universal, or widespread (e.g., "I do well in all of my classes because I check my agenda and do my homework after school") and the negative as specific (e.g., "I made a poor grade on my math test because I did not understand the ideas that were taught when I was out sick"). The final piece of explanatory style is *personalization.* Optimists take credit for positive events, as seen in the example, "I won the contest because of my effort and talent in creative writing." In contrast to self-blaming for positive events, optimistic thinkers consider the external forces that contributed to a negative event. An example of blaming other sources is reflected in "I lost the music video challenge on YouTube because I needed a higher-quality camera on my cell phone." During the session, practitioners help students generate such attributions to various positive and negative events through completion of a worksheet. They receive further practice in restructuring their thoughts to be optimistic through the homework assignment, which requires them to use and record optimistic thinking in response to a good or bad event at least one time each day for a week.

Hope

Snyder and colleagues (1991) have conceptualized hope as the perceived aptitude to set personal goals, identify pathways to achieve goals, and motivate oneself to use pathways through agency thinking. While children as young as 7 demonstrate hopeful thinking (Snyder, 2005), improvements in cognitive capacity across the course of development enhance students' ability to think more abstractly about their future ambitions and generate strategies to achieve them.

Students who have high levels of hope are more successful in obtaining their goals and subsequently experience more positive emotions and increased life satisfaction (Merkas & Brajsa-Zganec, 2011). Middle school students who participated in a five-session program intended to help them develop goals, create and pursue pathways, and reframe barriers, incurred lasting gains in hope as well as life satisfaction and self-worth (Marques et al., 2011). In light of the desire to address multiple targets in our intervention, we selected a shorter method of facilitating goal-directed thinking. Specifically, King (2001) found that college students who wrote about life goals in the form of an exercise termed one's "best-possible self" (i.e., a version of the future self having accomplished desired life goals) experienced increased life satisfaction, positive affect, and optimism. Thus, in Session 9, students visualize and write about their best-possible future self, including ways they will reach the specified goals. The focus on agentic thinking and personally valued goals is expected to increase positive thoughts and emotions about the future, and feelings of hope and optimism, which in turn leads to greater subjective well-being. As the imagined future self-concept is intentionally positive, benefits to self-esteem may also be expected.

Prior research has found that the best-possible self activity is most effective at harnessing self-regulatory behaviors toward a desired goal when the imagined future state is consistent with one's social identity, includes behavioral strategies for attaining the desired goals, and obstacles are anticipated (Oyserman, Bybee, & Terry, 2006). A comprehensive 13-meeting program focused on developing academic best-possible selves in the future had positive effects on middle school students' behavioral engagement in school (attendance, homework time, and fewer behavior problems) and academic performance (GPA), effects that maintained for 2 years. Thus, best-possible selves is an example of a relatively brief psychological intervention that improves students' school success not directly through academic skill interventions, but instead through improving students' subjective experiences in school, in this case, their hope—clear educational aspirations and self-directed activities toward meeting academic goals (Yeager & Walton, 2011). While conceptualization of mental health was limited to psychopathology, positive effects were apparent with the intervention group demonstrating fewer symptoms of depression, on average, 2 years later (Oyserman et al., 2006). Owens and Patterson (2013) implemented this activity with a sample of elementary school children and directed them to focus exclusively on positive futures (vs. also discussing negative or feared versions of one's future self). This study provided the first test of the best-possible self activity on youth outcomes beyond self-regulatory behavior, academic success, or mental health problems. Students were assigned to either a best-possible self condition or two comparison conditions: gratitude and active control. To ease the writing burden in this young sample, children were instructed to draw about things for which they were grateful and to depict their best-possible selves. Compared with children who drew about something that happened that day or specifically about something for which they were thankful for that happened that day, children who drew about their best-possible selves experienced significant increases in self-esteem. However, no improvements in indicators of subjective well-being were found. This is in contrast to trials with young adults; college students who wrote about their best-possible selves once per week for 4 weeks experienced a significant increase in positive affect, whether they completed the activity online or in person with an intervention facilitator (Layous, Nelson, et al., 2013).

Session 9 introduces Snyder and colleagues' (2005) definition of hope. Group leaders guide students through a discussion of how hope leads to positive outcomes in many domains of life as well as to feelings of happiness. Students are then provided with a concrete method for enacting goal-directed thinking through the best-possible future self activity. In this exercise, students visualize a positive version of themselves in the future that reflects attainment of personal goals. Students are asked to write for about 5 minutes about their desired life, and to describe ways they will reach the specified goals. For homework, they are instructed to revisit their best-possible future self and add new ideas each night for 1 week, encouraging them to think about specific ways in which they might accomplish goals. Examples of student goals have included having a big house, becoming a doctor/lawyer/sports star, traveling overseas, and having a spouse and children. Typical methods for achieving goals included working hard in school, going to college, and practicing athletics. In Session 10, student share their expanded best-possible self stories.

REVIEW AND TERMINATION—SESSION 10

The notion that students are ready for intervention termination begins during the review of homework assigned in the prior session. Specifically, the practitioner celebrates student success with independent practice of various positive psychology exercises. Then, the practitioner provides a review of concepts covered throughout the program, including relevant theory (e.g., determinants of happiness) and specific activities that enhance past, present, and future aspects of emotional well-being.

When preparing for this session, practitioners should keep in mind the phenomenon of the hedonic treadmill (see Chapter 4). In order to prevent the students from returning to the lower end of their happiness set point, students must continue to intentionally apply the positive activities they learned throughout the program. When the onus on use shifts from group leader prompts (such as in regularly scheduled meetings) to student responsibility, the concept of person–activity fit (Lyubomirsky & Layous, 2013) becomes vitally important. Rather than encouraging students to continue to practice *all* activities, they should leave the program feeling comfortable with retaining only those activities that have resonated the most with them. Throughout the intervention, group leaders have prompted students to reflect on any changes in personal happiness that have followed between-meeting applications of the various exercises. In this final session, practitioners want to lead students to consider which strategies they perceived to work the best in terms of increasing positive feelings and interpersonal connections. To capitalize on intrinsic motivation, students should plan to keep up those activities that felt natural and enjoyable and were consistent with their values. In contrast, those activities they completed primarily because "they had to" (e.g., to gain access to homework rewards or to please the group leader through compliance) may take a back seat. Thus, in this session, practitioners query students about which activities they felt gave them the biggest boost in happiness, and ensure that such clues pertinent to person–activity fit drive the strategies that students select to continue independently. Students must understand that a particular happiness-increasing strategy will work better if it feels natural to them and they are truly motivated to pursue it.

When planning future applications of the preferred activities, *variety* is key to preventing hedonic adaptation. Varying how one enacts a given positive psychology activity appears critical to determining whether the activity will continue to have positive effects on enhancing subjective well-being (Sheldon et al., 2013). In this vein, in addition to switching up the activities done with intentional effort, students must enact a selected activity in a way that prevents it from becoming monotonous. For example, rather than planning to incorporate an "Acts of Kindness Tuesday" into their week that features an admirable but common routine (e.g., walk sibling to the bus stop, compliment the homeroom teacher, carry a classmate's lunch tray, tutor after school, and help dad with the dishes), practitioners should encourage the student to vary the targets, timing, and nature of his or her kind acts (after, of course, reinforcing the *effort* and *intent* evident in the student's original plan). Student discussion of intent is a good sign that he or she understands the need to continue to incorporate the thoughts and activities from the program into daily life.

To this end, students receive a handout that summarizes the specific positive psychology exercises now in their repertoire. After reviewing the handout, the practitioner leads students in brainstorming situations when it would be particularly appropriate to use a given activity. After the leader guides students through a reflection on their intervention experience, students receive a congratulatory certificate of completion. Postintervention data collection should include qualitative and quantitative features to inform the practitioners' future implementations, as well as students' response to the intervention. Graphs that depict students' improved outcomes throughout the intervention period should be shared with key stakeholders, including parents, teachers, and school leadership. Demonstrating the effectiveness of any mental health intervention to educators in positions of power is one way to ensure continued support for implementation, particularly when student mental health gains are coupled with improvements in academic success, as reflected in indicators of skills, behaviors, and attitude (Suldo, Gormley, et al., 2014).

FOLLOW-UP CONTACT AND OTHER CONSIDERATIONS

These 10 sessions represent the core of the Well-Being Promotion Program, as originally developed and implemented with adolescents. In the intervening years, accumulating research has indicated that lasting and greater increases in subjective well-being follow: longer intervention periods, variety in use of multiple strategies, sustained motivation and effort to practice the positive activities, and perceived social support such as a team approach that encourages behavior change (Layous & Lyubomirsky, 2014). These researchers conclude that "studies offer persuasive evidence that increases to well-being garnered from a positive activity intervention can be sustained if people continue to muster effort into their practice" (p. 482). Curry (2014) recommends that adolescents treated for depression keep in regular contact with clinicians via follow-up sessions ("continuation treatment") to maintain remission.

In line with such findings, we have found it useful to hold follow-up group meetings with students to review the key concepts covered in the termination session, celebrate students' examples of independent application of the exercises, and prompt continued rehearsal of a variety of strategies. To that effect, two "booster sessions" that we used successfully in recent work with middle school students (Roth et al., 2016) are also included in the Appendix. Each of these follow-up sessions includes a general review of concepts followed by opportunities for students to discuss the strategies in which they had engaged since the termination session with a focus on how the activities impacted their well-being. The latter segment of each follow-up session focuses on rehearsal of specific strategies. The first booster session targets gratitude journaling, and the second booster session targets new uses of signature character strengths and optimistic thinking. Practitioners who anticipate holding more than two follow-up sessions can split the second session into two (one focused on strengths and the other on optimistic thinking) and/or create additional booster sessions with a similar update–celebrate–review beginning and then tailor the latter part of the session to rehearsal of additional targets, such as kindness, savoring, hope, and so on. Our initial evaluation of the utility of providing the two booster sessions presented in the Appendix provided evidence of promise for the notion that follow-up sessions in the 2 months after the termination session may help students maintain the gains in positive affect that were attributable to the core program.

Given this emerging research, practitioners should consider holding follow-up sessions with the entire group on a once-per-month basis or so for 2–3 months after the termination session, and/or encourage students to meet in pairs to build in social support for continued practice of the intentional thoughts and behaviors that facilitate happiness. Keeping in mind that perceived support may be more impactful than actual support (Layous & Lyubomirsky, 2014), simply reminding students that they are welcome to contact the practitioner as needed for future guidance or with updates relevant to their experiences with widespread application of the positive activities may help sustain students' program-related gains.

INTERVENTION DEVELOPMENT:
RATIONALE, FUNDING, AND EMPIRICAL SUPPORT

In 2007, we created and first tested the 10-session program described in this chapter, in close collaboration with a relatively affluent, suburban middle school that had a history of academic excellence. The school leadership had recently examined its student body, and found that a sizable minority of students had a vulnerable mental health status, as indicated by low subjective well-being but also low psychopathology. Compared with their peers with complete mental health (high subjective well-being, low psychopathology), the academic performance of vulnerable students was inferior across indicators of skills and school-related attitudes. In light of such data that made clear the benefits of subjective well-being, the school leadership requested guidance on appropriate intervention strategies their counselors could use. In the absence of published evaluations of psychological interventions intended to increase happiness in youth, we sought and received funding from the University of South Florida Collaborative for Children, Families, and Communities to conduct design and development research. The project culminated with a pilot study of this multitarget positive psychology intervention among sixth-grade students at the school.

As described in Suldo, Savage, and Mercer (2014), a quick grade-level screening of the 333 sixth-grade students indicated 132 students with less than optimal life satisfaction (average BMSLSS scores at or below 6 on the 1–7 response metric). Youth with scores in the top part of the metric (> 6.0) were excluded in line with the notion that "people who are already happy need not carry out happiness-increasing strategies intentionally—research shows that they are already practicing the behaviors and thought patterns that positive [psychology] interventions are meant to invoke" (Layous & Lyubomirsky, 2014, p. 490). All 132 students with BMSLSS scores between 1 and 6 were invited to take part in the free program offered at school. Sixty-seven of these students secured parent consent and student assent to participate. They were randomly assigned to immediate participation in the intervention ($n = 35$) or the delayed-intervention control group ($n = 32$). A total of 55 students (28 in the intervention group and 27 in the control group) participated in the project through the follow-up period. The sample was ethnically diverse, specifically, 36% were white, 24% Hispanic, 9% African American, 13% Asian, 9% multiracial, and 9% endorsed another identity. About half (53%) of the participants were female, and 46% of the student participants were eligible for the district's free or reduced-price school meals program.

The students who had been randomly assigned to the immediate intervention group participated in once-weekly sessions over 10 weeks during September–November of grade 6. Students completed the intervention sessions during an elective period (i.e., in lieu of art, physical education, etc.) in groups of seven students. We (Shannon and Jessica) led the groups, with the assistance of school psychology graduate students serving as co-leaders. We gathered data on students' subjective well-being and psychopathology at three time points: baseline, postintervention, and 6-month follow-up. Repeated measures analyses of a propensity score matched sample of students with equivalent life satisfaction scores at baseline indicated that the global life satisfaction of students in the intervention group increased significantly, while the control group showed a declining trend during the same period. At follow-up, both groups had higher SLSS scores than at baseline. We felt that these improvements in life satisfaction evidenced by students in the intervention group during the transition to middle school were important, given the adjustment difficulties that often appear during this sensitive developmental period that is often marked by biological and educational changes (Suldo, Savage, & Mercer, 2014).

The students who had been randomly assigned to the delayed-intervention control group were offered the opportunity to take part in the program the following school year, when they were approximately 1.5 years older (the intervention took place from March to May of grade 7). In this implementation, sessions were held twice per week and groups were smaller (three to five students per group). The group leaders were doctoral students in school psychology, who we supervised off-site during weekly meetings of the entire research group. To overcome barriers related to leaders' availability, the group leader position was split between two people, each responsible for 1 day/session of the week. Repeated measures analyses of the grade 7 students with complete data from this intervention period indicated significant gains in global life satisfaction (as assessed with the SLSS) from pre- to postintervention, $t(14) = -2.90$, $p = .01$, $d = 0.44$. The clinical significance of this gain is demonstrated by the stability of the control group's SLSS scores during grade 6, which averaged 4.589 across three time points (4.47, 4.35, and 4.95 in August, December, and May, respectively). Just prior to the intervention start in March of grade 7, student life satisfaction was still within this range (mean SLSS score = 4.59). At the end of the intervention, the mean SLSS score for the group had increased to 5.15. Analyses of the students' grade 7 pre- and postintervention BMSLSS scores indicated two domains of life that evidenced significant gains: self and family, both of moderate effect size, $t(14) = -2.78$, $p = .01$, $d = 0.55$ and $t(14) = -3.21$, $p = .01$, $d = 0.49$, respectively. Changes in the other domains of life were positive but somewhat smaller or not statistically significant, specifically: friends, $t(14) = -1.58$, $p = .14$, $d = 0.40$; school, $t(14) = -1.23$, $p = .24$, $d = 0.32$; and living environment, $t(14) = -2.09$, $p = .06$, $d = .21$.

Group leaders who directly served these students in the delayed-intervention group had served as our co-leaders during the school year prior. Anecdotally, the group leaders felt quite positive about the intervention modality (twice- vs. once-per-week sessions) as well as about the cognitive engagement of the seventh graders relative to their peers who had taken part during the prior school year (Friedrich, Thalji, Suldo, Chappel, & Fefer, 2010). The grade 7 students appeared to more readily comprehend the topics covered in sessions, as evident in the quality of participation in session-based activities and accuracy of completion of homework assignments. Possibly because less time passed between group meetings, students seemed better able to recall the content from the prior session, attended sessions regularly, and completed assigned homework. Such improved uptake was reflected in needing less time to review the previous session's objectives and catch up absent/tardy participants, which allowed more time to discuss new information. In sum, the continuous follow-up of students who began in the delayed-intervention control group suggested that participation in the 5-week small-group modality during grade 7 was associated with increases in global life satisfaction, and was possibly better suited for students' cognitive capacity to comprehend topics discussed in sessions.

CONCLUDING COMMENTS ON THE PROMISE OF THE WELL-BEING PROMOTION PROGRAM

The collaborative project described above, which yielded the manualized intervention presented in the Appendix, was grounded in theory regarding increasing positive emotions about the past, present, and future, and incorporated many evidence-based strategies for increasing happiness. The core intervention as well as modified versions that include supplemental components (teachers, classmates, parents, and student-focused booster sessions; see Chapters 6–8) has shown evidence of promise in increasing students' subjective well-being. We have confidence in practitioners' ability to use this book to provide evidence-based positive psychology interventions to students. A particular focus on vulnerable students may help increase the likelihood that all students in a school can experience maximum emotional and academic success. Thinking gratefully, performing acts of kindness and achieving gratifications through use of character strengths, and envisioning a better future create and direct focus to positive feelings about one's past, present, and future, respectively. Such positive emotions create an upward spiral, marked by increased cognitive capacity and behavioral flexibility that has positive impacts on life through enhancing social relationships and well-being.

In the years since we first advanced this intervention, the focus in positive psychology intervention research has shifted from *whether* these interventions work (research in Table 4.3 of Chapter 4 indicates "yes") to *how* the strategies work. Kristin Layous and Sonja Lyubomirsky (2014) summarize a number of key considerations when planning how to best implement evidence-based positive activities in a manner likely to maximize and maintain impact on subjective well-being. We are reassured that features of the core program developed in 2007 remain consistent with some of the recent research-based recommendations, including:

- *Begin with positive mood induction.* The Well-Being Promotion Program begins with a you at your best activity. This puts youth in a positive emotional state to receive ensuing instructions for how to complete positive psychology interventions.

- *Variety.* By design, the multitarget nature of the program arms students with many different methods for cultivating positive emotions. Within individual positive activities, students are directed to behave in ways intended to prevent the activity from becoming routine. For example, sessions on applications of signature strengths emphasize use of multiple strengths in novel and different ways, across life domains.

- *Timing and dosage.* Although gratitude journaling is initially assigned to occur daily in order to maximize intensity, the once-per-week recommendation for ongoing rehearsal of gratitude journaling as well as acts of kindness is consistent with recognition that many cultural routines ranging from household chores (e.g., laundry, grocery shopping) to worship to even viewing one's favorite television show tend to occur on a weekly basis.

- *Preference and choice.* As the program progresses, students are increasingly afforded choice in homework assignments (e.g., select from gratitude journaling *or* performing acts of kindness), and encouraged to continue use of the strategy they most prefer. Students are also provided with the opportunity to create and enact personally meaningful uses of their signature strengths. The termination session emphasizes such personal choice, homing in on continued use of those strategies with the greatest person–activity fit.

- *Rehearsal.* The interactive and activity-focused nature of sessions, as well as homework assignments that most often entail continued use of strategies learned in session, provide a natural means for practice of each exercise until mastery level is sufficient for continued successful use after the active intervention period.

- *Social support.* The small-group nature of the program may build bonds among youth drawn from a larger educational context. For instance, we were initially surprised but pleased to see some middle school students select another member of their group as the target of their gratitude visit; these students shared appreciation for the new friendship they had formed with a peer who shared their goal of increasing personal well-being. After the intervention conclusion, the group modality may provide some level of peer accountability for strategy rehearsal.

EXAMPLE SELECTIVE IMPLEMENTATION: CASE STUDY FROM A MIDDLE SCHOOL

Jamie Burch is a school psychologist, assigned to a large suburban middle school for 2.5 days a week. The school draws students from affluent neighborhoods as well as some more disadvantaged areas, and has a long history of academic excellence. The school principal often expresses a commitment to promoting the academic, social, and emotional well-being of all children in the school. As part of an annual needs assessment, in the second month of the school year, Dr. Burch distributed a brief survey to teachers to gather their perceptions of areas in greatest need of targeted psychological services throughout the school. This survey asked teachers to indicate (via checklists) the topics that they would like information about (e.g., attention-deficit/hyperactivity disorder [ADHD], depression/sadness, classroom management, grief/loss), as well as the greatest perceived need of students at the school (e.g., family stress, self-injury, friendship difficulties). Of the 12 options provided, the four topics that teachers indicated a desire to learn more about included two pertinent to promoting student wellness (positive psychology, promoting resilience) and two pertinent to managing student problems (anxiety, ADHD symptoms). The perceived student needs paralleled this, with the largest number of endorsements for positive psychology/feeling happier, developing resilience, anxiety/worrying, ADHD, and friendship difficulties.

Dr. Burch shared these results with the rest of the school's mental health team, which included two full-time guidance counselors (Ms. Jazz and Ms. Stonebrook), an itinerant social worker (Ms. Swift), and a part-time school psychology trainee (Rebecca) who assisted Dr. Burch on Tuesdays. In addition to the social skills and anxiety management groups they typically offer annually for students identified through a teacher nomination procedure, the team decided to further assess students' happiness and, if indicated, provide the Well-Being Promotion Program to students with room for growth in well-being. The team considered issues of parent consent and notification in psychological assessment and intervention, and consulted the relevant standards from the National Association of School Psychologists 2010 Principles for Professional Ethics. With regard to the screening process, even though the standard speaks specifically to universal assessment of mental health *problems* (as opposed to positive indicators, like life satisfaction), the team treated administration of universal screenings for mental health the same regardless of the indicator type (e.g., anxiety, depression, life satisfaction). Thus, parents received written notification of the upcoming schoolwide screening of happiness, and were directed to contact Dr. Burch if they wanted to remove their child from the screening.

During a before-school staff meeting, Dr. Burch briefly explained the goals of the Well-Being Promotion Program, and asked teachers to administer the BMSLSS to students in their homeroom that morning. Each teacher received a packet with a blank BMSLSS for each student, a cover letter instructing them to ask students to independently complete this "brief survey that asks about your happiness, both overall and in specific areas of life," and a large manila envelope for teachers to place completed surveys that were to be returned immediately to Dr. Burch. Dr. Burch spoke privately to the teacher of the one student whose mother had contacted her with a request to opt out, and informed the teacher of the name of the child who was not to complete the BMSLSS.

After students' circled responses on the surveys were entered into an Excel file, Dr. Burch computed students' average score across the six items and graphed the compiled averages by grade level. To illustrate, the results for the grade 7 students are presented in Figure 5.1.

To help teachers contextualize the numeric values, the response options on the BMSLSS were listed on the *x*-axis and student averages were rounded. The graph depicts that nearly 60% of grade 7 students reported they were *pleased* or even *delighted* with their lives (average scores above 6 on the 1–7 response metric). Just over one-quarter of students were *mostly satisfied* (scores around 5). Fortunately, no students expressed extreme negativity about their lives, in terms of feeling consistently terrible or unhappy across life domains. This skew toward high life satisfaction among most students was consistent with the positive school climate that featured caring and committed teachers and administration, a high level of parent involvement, and students who generally behaved in accordance with explicit schoolwide expectations for appropriate conduct. Nevertheless, a few students indicated feeling negatively about their lives (average scores corresponded to *mostly dissatisfied*) and about 10% of students were neutral or *mixed*. To help those students learn ways of thinking and behaving to increase their personal happiness, the mental health team decided to offer the Well-Being Promotion Program to any student in grade 7 or 8 whose life satisfaction level fell just at or below pleased (mean scores ≤ 6.0). Students in grade 6 were excluded because very few fell below that threshold. Students with average scores in this range were called to the guidance suite, where they learned about the Well-Being Promotion Program. The main points communicated to the students included:

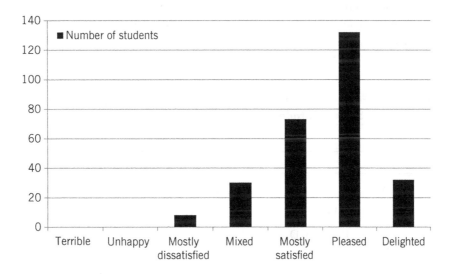

FIGURE 5.1. Average life satisfaction scores of seventh-grade students. Data from schoolwide administration of the BMSLSS.

- "Students who are happy and have little emotional distress often do better. They get better grades, get along better with people, and have the best attitudes toward school."
- "People can learn ways of thinking and acting that help them feel happier. We plan to offer a Well-Being Promotion Program at school to teach these ways. In the program, we will meet with small groups of students once a week during the school day, on a schedule approved by your teachers (for instance, the weekly group meetings may rotate through first, second, and third class periods, so that you will not miss a particular class more than once in 3 weeks). During those meetings, we do activities that teach these ways to think and act that are related to feeling happy. For instance, we practice grateful thinking, perform kind acts for others, and learn about our personal strengths."
- "We think you may be interested in this program because of a survey you filled out recently. Your answers showed that you have some room for growth in your satisfaction with life. You are not alone; many youth feel that one or more areas of life could be going better. That's why we teach students ways of thinking and acting that make them feel happier with their families, friends, school, and self. We aim for all students to feel delighted with their lives."
- "If you're interested in taking part in the Well-Being Promotion Program, please bring this letter that explains the program and gives my contact information to your parent. Only students with signed parent permission forms can take part."

For the next week, teachers of seventh- and eighth-grade homerooms issued brief classwide daily reminders for students who had spoken with someone in guidance *and* were interested in taking part in the Well-Being Promotion Program to return the signed parent consent form to school. Dr. Burch ultimately received written parent consent from 40 seventh-grade students and 35 eighth-grade students, which was about 40% of the number of students invited to take part. The mental health team decided to hold six small groups in the fall for the seventh-grade students, and then five groups in the spring to accommodate the eighth-grade students. Table 5.2 illustrates the fall implementation schedule. All groups were held on Tuesdays, when the mental health team had access to two conference rooms, as well as a particularly full staff. Dr. Burch and Rebecca implemented three groups (A–C) back-to-back in one conference room,

TABLE 5.2. Fall Schedule for Well-Being Promotion Groups Provided to Groups of Seventh-Grade Students

Class period	1	2	3	4	5	6	7	8	9	10
1	A/D				C/F	B/E	A/D			
2	B/E	A/D				C/F	B/E	A/D		
3	C/F	B/E	A/D				C/F	B/E	A/D	
5		C/F	B/E	A/D				C/F	B/E	A/D
6			C/F	B/E	A/D				C/F	B/E
7				C/F	B/E	A/D				C/F

while Ms. Jazz and Ms. Stonebrook implemented groups D–F in the other conference room. Rather than pull students from the same class each week, the team implemented a rotating schedule as depicted in Table 5.2. Period 4 was omitted from the rotation to avoid a complicated school lunch schedule, as some students had lunch at the beginning of Period 4 and others in the middle or end of the period.

The 40 seventh-grade students were then assigned mostly at random to a specific group (A–F), with the goal of having a heterogeneous group of students who were diverse in terms of baseline life satisfaction level, demographic features, and class schedule (e.g., honors vs. regular sections). To further illustrate, Table 5.3 presents the features of students in Group A.

Dr. Burch distributed two documents to seventh-grade teachers: (1) a list of the names of the students assigned to each group, and (2) the master schedule with the specific date each group would meet during which period (a matrix near identical to Table 5.2, except with "date" in place of "week number," and the specification of which conference room to direct students in Groups A–C vs. Groups D–F). The master group meeting schedule (but not the list of participating students) was also posted in the guidance suite.

To evaluate students' response to the Well-Being Promotion Program, the mental health team selected the SLSS as the primary tool to examine growth in global life satisfaction. Each dyad of implementers discussed how to coordinate leading and co-leading responsibilities in such a way that both were prepared each week (i.e., had read and rehearsed the session protocol in advance of Tuesday) while limiting redundancy (e.g., only one person photocopied the relevant materials like student handouts, secured a computer lab if needed, brought in supplies such as reinforcers for homework compliance). The leader took charge of creating a session agenda that included estimates of the amount of time she desired to allot for each procedure section in the protocol (e.g., about 5–7 minutes for "review homework assignment"), and typically facilitated the session activities from the front of the conference room. The co-leader typically sat interspersed between students; such proximity control helped redirect students to the leader as needed, and allowed the co-leader to provide more individual assistance to those students seated nearby. The co-leader was also responsible for ensuring fidelity of the leader's adherence to the intervention protocol by completing the corresponding one-page intervention integrity checklist. These forms, located in the online supplement to this book, provide a checklist of the primary elements (e.g., discussions, activities) intended for inclusion in a given session. The co-leader recorded "yes" when a planned session element was enacted. If the leader appeared to inadvertently skip over an intended element, the co-leader discreetly redirected the leader to that activity during a natural transition point. If an element was omitted completely (i.e., in the uncommon event that the leader intentionally omitted a planned activity due to insufficient time), the co-leader would record "no" for implementation of that element.

The guidance counselors chose to alternate primary responsibility for leading a given week's session, such that Ms. Jazz led all groups during the odd weeks (e.g., Sessions 1, 3, 5) and Ms. Stonebrook led all groups during the even weeks. In contrast, each week Dr. Burch served as the leader for the first two groups of the day with Rebecca taking a more active role in the third group. Each dyad set a regular time (i.e., before school each Tuesday morning) to plan how to verify responsibilities for implementing that week's session protocol in the manner detailed in the Appendix. At these meetings, the co-leaders reviewed the session agenda developed by the leader, and ensured they had all required session materials. Between Tuesdays, co-leaders communicated in person and e-mail regarding relevant ideas for the next session and logistical

TABLE 5.3. Features of Students Assigned to Group A

Name[a]	Track (number of advanced courses)	Sex	Exceptional student education status	Free or reduced-price school meals	Race	Parents' marital status	Average	Family	Friends	School	Self	Living environment	Global
			Demographic features				BMSLSS score (average and item-level)						
Renee	4	Female	None	No	White	Married	5.2	5	4	6	5	6	5
Katie	4	Female	Gifted	No	White	Married	5.5	6	4	4	7	7	5
Joel	4	Male	None	No	White	Divorced	6	6	6	6	6	6	6
Jamal	1	Male	None	Yes	Black	Never married	5.8	7	6	5	7	5	5
Ariana	2	Female	None	Yes	Hispanic	Divorced	5.8	5	6	6	6	6	6
Danielle	4	Female	Learning disability	No	White	Married	5.8	5	6	6	6	6	6
Chris	4	Male	None	No	White	Married	5.8	7	7	2	6	7	6

[a]All names are pseudonyms but reflect actual seventh-grade students who participated in the Well-Being Promotion Program, in the manner summarized in this case study.

issues—for instance, who might be available to meet on a Friday morning to hold a make-up session with a student who was absent from school that Tuesday. In general, such make-up sessions were rare because (1) attendance was generally high schoolwide, (2) distribution of the master schedule matrix and list of participating students ensured teachers were aware which children would miss their class each week, (3) students were reminded at the end of each session what period they should report to the conference room the following Tuesday, and (4) students who were unable to come to the conference room at their assigned time (with their typical group; e.g., because of an unavoidable class test in the affected period) were permitted to join a different group that day.

At the conclusion of the 10-week program, students completed the SLSS again. After the ratings were entered into an Excel file, Dr. Burch compared average SLSS scores from before and after the intervention. As shown in Figure 5.2, six of seven students in Group A experienced gains in life satisfaction over the course of the program. Whereas scores between 1 and 3 indicate dissatisfaction with life, average scores of 4–6 are in the positive range, with a score of 4 (corresponding to *mildly agree* on the metric) being the lowest threshold for endorsing at least mild satisfaction with life. Thus, when evaluating the clinical significance of Group A's postintervention scores, Dr. Burch was pleased that all students reported positive life satisfaction at the program's end; in contrast, prior to intervention nearly half of the group had reported global life satisfaction in the negative or neutral range on the SLSS. Dr. Burch noted that the consistently positive student outcomes in Group A co-occurred with exceptional implementation fidelity; Rebecca's completed intervention integrity checklists indicated that, on average across weeks, 98% of manualized tasks per session were ultimately implemented during a group meeting. Such implementation of the Well-Being Promotion Program with fidelity reflected Dr. Burch and Rebecca's planning and coordination efforts before, during, and between sessions.

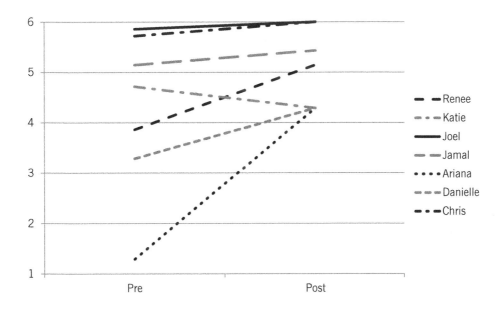

FIGURE 5.2. Baseline (Week 1) and postintervention (Week 10) life satisfaction of students in Group A. Data from repeat administration of the SLSS.

To help ensure that students' gains in happiness were maintained, the mental health team scheduled additional group meetings (for approximately 1 and 2 months after completion of the program) to provide two follow-up sessions using the protocols in the Appendix. At the end of the second follow-up session, students again completed the SLSS. In reviewing this follow-up data for Group A, Dr. Burch was pleased that life satisfaction remained high (average scores of 4.7–6.0) for five of the seven students. However, slight declines (although not to levels as low as at preintervention) were noted for Ariana (score = 3.1) and Danielle (score = 3.6). During various discussions in group meetings, comments from these two students suggested some particularly problematic parent–child relationships including rather low emotional support from their parents. During sessions, Ariana also displayed more internalizing symptoms than her peers, including a flat affect and lethargy. A review of these students' school records revealed a marked decline in school attendance throughout the past 2 months, particularly for Ariana. Whereas Danielle had not incurred any office discipline referrals (ODRs), Ariana was one of only two of the 40 seventh-grade students in the Well-Being Promotion Program who had received an ODR that fall. Dr. Burch recommended Ariana for consideration for additional mental health assessment and intervention services, and she was scheduled for discussion at the next Child Study Team Meeting. The mental health team agreed to monitor Danielle's academic data, and scheduled her for an individual follow-up meeting with Dr. Burch in approximately 1 month.

CHAPTER 6

Alternative Selective and Indicated Interventions for Promoting Youth Happiness

with Brittany Hearon

The 10-session Well-Being Promotion Program advanced in Chapter 5 has been evaluated most rigorously with samples of middle school students who took part in small groups during the school day. This program has also been piloted with different age groups and via different modalities. Other age groups include elementary school children as young as third grade, and preliminary work with high school-age youth both in school and in clinical settings. In this chapter, we discuss how to modify our multitarget positive psychology intervention for use with younger children in particular, followed by a summary of considerations when working with older adolescents.

In terms of modality, positive psychology interventions can be modified for use with targeted students with mental health needs in an indicated, individualized manner (discussed in this chapter), or implemented in a universal fashion (discussed in Chapter 7, with an emphasis on classwide and teacher-focused applications). The intervention protocols described in Chapter 5 and presented in the Appendix can be modified and adopted flexibly within an individual counseling relationship, by incorporating some but not necessarily all sessions into a comprehensive treatment plan that flows from a case conceptualization. In a similar vein, practitioners can select some but not all of the intervention protocols for group applications when students are not available for 10 meetings. In such situations, practitioners can select the activities they deem most relevant to the needs of their student(s), or the strategies they feel they can most feasibly include in their existing model of service delivery.

Practitioners who would like to assist specific students improve their subjective well-being have several options from which to choose. These options range in terms of theoretical frame-

Brittany Hearon, MA, is a doctoral candidate in the School Psychology Program at the University of South Florida.

work, clinical contact (minimal to extensive), and interventionist (teachers to mental health professionals). As alternatives to the multitarget positive psychology intervention for implementation by school mental health professionals (Chapter 5), this chapter directs practitioners to related approaches that have been advanced in the literature. These alternate interventions are relevant due to either their explicit focus on improving subjective well-being or theoretical compatibility with positive psychology. In particular, we describe self-administered positive psychology strategies, brief clinical interventions from a strengths-based approach, and lengthier interventions (coaching using positive psychology principles, positive psychotherapy). We conclude with a more detailed description of our work applying the full Well-Being Promotion Program with individual students in a more traditional counseling capacity.

Consistent with a positive psychology perspective, the target population of interventions discussed within this chapter is not limited to troubled students. Less intensive interventions like motivational interviewing and self-administered positive psychology applications may be appropriate for vulnerable students who may have no or subthreshold symptom levels but who have room for growth in subjective well-being. Intensive approaches like positive psychotherapy may be well-matched to the treatment of students with mental health diagnoses. This notion remains logical but untested in youth; however, research with adults supports the feasibility of positive interventions with clinical populations. Case in point, qualitative study of nearly 40 adults with psychosis (diagnoses of schizophrenia, bipolar, and psychotic depression) who had participated in small-group positive psychotherapy indicated satisfaction with many activities, including savoring, gratitude, and personal strengths exercises (Brownell, Schrank, Jakaite, Larkin, & Slade, 2015). As summarized by Brownell and colleagues (2015), "Almost all participants reported that the intervention helped them to focus on the positive things in life rather than ruminating on the negative, helping them to become more confident and to develop their strengths to increase enjoyment of life" (p. 87). Such sentiments by individuals with mental illness support the relevance of positive psychology interventions to indicated services.

DEVELOPMENTAL CONSIDERATIONS WHEN IMPLEMENTING THE WELL-BEING PROMOTION PROGRAM

Elementary School

In partnership with a suburban elementary school, we adapted the Well-Being Promotion Program to be accessible to students in Grades 3–5 (Suldo, Hearon, Dickinson, et al., 2015). Modification strategies were sensitive to these children's reduced attention spans, concrete thinking, limited vocabulary, and educational context (frequent contact with a primary classroom teacher vs. multiple educators throughout the day). Additionally, some but not all students had challenges with various instructional methods built into the group procedures, including writing, reading aloud, sharing personal experiences, and completing activities between group meetings. For example, on the whole we found that elementary school students were less likely than middle school students to remember to do homework assignments or bring completed homework to sessions. Direct instruction in study and organizational skills was outside the scope of the program goals; instead, we employed strategies (see Table 6.1) that were moderately successful in increasing compliance with the assignments that provide essential opportunities for rehearsal

TABLE 6.1. Intervention Modifications for Use with Elementary School Students

Goal	Example strategies
Increase student participation in session	• Use the session protocols flexibly. Rather than adhering to example scripts verbatim, internalize the main points to cover. Create agendas with bulleted points to accomplish. Cover key points in natural conversations about the material throughout the session.
	• When reviewing the homework assigned the session prior, routinely ask all students (including those who did not complete the task at home) to share their pertinent experiences.
	• Incorporate a structured behavior management system. Develop, post, and review (start of each session) a detailed description of behavioral expectations for in-session behavior.
	• Increase extrinsic motivation to participate or maintain attention. Provide encouragement, praise, and tangible reinforcers contingent on compliance with in-session rules, including participation (e.g., reading aloud, sharing stories) and on-task behavior.
	• When forming groups, aim to keep size small and include pairs of students who are familiar with each other, like are in the same class.
	• When/if students appear reluctant to share experiences in front of peers, include team-building activities.
	• If off-task behavior is more frequent in large-group discussions, break students into smaller groups *or* ask students to take turns (when reading aloud, answering questions, etc.) to distribute engagement opportunities. For example, during introduction of VIA strengths, children can take turns reading aloud definitions and providing examples of relevant people and situations.
	• Provide alternatives to written communication in story-based exercises. For example, permit students to dictate to the practitioner their "you at your best" or gratitude letter, and/or to draw responses to applicable prompts (e.g., for gratitude journaling, you at your best, best-possible future self).
Ensure discussions are developmentally appropriate	• Explain gratitude in simpler terms (e.g., thankful) and through use of a graphic organizer in which thankful is written in the middle with reasons for thankfulness written around the word.
	• To describe the idea of a genetic set point, offer a simpler explanation like "About half of your happiness is determined by what you're born with. Some people are born with the ability to be happier than others."
	• Omit cognitively complex protocols that require abstract thinking, specifically those targeting optimistic thinking, savoring, and hope.[a]

(continued)

TABLE 6.1. *(continued)*

Goal	Example strategies
Increase fidelity of the identify and use signature character strengths activity	• Create a "child-friendly" list of terms appropriate for explanation of the VIA strengths, and provide additional synonyms as needed. In subsequent sessions, review the definitions (with more synonyms and examples) of strengths that continue to prove challenging for children to understand (e.g., prudence, zest, authenticity).
	• Split the typically single session on "Assessment of Signature Character Strengths" into two meetings. In the first meeting, focus on completing the VIA-IS-Youth (for homework, students can continue acts of kindness). In the second meeting, compare expected versus VIA-identified strengths, and develop the plan for how to use one's first signature strength in new ways.
	• Provide intensive guidance (near one-on-one assistance) when students develop lists of novel ways to use their strengths. Between group meetings, compile ideas for developmentally appropriate ways that children may use specific strengths, including by consulting web-based resources from practitioners who previously helped individuals identify ways to use their VIA strengths.
	• Use "New Uses of My Signature Strength (Child)" homework form (see the Appendix). This version has space for the practitioner to specify one to three concrete ways for using the strength, capturing the feasible and new ways developed in group.
Increase rehearsal of exercises between sessions	• As part of the behavior management system, provide tangible reinforcers (e.g., candy, stickers, school supplies) contingent on homework completion.
	• In later sessions, restrict the focus of homework assignments to application of signature strengths in new ways, thereby omitting the prompt to ask students to complete a second assignment.
	• Increase involvement of the classroom teacher, starting with sharing an overview of the intervention schedule and intended session content in advance of program initiation.
	• When possible, include teachers in the session, perhaps to serve as co-leaders. When schedules preclude in-session participation, provide written summaries of the session content with guidance on how to integrate topics covered in group into class discussions and follow-up assignment completion (see Chapter 7).
	• Solicit assistance from the student's teacher, for example, via an e-mail asking the teacher to remind students to complete homework prior to the session and to bring materials (e.g., notebooks, previous session handouts and homework) to sessions.

[a]Findings are mixed regarding the applicability of strategies targeting hope for elementary-age students. McDermott and Hastings (2000) concluded that a lengthy intervention period (i.e., more than eight sessions) was needed to instill high hope in children. In contrast, elementary school students who participated in a "best-possible future self" activity through drawing on a weekly basis for 4–6 weeks incurred gains in self-esteem (Owens & Patterson, 2013). This provides some support for positive effects on children who visualize and draw a future version of themselves as happy and interested.

of strategies between sessions. During sessions, we sometimes encountered challenges with student engagement, focus, and participation in group discussions. Behavioral management and active instructional strategies were helpful in maintaining student involvement. Challenges with vocabulary and abstract thinking were particularly apparent during sessions that focused on the VIA classification system of character strengths; children had greater difficulty grasping definitions of many strengths (e.g., authenticity, zest, prudence) and then struggled to generate new and feasible uses for their identified strengths. Comprehension of the primary determinants of happiness was also hampered by children's prior knowledge, as they had not yet learned how to read a pie chart (which we often use to contrast the amount of variance in happiness explained by genetic factors, life circumstances, and purposeful behaviors and thoughts) and struggled with the idea of a genetic set point. To accommodate such concerns, in Table 6.1 we offer several strategies and intervention modifications for consideration by practitioners planning to serve elementary school students.

High School

As part of an agency's comprehensive system of mental health services, we have provided the Well-Being Promotion Program to individual students and small groups of youth ages 14–19 in high school and clinical settings. Through various identification mechanisms, such as referral by educators, parents, or physicians or students' self-referral, all teenagers were receiving this indicated intervention with the goal of improving mental health. The multitarget intervention was originally developed with middle school-age youth in mind, but we have not had older adolescents express perceiving the materials or content as too juvenile; instead, anecdotally we have observed high school students to resonate with the activities quite well. In our most recent small-group implementation with seven students in grades 9–12 in a suburban high school (program abbreviated to six sessions due to time constraints caused by the end-of-the-year testing requirements), students' ratings on the BMSLSS reflected growth improved from pre- to postintervention in every domain of life except family (the item with the highest score at baseline). Also, the global life satisfaction item improved an average of 1 full point on the response metric (specifically, the average score for the group was 2.75 [*mostly dissatisfied*] at baseline, and 3.75 [*mixed*] at postintervention) indicating a forward trajectory away from the clearly negative range after just six sessions. The domain that evidenced the most growth was satisfaction with friends ($M = 2.75$ moved to 5.0 [*mostly satisfied*]); at postintervention, the average satisfaction ratings for all domains were above 4.0, and highest for school ($M = 5.5$).

Although no modifications to intervention content or procedures have been necessary for these teenagers, their enhanced cognitive capacity warranted unique considerations. For example, some high school students expressed concern with the motives behind some prescribed behaviors. In particular, performing acts of kindness in a purposeful manner rather than at random struck some students as inauthentic. Nevertheless, students reported back that they still experienced higher levels of happiness despite the deliberate nature of their efforts to benefit others. To address students' concerns, we engaged in a discussion of person–activity fit. Students were able to identify at least one intervention activity that felt personally meaningful, while also recognizing every activity was beneficial to someone in the group. Also pertinent to fit, some male teenagers have reported experiencing discomfort completing emotionally expressive activities such as reading their gratitude letter aloud to the recipient. In such cases, we asked students to simply deliver the letter without reading it. Logistical issues related to scheduling have also proven to be particularly challenging with groups inclusive of students across grades 9–12. We have condensed and combined some session protocols to reduce the total number of meetings, which has helped accommodate students.

Intervention implementation with high school youth has also yielded advantages. Specifically, these older students have provided more detailed self-reflections of their experiences completing intervention exercises, and demonstrated greater comprehension of advanced topics, such as optimism. Since teenagers tend to understand and complete the in-session activities a bit quicker, some of our colleagues have used the remaining time during a meeting period to include a breathing meditation exercise, in line with Fredrickson's (2009) recommended strategies for facilitating positive emotions. Furthermore, heightened cognitive abilities of high school youth have permitted them to successfully complete brief assessments of signature strengths developed for adults, such as the Brief Strengths Test (available online via *www. authentichappiness.org*). Teenagers have also been particularly appreciative of the intervention focus on strengths as opposed to the myriad of problems they have become accustomed to speaking about with adults.

SUPPORTING TARGETED STUDENTS
WITH OTHER POSITIVE PSYCHOLOGY APPROACHES

Self-Administered Programs

Interest in self-help-style positive psychology interventions, including those delivered online, has grown in recent years in accordance with their vast potential in terms of increased accessibility, cost-effectiveness, and enhanced treatment fidelity in that activities are programmed electronically thus removing variability between interventionists (Layous, Nelson, et al., 2013). Research demonstrates that self-administered positive psychology interventions have small to moderate effects on reducing symptoms of psychopathology and enhancing well-being among samples of adults (Seligman et al., 2005; Shapira & Mongrain, 2010) and, more recently, youth (Manicavasagar et al., 2014). There are few evidence-based self-administered positive psychology interventions appropriate for youth. One promising option is an online multitarget program, Bite Back, developed by the Black Dog Institute in Australia. Bite Back is a website that provides adolescents with self-guided interactive exercises and information relevant to nine positive psychology targets (e.g., gratitude, mindfulness, and character strengths). Users learn the benefits of happiness, access positive exercises within each of the nine targets, and engage in virtual discussions with other adolescent users. In a randomized controlled trial, 235 Australian youth (ages 12–18) were instructed to visit either Bite Back (intervention) or another entertainment website (control) for at least 1 hour per week over 6 consecutive weeks (Manicavasagar et al., 2014). Youth in the Bite Back condition with high levels of participation (website usage > 30 minutes per week) and who visited the site more frequently (three or more times per week) reported significant decreases in symptoms of depression, anxiety, and stress, as well as improvements in well-being as assessed by the Short Warwick–Edinburgh Mental Well-Being Scale (Stewart-Brown et al., 2009). Findings indicate that online positive psychology interventions hold promise as an alternative or supplemental method of increasing well-being and decreasing psychopathology among youth. However, a relatively high number of youth either dropped out or did not use the website for the weekly 1-hour interval as instructed. Therefore, issues of intervention adherence may need to be addressed to ensure adolescent users experience optimal outcomes.

In general, self-administered programs tend to be less effective compared with individual and group-administered positive psychology interventions (Mitchell, Vella-Brodrick, & Klein, 2010; Sin & Lyubomirsky, 2009). Face-to-face modalities offer contact and feedback. The lack of such social support may contribute to the higher attrition rates and lower effect sizes observed in studies of self-administered positive psychology interventions. Additionally, self-administered programs can present logistical (e.g., user prerequisite of basic computer and literacy skills) and ethical (e.g., confidentiality of online information) challenges that are less evident during face-to-face implementation (Mitchell et al., 2010). As such, self-administered approaches may be best positioned as a supplement to traditional face-to-face delivery formats, or may eventually prove useful as a Tier 1 intervention in a multi-tiered framework of mental health services.

Brief Strengths-Based Counseling Interventions

Time-limited counseling approaches that are compatible with the goals of positive psychology include solution-focused brief therapy and motivational interviewing. These predated the modern positive psychology interventions that surfaced in the early 2000s. Both approaches are strengths-based, client-centered practices that facilitate the identification and utilization of personal strengths and resources to achieve psychotherapeutic goals that improve the individual's quality of life. Solution-focused therapy, introduced by Steve de Shazer, Insoo Kim Berg, and their colleagues at the Milwaukee Brief Family Therapy Center in the 1980s, is aimed at constructing solutions, rather than ameliorating problems, as its name suggests (Bavelas et al., 2013). Through a number of specific techniques (e.g., questions that identify when a problem does not occur; compliments; scaling), solution-focused therapists assist people envision how things could be better and take subsequent steps to make this vision a reality. Such therapists assume people are striving to make positive changes happen and already have solution behaviors in their repertoire (Bavelas et al., 2013). Because of the short-term (e.g., six or fewer sessions) and flexible nature of solution-focused brief therapy, it is a popular intervention approach for helping students with various academic and behavioral problems. However, few well-designed impact studies have been advanced, leading Kim and Franklin (2009) to suggest that further research is necessary to determine the efficacy of solution-focused strategies in educational settings. Existing research provides evidence of the promise that a solution-focused approach may help students manage various conduct or internalizing problems, particularly when implemented as an early intervention with students with mild to moderate symptom levels (Bond, Woods, Humphrey, Symes, & Green, 2013).

Motivational interviewing is a widely disseminated, evidence-based approach to helping individuals approach positive changes in their lives, in part by resolving ambivalence about change through considering discrepancies between personal values and behaviors (Miller & Rollnick, 2013). Central to this approach is the idea that individuals are more likely to accomplish things that they say they will do, rather than things they are told to do. Motivational interviewing entails four overlapping and sequential processes: (1) *engaging* the client in the therapeutic process, (2) *focusing* conversation on narrow goals, (3) *evoking* change talk to promote readiness for change, and (4) *planning* to use client-developed steps to achieve goals (Miller &

Rollnick, 2013). Applications of motivational interviewing in educational settings have shown promising effects on students' academic and mental health outcomes, including via consultative interactions with educators and parents, and through brief individual counseling interventions (Herman, Reinke, Frey, & Shepard, 2014). Regarding the latter, in efficacy studies using random assignment to intervention or control conditions, middle school students who took part in a single 45-minute motivational interviewing session demonstrated significantly higher class participation, positive academic behavior, and grades in math (Strait et al., 2012; Terry, Strait, McQuillin, & Smith, 2014). More recent study of dosage effects suggests that participation in two motivational interviewing sessions may have a greater and broader impact on academic performance (math, science, and history grades) in comparison to a single session (Terry et al., 2014). In sum, accumulating evidence supports motivational interviewing as a promising brief method for improving student success. Current directions in clinical applications of motivational interviewing involve integrating this approach with positive psychology interventions. As described by Csillik (2015), the two theoretical frameworks are complementary. For instance, motivational interviewing may be useful in building students' intention and efficacy to practice the positive psychology exercises presented in Chapter 5.

Intensive Positive Psychology Interventions

The lengthier interventions in this category entail meeting regularly with a practitioner in the context of a coaching or psychotherapeutic relationship for around eight or more planned contacts. While this sometimes occurs with nonclinical individuals seeking to attain personal goals or simply enhance well-being, intensive interventions may be particularly appropriate for individuals who have elevated levels of psychopathology. Quality of Life Therapy and Coaching (QOLTC; Frisch, 2013) is one of the first such comprehensive counseling applications from a positive psychology perspective. QOLTC provides subclinical adults with tools to boost satisfaction in one of 16 specific domains of life (e.g., relationships with family and friends, goals and values, health) to enhance overall quality of life. Coaching is an applied subdiscipline of psychology, in which practitioners support individuals in creating and following their own path for personal success, primarily by developing insight and skill in tapping their personal resources in goal-directed activities. Congruent with aims of positive psychology, coaching entails a systematic approach to promoting positive change and enhanced well-being in the lives of nonclinical populations (Green, Oades, & Grant, 2006). Coaching has garnered support within the past decade due to emerging empirical evidence demonstrating its effectiveness with samples ranging from high school seniors to adult professionals (Grant, 2014). Although relatively few randomized controlled trials have investigated the efficacy of coaching, extant research findings (primarily from studies of adults) support its use for the improvement of cognitive hardiness, hope, goal striving, subjective well-being, self-efficacy, and resilience (Franklin & Doran, 2009; Green, Grant, & Rynsaardt, 2007; Green et al., 2006). Such findings warrant greater comprehension of the potential benefits of applying systematic coaching positive psychological interventions with students in educational settings.

Suzy Green and colleagues (2007) have advanced school-based coaching interventions that are aligned with hope theory, as discussed in Chapter 5. Green and colleagues conducted a randomized controlled trial to investigate the efficacy of a 10-session teacher-led life coaching program. The sample included 56 nonclinical female high school students (mean age 16) in

Australia. Ten teacher-coaches participated in two half-day coaching workshops provided by the school counselor. The solution-focused, cognitive-behavioral coaching program consisted of 10 face-to-face individual coaching sessions over the period of two semesters (28 weeks). Students generated two issues (one school, one personal) to improve. Teachers coached students to identify personal resources to achieve goals, develop self-generated solutions and specific action steps, and monitor and evaluate progress; students systematically worked through the problem-solving process to continuously obtain new goals. Relative to their peers in the wait-list control group, students who were coached experienced significant increases in hope and cognitive hardiness, as well as a significant decrease in depression. More recent applications of coaching interventions have explicitly incorporated use of students' character strengths in facilitating goal attainment. Madden, Green, and Grant (2011) piloted a strengths-coaching program with 38 Australian male students in fifth grade at a private primary school. Students were identified for program participation due to elevated symptoms of psychopathology, per self-report on a screening measure. The teacher-coach was a primary school teacher who also had extensive training in coaching, including an advanced degree in coaching psychology and previous applied experience coaching children and adults. The program consisted of eight 45-minute coaching sessions over the course of two school terms (totaling 6 months). Discussions with the coach were individualized, but occurred in the context of small groups. The program consisted of three phases: (1) increasing self-awareness and identification of strengths using the VIA framework; (2) coaching to identify and use personal resources to achieve goals tied to applications of character strengths; and (3) developing individualized action plans, then monitoring and evaluating progress. Students also completed a writing activity akin to best-possible future self. Students experienced statistically significant increases in hope and engagement from pre- to postintervention. Such outcomes provide evidence of promise that coaching can enhance the well-being of children and adolescents served in school settings, with teachers providing the coaching.

Grounded in Chris Peterson's (Peterson & Seligman, 2004) seminal work on character strengths, positive psychotherapy is a therapeutic treatment approach designed to reduce symptoms of psychological distress by identifying and emphasizing individuals' positive resources (Rashid, 2015). Positive psychotherapy operationalizes Seligman's (2002, 2011) conceptualization of well-being through activities targeting individuals' positive emotions, engagement, relationships, meaning, and accomplishment (PERMA). The three phases of treatment include (1) explore strengths and develop personally meaningful goals; (2) create positive emotions and cope with negative memories; and (3) foster positive relationships, as well as meaning and purpose (Rashid, 2015). Throughout the course of therapy, individuals engage in a variety of positive psychology interventions also contained in our Well-Being Promotion Program, including you at your best, identifying and cultivating signature character strengths, gratitude journaling, and savoring. In additional exercises, people learn how to encounter negative experiences with a more positive mind-set and reframe those experiences into those that are more adaptive, such as forgiving a transgressor and increasing satisficing (instead of maximizing). As such, positive psychotherapy does not deny negative emotions and experiences, but emphasizes individuals' use of personal strengths to overcome challenges (Rashid, 2015). In several pilot studies, positive psychotherapy has been implemented with diverse samples using individual and group delivery formats with varying numbers of sessions. Overall, these studies provide evidence of promise with respect to reductions in depressive symptoms, and greater subjective well-being compared with control groups or preintervention scores; in adult samples, effect sizes have been medium to large (Rashid, 2015). When compared with other evidence-based treatments, such as cognitive behavior therapy or dialectical behavior therapy, positive psychotherapy performs as well or significantly better on measures of well-being (e.g., Asgharipoor, Farid, Arshadi, & Sahebi, 2010).

Although few investigations have explored the utility of positive psychotherapy with youth in schools, preliminary findings from Rashid and colleagues' (2008, 2013) research suggest that this strengths-based treatment may also be viable in educational settings. For instance, sixth-grade students randomly assigned to eight weekly 90-minute sessions of positive psychotherapy experienced lasting improvements in well-being (as assessed by the Positive Psychotherapy Inventory [PPTI] developed by Rashid, 2005) relative to their peers in a control group (Rashid et al., 2013). In contrast, no effects of intervention were seen in a different sample of sixth-grade students with academic and behavioral challenges at an inner-city school, who participated in positive psychotherapy (modified to include exercises targeting students' negativity bias) for eight weekly 60-minute sessions. Rashid and colleagues speculated that the intervention brevity, teacher's limited participation, and lack of parental involvement may have contributed to the nonsignificant findings. Accordingly, they reported more positive outcomes from a subsequent application with elementary school students that included a relatively extensive parent component (i.e., workshops on character strengths and how to facilitate their child's well-being, participation in exercises to cultivate students' strengths) and teacher component (i.e., integration of strengths into the curriculum). This multicomponent version of positive psychotherapy was associated with improved academic performance and social skills, as well as reduced problem behavior, but no change in student well-being (PPTI scores; Rashid et al., 2013). In spite of somewhat inconsistent impacts on outcomes, across samples these findings provide support for promise that positive psychotherapy may improve students' social skills, academic performance, and well-being. More studies are necessary to determine if such findings are replicated in larger samples of diverse youth across different educational levels. Future directions in research also involve studies geared toward clinical applications. Such studies should determine if positive psychology interventions may be particularly effective for treating specific forms of psychopathology, such as adolescent depression (Curry, 2014) or if specific targets are particularly beneficial among clinical populations, such as gratitude (Emmons & Stern, 2013) or mindfulness meditation (Shonin, Gordon, Compare, Zangeneh, & Griffiths, 2015).

INDIVIDUALIZED APPLICATIONS OF THE WELL-BEING PROMOTION PROGRAM WITH TARGETED STUDENTS

In the years since advancing the Well-Being Promotion Program in a selective way for small groups of youth (Chapter 5), we have adapted it for use with individual students in a more traditional counseling capacity. The specific protocols implemented stemmed first from issues of feasibility—namely, students' developmental level—we omitted more abstract targets as a general rule of thumb when working with students in elementary school or as indicated when serving older students with cognitive limitations. Then, target selection was matched to level and type of student need in consideration of the complexity of a given students' mental health concerns, akin to Tier 2 (selective) or Tier 3 (indicated) services in a multi-tiered system of supports.

Selective Level

We conceptualize the well-being program as a selective-level intervention when offered to students who are identified through a universal screening of subjective well-being, such as with the BMSLSS. When we have had sufficient professional resources (i.e., counselor trainees supervised by experienced clinicians) to support these students individually or in dyads, as opposed to in larger groups of six to eight students, we have typically implemented all developmentally appropriate protocols in the Well-Being Promotion Program in a sequential manner. This modality is identical to what is described in Chapter 5, with the exception of starting with the two individualized sessions described next. The application of the complete set of core positive psychology intervention protocols in this uniform manner is consistent with the reason why these students were selected for mental health services in the first place—specifically due to diminished life satisfaction. All activities in the Well-Being Promotion Program target different correlates of life satisfaction, and as such are matched to the "referral concern" and corresponding intervention goal: increase student subjective well-being.

The Appendix contains the protocols for the two supplementary sessions intended to initiate and enhance the counseling relationship by providing the practitioner and student with an opportunity to get to know each other better. In the first individual session, the practitioner acquaints him- or herself with the student by explaining the role of a counselor and the goal of meeting: to help the student become and stay happier. The practitioner makes clear how the student was selected for the program; we find it helpful to reference a blank copy of the measure completed during the screening process (i.e., the BMSLSS) to jog the student's memory. After getting to know the student's general interests, the practitioner begins exploration of the student's level of subjective well-being and factors that may boost or hamper it. When working with younger or reticent youth (particularly elementary school students), engaging the student in a brief card or board game to facilitate rapport may help transition to this personal discussion. Completion of the SLSS and MSLSS (described in Chapter 2) directs students' attention to thoughts about their quality of life, and provides preintervention levels of life satisfaction both globally and in various domains. When exploring the student's unique determinants of happiness, the practitioner references a global item and asks the student what he or she was thinking about when answering this question. When working with students who can handle abstract questions, the practitioner can also ask what would need to change in the student's life in order to increase happiness by 1 point on the scale, probing specifically for environmental or interpersonal influences. The goal of the second individual session is to better understand the student's unique behaviors and circumstances that may influence his or her life satisfaction. In the semistructured interview that follows, the student describes (1) features of his or her personality; (2) perceived well-being level of each person living in the home; (3) additional people and events that may affect personal happiness; and (4) what he or she does to regulate mood, including in the face of challenges. The practitioner can refer back to information shared in these individual meetings when tailoring discussions throughout the core sessions of the Well-Being Promotion Program to the student's specific situation.

Many students with whom we have worked in this manner have started out mildly to moderately happy, and progress to flourishing throughout the program. However, other students show signs of mental health problems and/or discuss significant environmental stressors, often early in the counseling relationship. As with any school mental health intervention, crisis services are provided and referrals for additional services are initiated as warranted. As a general practice, though, we continue to implement the core Well-Being Promotion Program as planned, rather than switching to an alternative intervention for (suspected) depression, anxiety, ADHD, and so forth. In this continued implementation, we couple empathy with reframing a negative situation to draw attention to students' strength(s). For example, one regular education middle school student noted at the onset of a session that her grandmother had died. While providing her with emotional support, we discussed that this might be a particularly good time to use her character strength of humor to help other family members, as well as cheer up herself. She integrated those ideas into her "new uses of my signature strength" activity. In another example, a high school student with a likely mood disorder got into a fight with another student who called her sister a derogatory name due to her sexual identity. We pointed out how she used her strengths of fairness and bravery in standing up for her sister, but also discussed how those strengths could be used in a more prosocial manner (using Martin Luther King Jr. and peaceful protesting as an example). The progress and well-being for each student is reviewed at the end of the intervention. Students who continue to report low life satisfaction or who display concerning symptoms of mental health problems are referred to the school mental health team for additional services. In contrast, most students cease care or reduce to intermittent contact, such as in the form of periodic follow-up sessions to review strategies learned for promoting happiness.

Indicated Level

We conceptualize the Well-Being Promotion Program as an indicated-level intervention when provided to students receiving psychological services due to significant mental health problems. This includes students who have been referred for mental health services due to emotional symptoms displayed at school or home, or students previously identified with emotional/behavioral disabilities. No surprise given our school psychology backgrounds, we have extensive experience with such subgroups. When designing treatment plans for students with significant mental health needs, some of whom have counseling services specified on individualized education plans (IEPs), we have increasingly incorporated various evidence-based positive psychology interventions that are consistent with a case conceptualization. The supplemental sessions described above are not often applicable because our aforementioned case conceptualization flows from a more traditional intake assessment that routinely uses comprehensive data collection procedures, including quantitative indicators of mental health (e.g., self-report surveys of life satisfaction and psychopathology), as well as observations and interviews that shed light on factors correlated with subjective well-being.

EXAMPLE INDICATED IMPLEMENTATION: CASE STUDY FROM A HIGH SCHOOL

We have found various intervention protocols described in Chapter 5 to provide logical methods for addressing a host of student problems, such as negative view of self, low connectedness to school, and poor relationships with family and friends. By way of example, we summarize the case of Jill (pseudonym), a high school female who received exceptional student education services due to an emotional/behavioral disability. When we met Jill early in her 10th-grade school year to initiate counseling services in accordance with her IEP, she was participating in general education courses, had incurred several ODRs for disruptive and aggressive behavior, and was taking psychotropic medication to manage symptoms of ADHD and bipolar disorder. A records review indicated she had incurred a number of traumatic experiences during childhood, including abuse that led to temporary removal from the family home. Strengths evident in the intake process included high academic motivation and educational aspirations, engagement in extracurricular activities at school and in the community, and many hobbies that utilized her vocal and athletic talents. She also demonstrated remarkable self-awareness and motivation to improve her mental health. The intake process indicated three primary target problems: family discord, irritability and aggressive behavior, and low self-esteem. For the first two areas, therapeutic interventions planned to achieve goals (i.e., improve family communication, implement anger management and conflict resolution strategies) entailed traditional cognitive-behavioral strategies to develop social and communication skills coupled with behavioral parent consultation. Regarding the third area, Jill's low self-esteem was reflected in frequent descriptions of herself as unattractive and unimportant, inability to identify positive personal traits, and fears of interpersonal rejection. The broad counseling goal for this area was to increase self-confidence through recognizing her positive qualities and increasing statements of self-acceptance, increasing contact with individuals who valued her positive qualities, and eliminating self-disparaging remarks. To accomplish the latter objective, the treatment plan included cognitive-behavioral strategies pertinent to identifying, evaluating, and modifying negative automatic thoughts, and replacing them with positive self-talk messages. This was complemented by beginning with many positive psychology interventions in the Well-Being Promotion Program. We selected protocols intended to focus her attention to the positive features of herself (i.e., character strengths) and life circumstances that were going well or held potential. To develop Jill's awareness of her positive qualities, sessions consisted of activities in the protocols for the core student Sessions 1, 5, 6, and 7 (i.e., you at your best, identification and use of character strengths from the VIA framework). To help Jill identify positive aspects of her environment, including examples of displays of kindness by others, we adapted the Session 2 protocol (gratitude journaling) for use with an individual student. To spur positive interactions with key people in her life and otherwise cultivate positive relationships, the protocols for Sessions 3 (gratitude visit) and 4 (acts of kindness) served as session guides. To monitor response to such interventions, we periodically administered the MSLSS and reviewed scores from the relevant domains to gauge improvements from the low levels at baseline, such as an average score of 3.6 on the self scale of the MSLSS during the intake process.

This treatment plan that ultimately included a mix of strategies across cognitive-behavioral, motivational, humanistic, and positive psychology frameworks was well received by Jill and provided a comprehensive road map for subsequent session content and focus. Likely expected given her complicated family and psychiatric history, Jill's progress in session and at school was not without hurdles. For instance, completion of the "you at your best" activity was hampered by her inability to identify a situation to write about. To overcome this, we encouraged Jill to reflect on her participation in a school club that facilitates close friendships between students with and without intellectual disabilities, an activity discussed and observed during the intake process. At school, exclusionary consequences for fighting posed obvious logistical barriers to learning anger management strategies. The focus of counseling sessions could have easily turned to her experiences with these suspensions as well as a later arrest and ongoing challenges with an alcoholic parent. Fortunately, the positive psychology strategies built into the treatment plan provided a basis for maintaining relatively balanced attention to strengths and hope throughout therapy. At the end of the school year, her average score on the self scale of the MSLSS had improved to 4.0, just at the threshold that corresponds to (mild) satisfaction in this domain. Jill's global life satisfaction also improved from baseline, as did satisfaction with every domain of life except for school (no surprise given ongoing reports of conflict with educators and classmates within her classes that had an additional aide to support the numerous students with emotional and behavioral disorders). Also notable, at intake her levels of psychopathology (as measured by the Youth Self-Report Form of the ASEBA; Achenbach, & Rescorla, 2001) were in the clinical ranges for both internalizing and externalizing symptoms. At the end of the school year, only externalizing symptoms remained clinically elevated.

PART III

ECOLOGICAL STRATEGIES FOR PROMOTING YOUTH HAPPINESS

CHAPTER 7

Universal Strategies for Promoting Student Happiness

with Mollie McCullough and Denise Quinlan

The impact of the emotional climate in a classroom on students' academic and psychological success cannot be overstated. As described in Chapters 1 and 3, the quality of students' interpersonal relationships is a primary predictor and consequence of youth subjective well-being. Students with complete mental health perceive greater social support from parents, classmates, and teachers (Antaramian et al., 2010; Suldo & Shaffer, 2008). Supportive relationships with family and teachers are also key to maintaining a flourishing mental health status characterized by elevated subjective well-being (Kelly, Hills, Huebner, & McQuillin, 2012). Accordingly, attempts to improve youth subjective well-being should target strengthening of relationships with a variety of sources at home and school.

This chapter focuses on (1) interventions directed toward the well-being of the key adults at school, who have the ability to positively or negatively impact a given student; and (2) classroom-based strategies that target students' interpersonal relationships or subjective well-being. First, we discuss the influence of teachers' well-being on the classroom climate and student outcomes, followed by a summary of the applicability of positive psychology interventions to improving teacher well-being. Then, we discuss the promise of universal positive psychology interventions implemented classwide, primarily evaluated in terms of impact on students' happiness. We describe in detail two promising classwide positive psychology programs recently implemented in elementary schools. One focuses on teaching students to recognize activity strengths and character strengths in themselves and others, and to use their character strengths to support

Mollie McCullough, MA, is a doctoral candidate in the School Psychology Program at the University of South Florida.

Denise Quinlan, PhD, is an independent consultant on Well-Being in Education and is part of a University of Otago–led research group studying successful transition from high school to university.

meaningful goals (Quinlan, Swain, et al., 2015). In that program, teachers and students are also encouraged to practice strengths spotting (i.e., noticing strengths in others) on a daily basis. The other program is a version of the Well-Being Promotion Program presented in Chapter 5 that we modified to include supplemental components targeting the larger classroom context through activities intended to strengthen classroom relationships; the core student-focused sessions retained target gratitude, kindness, and application of signature strengths (Suldo, Hearon, Bander, et al., 2015). These programs illustrate teachers' potential roles in the implementation of positive psychology interventions, ranging from co-participant (e.g., another person in the classroom to help spot the character strengths we all display) to co-interventionist (e.g., individual charged with teaching youth about positive psychology or reinforcing content first introduced by a school mental health provider) to informed consultant (e.g., being kept abreast of the student-focused intervention strategies).

THE IMPORTANCE OF TEACHERS' WELL-BEING

Applying positive psychology to the classroom can have dramatic effects on a climate that reflects improved well-being on the part of students and teachers alike. Teachers play a pivotal role in promoting students' social–emotional well-being, often serving as gatekeepers for the implementation of positive activities within the classroom. Unfortunately, the importance of well-being for teachers and other school professionals has often taken a backseat in consideration of mental health (Fleming, Mackrain, & LeBuffe, 2013; Miller, Nickerson, Chafouleas, & Osborne, 2008). This is surprising given the reality of teachers' intense job demands and workloads. Teachers are under increased pressure to ensure that students attain proficiency in reading and math as measured through annual high-stakes testing. Rigorous teacher evaluation procedures are implemented to guarantee that teachers are held more responsible to student performance (Fleming et al., 2013). This accountability focus likely contributes to the growing epidemic in teacher attrition and migration—for example, 17.3% of beginning public school teachers leave the profession within 5 years (Gray & Taie, 2015). The chronic stress that teachers endure has resulted in diminished work performance, reduced motivation, and increased physical symptoms that ultimately cascade into burnout with the profession (Montgomery & Rupp, 2005). Without a more direct focus on teacher well-being, the proposed strategies for promoting youth happiness may be futile, especially if the adults with whom they interact most during the school day feel emotionally exhausted and overworked. Accordingly, Hills and Robinson (2010) emphasized that teachers need to be the first to put on their oxygen masks prior to supporting their students' social–emotional wellness.

Defining Teacher Well-Being

For many decades, the well-being of teachers was examined through the lens of stress and burnout indicators. Chronic exposure to workplace stressors (e.g., administrative work demands, student behavior problems, and negative interactions with parents or colleagues; Montgomery & Rupp, 2005) without adaptive coping mechanisms can lead to dissatisfaction at work and ultimately teacher burnout. Teacher burnout consists of emotional exhaustion, depersonalization, and diminished personal accomplishment (Maslach & Goldberg, 1999). Attention to teacher stress and burnout has afforded understanding of the extent of the problem, but has provided minimal insight regarding how to solve it or how to support teachers' well-being. More recently, researchers have homed in on positive indicators of teacher well-being in order to understand what facilitates healthy functioning for educators at work. Such positive constructs include teacher self-efficacy, emotional intelligence, academic optimism, job satisfaction, and grit (Duckworth, Quinn, & Seligman, 2009; Jennings & Greenberg, 2009; Spilt, Koomen, & Thijs, 2011; Stansberry Beard, Hoy, Woolfolk Hoy, 2010; Tschannen-Moran & Woolfolk Hoy, 2001). Jennings and Greenberg's (2009) prosocial classroom theoretical model illustrates the contribution of teachers' social–emotional competence and well-being to healthy student–teacher relationships, effective classroom management practices, and quality social–emotional learning (SEL) for students. Van Horn, Taris, Schaufeli, and Schreurs (2004) asserted that *teacher occupational well-being* includes five dimensions: (1) *affective* (emotional exhaustion, job satisfaction, organization commitment), (2) *professional* (self-efficacy, professional competence), (3) *social* (depersonalization, relationships at work), (4) *cognitive* (cognitive weariness, functioning at work), and (5) *psychosomatic* (psychosomatic complaints and/or physical ailments). This multifaceted consideration of teacher well-being is consistent with a conceptualization of complete mental health as entailing the absence of psychopathology (e.g., stress, fatigue, absenteeism) and presence of thriving (e.g., job satisfaction, positive emotions).

The Influence of Teachers' Well-Being on the Classroom Climate and Student Outcomes

A growing body of research indicates that teachers significantly impact student outcomes through their personal attributes, changes in behavior, and improved well-being. Teacher stress and burnout (the indicators examined in most studies) are linked to a multitude of detrimental outcomes including teachers' reduced tolerance for challenging behaviors, impaired student–teacher relationships, and poor student performance (Fleming et al., 2013; Montgomery & Rupp, 2005). Teacher stress and burnout significantly predicts reduced teacher effectiveness in classroom management (Long, Renshaw, Hamilton, Bolognino, & Lark, 2015), while also contributing to the depersonalization and distancing of teachers from their students (Lambert, McCarthy, O'Donnell, & Wang, 2009). Teacher stress has also been associated with higher levels of student misbehavior resulting in increased teacher emotional exhaustion and use of harsher and more reactive discipline further exacerbating the burnout cycle (Clunies-Ross, Little, & Kienhuis, 2008; Reinke, Herman, & Stormont, 2013). No surprise given humans' basic needs for relatedness, as well as the saliency and frequency of interactions between teachers and their students, conflictual relationships with students exacerbate teacher stress (Spilt et al., 2011). While student misbehavior matters, teachers who tend to provide minimal emotional support to their students contribute to such conflict (Hamre, Pianta, Downer, & Mashburn, 2008). Teachers who report higher levels of classroom stress from student misbehavior also report reduced self-efficacy in approaching classroom management (Klassen & Chiu, 2010). Such depletion in self-efficacy exacerbated by professional stress impairs effective teaching practices, thereby negatively impacting student academic performance (Tschannen-Moran & Woolfolk Hoy, 2001). Jennings and Greenberg (2009) suggest that teachers overwhelmed by the exhaustive demands of their work may also find it difficult to display socially appropriate behavior and disengage from their students, further impairing students' social–emotional competence.

Recent research draws attention to the benefits of the positive features of teacher well-being. Greater self-efficacy beliefs pertinent to classroom management and instructional strategies are tied to higher satisfaction with the profession (Klassen & Chiu, 2010) and increased student achievement (Caprara, Barbaranelli, Steca, & Malone, 2006). Teachers with high levels of academic optimism (i.e., beliefs that one can effectively teach, one's students can learn, and one has established trust with both parents and students) may also be more highly motivating to their students through demonstrations of social support and constructive feedback (Stansberry Beard et al., 2010). Duckworth and colleagues (2009) found that high levels of teacher grit (i.e., intrinsic determination) and global life satisfaction were even stronger predictors of effectiveness in terms of student academic gains among new teachers within a low-income school. Further examination of teacher grit (as evidenced through academic credentials and ratings of leadership potential) indicated that teachers with higher ratings of perseverance and dedication were more effective teachers and less likely to leave the classroom during the middle of the school year (Robertson-Kraft & Duckworth, 2014). The aforementioned positive effect of teachers' global life satisfaction on student academic outcomes is consistent with a host of studies of other employment settings that found happier employees tend to be much more productive, successful, and satisfied at work (Boehm & Lyubomirsky, 2008).

POSITIVE PSYCHOLOGY INTERVENTIONS FOCUSED ON TEACHER WELL-BEING

Clearly, supporting teachers' complete mental health is essential to ensuring optimal academic, behavioral, and social–emotional outcomes among students. Gibbs and Miller (2014) suggested that interventions targeting teacher wellness may be best driven by the positive psychology field. However, interventions supporting teachers' well-being are sparse, with a majority explored outside of the United States (e.g., England, Australia, and China). The dimensions of well-being most often examined in relevant studies have entailed cognitive and psychosomatic indicators (e.g., physical health, efficacy beliefs), as well as reductions in teacher stress and burnout, with minimal attention to indicators of happiness. Although research on the efficacy of positive psychology interventions for improving teachers' well-being is in the early stages, findings to date provide evidence of promise with regard to the targets described next.

Mindfulness

In recent years, the predominant focus of methods intended to increase teacher well-being (i.e., reducing occupational stress and burnout) has centered on mindfulness activities (Jennings, Frank, Snowberg, Coccia, & Greenberg, 2013; Roeser et al., 2013). Buddhist meditation practices and other Eastern religious traditions culminated into Jon Kabat-Zinn's modernized purposeful activities that are reflected in current mindfulness interventions (Albrecht, Albrecht, & Cohen, 2012; Kabat-Zinn, 2003). Such activities can include body scanning (similar to progressive muscle relaxation), forms of meditation (e.g., loving-kindness meditation), and yoga. Programs targeting teachers that have been evaluated recently include Stress Management and Relaxation Techniques in Education (Benn, Akiva, Arel, & Roeser, 2012; Roeser et al., 2013) and Cultivating Awareness and Resilience in Education (CARE; Jennings et al., 2013). Such programs have demonstrated utility in reducing occupational stress and burnout, while also improving teacher efficacy (Benn et al., 2012; Jennings et al., 2013). Acceptability for mindfulness programs is generally high; teachers have emphasized benefits to their teaching practices and ease of implementation.

Gratitude

Other attempts to improve teacher well-being have targeted gratitude among international samples. In Hong Kong, teachers listed three specific things for which they were thankful, and reflected on the reason for their good fortunes, during eight weekly sessions. After the intervention concluded, teachers showed significant increases in life satisfaction and positive affect, and reduced burnout, especially those teachers who began with low levels of gratitude (Chan, 2010) or a greater tendency to seek meaning in life (Chan, 2011). Findings from a mixed-methods study suggested that teachers in England who participated in the "Three Good Things" intervention improved their efficacy beliefs regarding perceived ability to work effectively with colleagues, be an effective leader, and maintain flexibility at school (Critchley & Gibbs, 2012).

Multitarget Intervention

A modern psychoeducational program intended to prevent burnout and improve well-being among Chinese teachers includes instruction on how to apply positive psychology principles (benefits of happiness, character strengths, hope) to the workplace (Siu, Cooper, & Phillips, 2014). This stress management program takes place over a 2.5-day professional development training. The primary effect of this program was observed in teachers' feelings of mastery experiences outside of work (e.g., greater involvement in challenging activities); no improvements were detected in the positive emotions or burnout of teachers in the intervention versus control groups. It is possible that following up on such didactic training with opportunities to put the learned strategies into practice would yield greater benefits.

Character Strengths

As described earlier in this book, research with community samples of adults suggests that cultivating use of character strengths is among the most impactful positive psychology interventions, associated with lasting improvements in well-being (Seligman et al., 2005). Given the promise of this practice, we recently conducted a pilot study with elementary school teachers to determine the impact of a brief school-based application in which a practitioner guides the teacher to identify and use character strengths in the classroom. In Table 7.1, we summarize the primary activities in each of the four individual meetings between the practitioner and teacher.

Before, during, and after the intervention, teacher participants reported their subjective well-being via completion of the Satisfaction with Life Scale (Diener, Emmons, Larsen, & Griffin, 1985) and the Positive and Negative Affect Schedule (Watson, Clark, & Tellegan, 1988). The eight participants ranged in classroom teaching experience from 2 to 27 years ($M = 11.4$ years), and represented most levels of elementary school, from kindergarten through grade 5. Data from these participants were analyzed in three ways: (1) examining change over time (pre, post, follow-up) through use of nonparametric statistics to analyze data collapsed across the small

TABLE 7.1. Intervention Procedures to Cultivate Elementary School Teachers' Use of Character Strengths in the Classroom

Meeting	Activities
1	• Introduce the 24 character strengths within the VIA Classification System. • Teacher generates a list of strengths that he or she believes he or she possesses and discusses reasoning. • Describe how character strengths are related to happiness. • Teacher completes the VIA online, learns top five "signature" strengths.
2	• Review signature strengths; evaluate them in terms of compatibility and recent uses across primary domains of life (family, friends, work). • Select signature strength to use in new and different ways for 5 work days. • Brainstorm ways to apply the selected strength within the classroom and/or school context. • Show how to complete a journal to track use of signature strength in new and different ways.
3	• Discuss progress in completing daily intervention task (use a signature strength in a new and different way at school). • As needed, problem solve any barriers to strengths application. • Reflection on experience; share success with application of strength. • Develop a plan for using a second signature strength in new and different ways during this second week of the intervention period.
4	• Discuss progress in completing daily intervention task (use second signature strength in a new and different way at school). • As needed, problem solve any barriers to strengths application. • Reflection on experience; share success with application of strength. • Describe concepts of happiness set point and hedonic treadmill to emphasize importance of continued use of signature strengths. • Plan for continued application of strengths at work. • Receive a celebratory certificate of intervention completion. • Complete measures of intervention acceptability and well-being.

sample, (2) applying single-case analytic strategies to time series data obtained from a multiple baseline design, and (3) examining qualitative feedback regarding intervention feasibility (McCullough, 2015). The teachers experienced significant gains in life satisfaction and reductions in negative affect from pre- to postintervention, improvements in subjective well-being that were still evident at 1-month follow-up. While positive affect did not change significantly from pre- to postintervention, a significant gain was evident at the follow-up point. To further isolate the effect of the intervention on change in subjective well-being, single-case analytic strategies were applied to time series data to evaluate near daily ratings of subjective well-being at different phases of intervention implementation (baseline, intervention, follow-up). In terms of overall subjective well-being (composite of standardized life satisfaction, positive affect, and negative affect scores), results of visual analysis (i.e., within and between phases patterns and data overlap), masked visual analysis, and hierarchical linear modeling supported the conclusion that the intervention positively impacted subjective well-being. Of the three variables that contributed to this composite score, the effect of treatment was particularly apparent in life satisfaction (as indicated by a four-item version of the Satisfaction with Life Scale). Some variability in treatment effects on individuals were apparent, in that some teachers benefited more than others (with effects particularly apparent on different aspects of subjective well-being) in line with the person–activity fit described by Lyubomirsky and Layous (2013).

Regarding intervention feasibility, it was well received by all eight teacher participants. In response to open-ended questions on an adapted version of the Intervention Rating Profile for Teachers (Martens, Witt, Elliott, & Darveaux, 1985), teachers unanimously reported the intervention to be rewarding and fulfilling in terms of improving their happiness within the classroom and school context, while also improving their interactions with both students and colleagues. When asked about the most important things learned in the intervention, participant responses included:

> "That I have control over my happiness and that I can do specific, concrete interventions to influence my happiness."
> "I was reminded of my personal attributes and learned how I can use those natural strengths to improve my own happiness and my students' engagement."
> "Just to take a couple of minutes to purposefully plan can change [my] whole day."
> "Learning which signature strengths lend themselves to my personal happiness."
> "Taking the stress off of both the students and teacher makes the classroom a happier place to be."
> "Did not realize what my key strengths were . . . I will continue to emphasize them as I teach."

Responses to the question "What did you like best about the intervention?" included:

> "I like that it helped me to focus on my strengths. For example, I am a naturally playful and grateful person, but I can often lose sight of that. Doing activities that helped me focus on my strengths was refreshing."
> "I loved finding out my strengths and using them to influence my happiness."
> "The reflecting; it helped me see how much happiness is occurring."
> "I enjoyed sharing my trials and activities with [the researcher] and discussing/reflecting on the parts that were successful. Reflecting online was helpful, but it was the one-to-one support that really encouraged me to stretch my limits and explore myself as a teacher. Upon further reflection, I think of the interactions with my students and colleagues that were fueled by this study. I am happy to think of some of my students' successes and how I was able to encourage them because I was happier myself."
> "My students showed more kindness to others and myself."

Given the salience of teacher well-being to positive student outcomes, practitioners are in need of evidence-based methods to promote and monitor teacher happiness. Our future work includes refining teacher-focused interventions such as this one that targets character strengths;

it warrants more rigorous evaluations of efficacy in larger samples. We are excited about the development of new tools to assess teacher well-being that are aligned with a positive psychology framework, such as the Teacher Subjective Wellbeing Questionnaire (Renshaw, Long, & Cook, 2015), in which feelings of excitement, interest, and joy while teaching are reflected in teaching efficacy beliefs and connectedness to one's school.

THE IMPORTANCE OF RELATIONSHIPS IN THE CLASSROOM TO STUDENTS' WELL-BEING

Positive relationships with peers and teachers create a sense of school connectedness. Children and early adolescents who experience positive social relationships have greater life satisfaction (Oberle, Schonert-Reichl, & Zumbo, 2011). The influence of positive peer relations and feelings of school connectedness on students' life satisfaction is significant even after considering the strong influences of parent support and students' internal assets, such as optimism. Students who report dissatisfaction with school refer to poor student–teacher relationships and diminished feelings of school relatedness as reasons for their overall disconnect from school, producing detrimental effects on academic outcomes (Baker, 1999). Such findings provide a strong rationale for targeting the school context as a logical setting to cultivate students' subjective well-being, either by directly teaching strategies that stem from the positive psychology literature (discussed in the next section), or through classroom-level programs that nurture quality relationships with both teachers and peers. A full discussion of strategies for strengthening students' relationships in the classroom is beyond the scope of this chapter. Instead, we refer the interested reader to *Resilient Classrooms: Creating Healthy Environments for Learning* (Doll, Brehm, & Zucker, 2014), an influential and recently updated resource for practitioners that provides concrete guidance for building effective student–teacher relationships, peer relationships, and home–school relationships, which are key school-based relational correlates of youth subjective well-being.

SCHOOLWIDE AND CLASSWIDE POSITIVE PSYCHOLOGY INTERVENTIONS

As suggested by research summarized in Chapter 4, recent advancements in applications of positive psychology to youth include universal strategies implemented either throughout a school or in specific classrooms. Schoolwide approaches include multitarget programs (Shoshani & Steinmetz, 2014), as well as those focused on a specific target such as character strengths (White & Waters, 2015) or kindness (Lawson, Moore, Portman-Marsh, & Lynn, 2013). Classwide applications range from multitarget programs for high school freshmen (Gillham et al., 2013; Seligman et al., 2009) to classroom curricula that target grateful thinking among elementary school children (Froh et al., 2014), character strengths among middle school students (Proctor et al., 2011; Rashid et al., 2013), and mindfulness among students in elementary and middle school (Schonert-Reichl & Lawlor, 2010; Schonert-Reichl et al., 2015). Next, we discuss two such examples of universal positive psychology interventions applied in elementary schools in New Zealand, and America; the former program focuses on the target of character strengths (Quinlan, Swain, et al., 2015) and the latter reflects a multitarget, multicomponent approach (Suldo, Hearon, Bander, et al., 2015).

Classroom Application of a Strengths-Based Positive Psychology Intervention

We (Denise, with Nicola Swain in New Zealand and Dianne Vella-Brodrick in Australia) developed the Awesome Us strengths program to (1) foster student awareness of strengths in themselves and others, (2) encourage strengths spotting by teachers and students, and (3) support students' intrinsic goal setting along with identifying how particular strengths could support those goals. The program has been evaluated with nearly 200 students (9–12 years old), in low to mid socioeconomic status schools (Quinlan, Swain, et al., 2015). In that trial, the intervention included six weekly 90-minute sessions led by a facilitator (Denise) who was supported by the classroom teacher and another educator at the school. Including teachers as co-facilitators was intended to develop their knowledge and skills in positive psychology to make possible larger intervention roles in later applications.

Overview of Intervention Activities

In the first two sessions, students create and share a photo collage of "me at my best." Using set prompts, pairs of students identify and label the strengths they see in each other's collage. These strengths are not constrained by a classification framework and are called *activity strengths*. Student examples have included designing skateboard tricks, making craft gifts for my family, being a patient fisherman, and hugging my mom. In an exercise adapted from Fox (2008), students identify "the best thing" about their favorite subject, hobby, and sport. Then, they create a new activity that includes all of the "best things." Example new activities have included designing and building a gingerbread go-cart with friends, riding it fast downhill, crashing it, and eating it. This activity has been especially popular with students. Again working in pairs, students identify and label the strengths they observe in each other's work. They also explore where and how else they could use these strengths. In the next two sessions, students learn about *character strengths* as specified in the VIA Classification System. They consider character strengths as ingredients that help them perform their activity strengths or pillars that support them. Working together, students consider "What does it take to . . . [e.g., design new skateboard tricks]?" and identify the character strengths that enable and support them to perform these activities. Then, they use a card sort of character strengths to pick out the ones they feel they use most often. They rank their strengths on a wheel rather than in a list to minimize focusing on lower strengths as absences or weaknesses. Students also explore how they can use their strengths to help deal with a current challenge and map the class's "most used strengths" onto strengths posters (and create graphs in mathematics to display this). In the remaining sessions, facilitators emphasize that the purpose of having strengths is to use them. Students create a strengths superhero based on their favorite strength. They consider the strength's everyday "powers" and uses, then decide on its superpowers. Students learn about intrinsic goal setting and strategies to support goal-directed behavior. They also discuss the benefits and challenges of friendship. Students select two personally important short-term goals: one general and one dedicated to developing a friendship. They identify the strengths and other resources, like people, that could help them with their goals. Last, they create strengths posters or shields that display their favorite strengths, and how and where they most often use them.

Strengths Spotting

Strengths spotting encourages people to look at behaviors and notice the strengths displayed (Linley et al., 2010). This strengths program deliberately starts with asking children to identify strengths used in the activities they most enjoy doing. Students notice their strengths and those of their peers in concrete activities. Such discussions provide practice in strengths spotting, promote a sense of ownership of their strengths, and underscore that everyone has strengths. Strengths spotting was revisited at the start of each session, through discussions of current affairs (e.g., "What strengths would you need to cope with an earthquake?") and in the very popular video clips played each session. Video clip topics ranged from base jumpers to injured robots, and wheelchair extreme sports to lion cubs. This intervention's emphasis on strengths spotting in self and others contrasts with other interventions' emphasis on use of top strengths (e.g., "signature strengths" identified after completing the VIA Youth Survey). It promotes the view that all of us demonstrate strengths at various times, even if they are not our "top strengths" (explained as the strengths we recognize ourselves as using most frequently). Rather than labeling a student as owning some strengths (and not owning others), this approach encourages teachers and peers to spot a student doing something right, and remains flexible and open as to what strengths a child may display. This growth mind-set approach to strengths is well-matched to interventions with children, who are by definition still developing.

Classroom Climate

Strengths were originally hypothesized to effect well-being by providing a sense of mastery and self-efficacy (Seligman, 2002). This individual perspective carried through to strengths research that has focused on individual factors, including engagement and achievement (Gillham, 2011; Seligman et al., 2009), academic self-efficacy (Austin, 2005), and well-being (Proctor et al., 2011; Rust, Diessner, & Reade, 2009). When developing Awesome Us, we hypothesized that having one's strengths noticed and recognized by teachers, family, friends, or peers would enhance relatedness, thereby supporting engagement and class climate, and ultimately well-being. This notion is consistent with prior research linking relatedness to engagement and class climate (Furrer & Skinner, 2003), and satisfaction of relatedness to subjective well-being (Veronneau, Koestner, & Abela, 2005). Strengths spotting was therefore considered as a separate pathway through which strengths could support relatedness and well-being—perhaps as effectively as identifying and using one's own strengths.

Teacher Involvement

In line with the anticipated intervention effects on classroom relationships and climate, we expected the teacher to play a pivotal role in creating class norms for noticing strengths. Teachers are well positioned to model and encourage this behavior in students. Therefore, in Awesome Us they are trained and involved as co-interventionists, and given activities to use between and after program sessions. In the school year prior to the start of the initial implementation trial

(Quinlan, Swain, et al., 2015), the teachers took part in a 1-day strengths training of all staff (which included administrators, teachers, teacher aides, and custodial staff) to become familiar with the VIA Classification System (Peterson & Seligman, 2004). Throughout the Awesome Us classwide implementation, teachers increased their strengths spotting over a greater domain range, enjoyed strengths spotting more, and felt more motivated to strengths spot. Providing strengths training for teachers prior to the classwide implementation is likely to increase engagement with the program, support teachers' well-being, and enhance intervention outcomes.

Preliminary Support for Intervention Efficacy

From pre-intervention to follow-up (3 months after the intervention concluded), the elementary school children who took part in the initial trial of Awesome Us experienced significant growth in positive affect, emotional and behavioral classroom engagement, perceptions of classroom emotional climate (cohesion and friction, satisfaction of intrinsic needs for autonomy and relatedness), and personal strengths use, as compared with their peers in a control condition (Quinlan, Swain, et al., 2015). Teachers completed the Strengthspotting Scale (Linley et al., 2010), which assesses attitudes toward recognizing strengths across five domains: ability, frequency, motivation, positive emotion, and application (i.e., range of domains across which strengths are noticed). Positive change in teacher strengths-spotting scores was observed across all domains, suggesting that teachers' enjoyment of strengths spotting and motivation to do it increased along with their skill and practice. Teachers' change in strengths-spotting scores was shown to mediate student outcomes of positive affect; autonomy, relatedness, and competence need satisfaction; and classroom engagement (Quinlan, Vella-Brodrick, Gray, & Swain, 2016). In contrast, teachers' own level of subjective well-being and frequency of use of personal strengths did not contribute significantly to student outcomes. Although these results constitute a weak pilot (sample of nine teachers in a nonrandomized study), the trends in the data suggest that the tendency of a teacher to spot strengths may impact student outcomes more than teachers' personal well-being or strengths use. Implications of these results include that with practice, strengths spotting is a skill teachers can develop. Also, to maximize intervention impact, practitioners should fully consider how they can support teachers' intervention implementation and personal growth in strengths.

Qualitative Findings

After the initial trial concluded, we conducted qualitative research to examine the students' experience of identifying and using strengths, and to gather teacher feedback on intervention acceptability. When interviewed, all students were able to define strengths, most often as "things an individual does and enjoys doing or is good at" (Quinlan, Vella-Brodrick, Caldwell, & Swain, 2016). They viewed strengths as valued personal resources, available for use at any time. When asked "If strengths were a thing, where would you keep yours?" students described keeping them safe and close so they could use them at any moment. Students expressed a strong sense of ownership of one to three strengths. Identifying their strengths enabled many students to view themselves more favorably: "It was exciting knowing that I had strengths. More strengths than I thought I did. It means that I am capable of doing more than I do . . . I can keep on going and try, and not giving up on it."

Interestingly, virtually all students reported not noticing their strengths while they were using them. Students reported being able to think about their strengths before or after using them, but in the moment, they just "get on and do it." In fact, many students noted that a deliberate attempt to use a strength during an activity (e.g., explicitly trying to use creativity while painting) actually got in the way of carrying out the activity, perhaps because they got bogged down by overthinking the strengths use in the moment. When putting a clear focus on a strength, they may have become uncharacteristically aware of doing something that typically worked well for them at times when they were not self-conscious about it. This finding suggests that children in this age group (9–12 years) may benefit from advice beyond simply to "use your strengths more often" as has been done in prior interventions with adults (e.g., Seligman et al., 2005). As might be expected, children's ability to plan or reflect on strengths use varied widely. Some students reported noticing strengths use after an event, such as "when I'm having dinner or when I'm in bed thinking about the day." Others said they would be unlikely to ever think about it. It may be challenging for 10-year-olds to believe they have strengths if they never notice themselves using a strength or reflect on their own strengths use.

These findings suggest that teachers (and parents) have specific opportunities to help children see where they can use their strengths (planning), notice when they are using them (strengths spotting), and to think about what strengths they may have used in a situation (reflection). Planning and reflection already take place in many classrooms before and after projects, assessments, and other activities such as a cross-country run or a "mathalon." As part of planning, students could be encouraged to identify the strengths that might help them, and as part of reflection, to consider which strengths they have demonstrated. While children are engaged in playing, interacting, creating, or responding, it seems likely that they will need to rely on their teachers, family, or peers to notice their strengths. For teachers, this can be likened to holding a mirror up for the child so that he or she can see his or her strengths, in effect becoming a "strengths mirror" for their students. Together these practices are likely to help students know themselves as valuable people capable of displaying a range of strengths.

During the postintervention interviews, teachers reported that students appeared more receptive to class participation; particularly at times when strengths were discussed (Quinlan, Vella-Brodrick, Caldwell, et al., 2015). They described their classes as less cliquish, with students displaying a more caring or protective attitude toward less able classmates. Teachers believed that the students who benefited most were the less confident or more negative students. Teachers also noted changes in their teaching practices, including more use of strengths language, noticing a broader range of strengths in students, and using strengths to praise or provide corrective feedback. Teachers also noted that strengths relevant to the classroom setting (e.g., interpersonal strengths) were discussed more often. Rarely mentioned strengths included spirituality, modesty, prudence, wisdom, and gratitude. Teachers said this was due in part to student challenges with comprehension of the meaning of those strengths, and/or teachers feeling less comfortable discussing strengths that were not characteristic of themselves.

This variation in how easily or often strengths are noticed in a classroom was an area of interest throughout the project. Before the program began, teachers were asked to "rank the strengths in order of the importance you place on them in the classroom, i.e., how much you value them." These rankings were used to create two groups of students: high match (students' top strengths matched those of their teacher's highest-ranked strengths), and low match (students' top strengths matched their teacher's lowest-ranked strengths). The groups were very small ($n = 10$ and $n = 6$ for high and low groups, respectively) and analyses of differences in student outcomes were not statistically significant. However, some interesting trends in the data were observed. Specifically, low-match students began the study with lower scores on engagement, positive affect, class climate, relatedness, and strengths use, but increased their scores on almost all indicators by the end of the program. Three months later their scores were still above baseline levels for positive affect and engagement. In contrast, high-match students began the study with better functioning on all indicators, but their levels of engagement, strengths use, and perception of class climate actually fell during the program. One possible explanation is that students whose strengths were not typically noticed in class received increased attention and acknowledgement during the program. In contrast, students whose strengths were historically acknowledged may have experienced comparatively less positive attention. Independent of these analyses, teacher comments indicated that not all strengths were noticed equally in the classroom, and this may potentially influence program effectiveness for some students. Although teachers were familiar with the VIA Classification System, they were not explicitly encouraged to notice strengths they did not value. Practitioners may consider encouraging teachers to form a "strengths buddy" with a teacher colleague who has complementary strengths, in order to learn about and appreciate other strengths.

Classroom Application of a Multitarget Positive Psychology Intervention

We (Shannon, Mollie, and several graduate students in school psychology at the University of South Florida) developed and piloted an 11-session classwide intervention designed to strengthen elementary school (i.e., third- to fifth-grade) students' relationships in the classroom, as well as their novel use of personal character strengths, gratitude, and kindness (Suldo, Hearon, Bander, et al., 2015). The small-group multitarget positive psychology intervention described in Chapter 5 was modified to exclude activities targeting optimistic and hopeful thinking. These omissions were made in consideration of the cognitive complexity of future-oriented strategies and elementary school children's concrete thinking, in line with developmentally appropriate recommendations detailed in Chapter 6. Activities targeting gratitude, acts of kindness, and identification and use of signature character strengths were retained. Two new sessions targeting positive relations with peers and teachers were developed; protocols for these supplemental sessions are presented in the Appendix. Student–teacher relationships were the focus of the first supplemental session, and student–student (classmate) relationships the focus of the second; both targets were revisited throughout the subsequent sessions, which marked a return to the core student-focused protocols. Student–teacher relations were strengthened by directing children's attention to their teachers' positive behaviors, and by encouraging teachers to convey emotional support and reinforce the student-focused positive psychology intervention content through classroom activities. Positive relations with classmates were fostered through team-building activities and purposeful attention to peers' strengths and kind actions. Table 7.2 summarizes the primary focus of each session in this classwide intervention for elementary school students, and illustrates the correspondence with sessions in the core program (see Chapter 5).

TABLE 7.2. Overview of Classwide Well-Being Promotion Program for Elementary School Students

Session Classwide program	Core program	Target	Strategies
1	N/A	Positive relationships: Student–teacher	Teacher psychoeducation: Strategies for conveying social support to students
2	N/A	Positive relationships: Student–student	Team building
3	1	Positive introduction; character strengths	You at your best
4	2	Gratitude	Gratitude journals
5	3	Gratitude	Gratitude visit
6	4	Kindness	Acts of kindness
7	5	Character strengths	Introduction to character strengths
8	6	Character strengths	Character strengths assessment
9	6 (cont'd)	Character strengths	Apply signature strength 1 in new ways
10	7	Character strengths	Apply signature strength 2 in new ways
11	10	All	Termination; review of strategies and plan for future use

Student–Teacher Relationships

The goals of this session are to establish rapport with the teacher, introduce key concepts within positive psychology, share strategies the teacher can use to communicate social support, and explain the positive psychology intervention curriculum and schedule for the subsequent student-focused sessions. The meeting is intended to occur during a period the teacher does not have responsibility for supervising students in the classroom, so that the teacher's attention can be focused on the discussion with the school mental health provider who has primary responsibility for intervention implementation.

The general introduction to the purpose and methods in the positive psychology intervention can be facilitated with reference to a handout (see "Overview of Program Activities" in the Appendix). We have found it useful to present a brief PowerPoint presentation that defines key terms within positive psychology (e.g., *happiness, character strengths*), as well as communicates the specific importance of student–teacher relationships in students' subjective well-being. Takeaway points gleaned from earlier chapters in this book can be included in this presentation. The practitioner should make sure to explain the research-based ties between teacher social support and student subjective well-being, and suggest strategies for conveying support as suggested by prior research (see specifically Suldo et al., 2009), as summarized in the handout "Building Strong Student–Teacher Relationships" in the Appendix.

The conversation then turns to applications of positive psychology to the teacher's classroom. Regarding class-specific mental health status, the practitioner describes baseline levels of life satisfaction averaged across students who completed preintervention surveys, communicated with enough detail to interpret the class averages. For example, Ms. Smith (pseudonym for the teacher who took part in the pilot described in Suldo, Hearon, Bander, et al., 2015) received the graph in Figure 7.1 that summarized the average levels of life satisfaction that her fourth-grade students reported on the SLSS and MSLSS (described in Chapter 2). Ms. Smith commented on the areas of relative strength and concern as rated by her students, including the children's room for growth in their feelings of satisfaction with school.

The practitioner underscores that the purpose of the intervention is to raise the current levels of happiness in the classroom through the classwide positive psychology intervention, with the assistance of the teacher as co-facilitator during each of the student sessions. The teacher is provided with an intervention manual to review in advance of the corresponding session, and encouraged to communicate with the practitioner between sessions to clarify any questions and confirm how the planned material will be divvied up between co-facilitators. The teacher's level of activity involvement should correspond directly to his or her levels of interest and prior experience with universal wellness initiatives, such as SEL curricula. Teachers have a long history as successful interventionists in programs that promote social–emotional skill development, especially through the integration of such practices within the classroom context (Durlak, Weissberg, Dymnicki, Taylor, & Schellinger, 2011). Ms. Smith, a relatively new teacher, asked the practitioner to take primary responsibility for planning and leading implementation of whole-class discussions and activities. Ms. Smith planned to support the practitioner through her physical proximity near the front of the room, implementation of behavior management strategies (e.g., rule checks at the agreed-upon intervals, delivery of tangible reinforcers and verbal praise contingent on student participation), and facilitation of small-group activities that the practitioner set up such that each co-facilitator would supervise a group. Ms. Smith was encouraged to purposefully revisit positive psychology topics between sessions, for instance, by taking advantage of natural teaching opportunities to prompt students to use a given character strength to address a classroom need, or by calling attention to acts of kindness she witnessed among students.

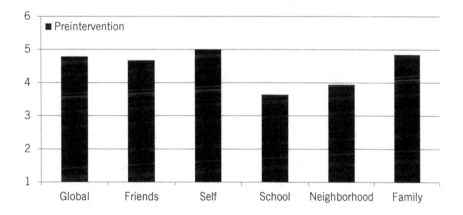

FIGURE 7.1. Baseline life satisfaction of Ms. Smith's students (January 2014). Score range: 1 (*very dissatisfied*) to 6 (*very satisfied*).

In subsequent sessions of this classwide intervention, student–teacher relationships are targeted through follow-up discussions of teacher support. Between student-focused sessions, the practitioner revisits the importance of teacher demonstrations of support and care toward students, prompts the teacher to share how he or she has communicated support to students recently, and facilitates reflection on how such teacher behaviors seem to have impacted the classroom climate and/or the teacher's relationships with specific students. Also, at the beginning of most sessions, the practitioner asks the students to share instances in which their teacher conveyed support to them or ways in which they were kind to their teacher. Students are similarly guided to reflect on the impact of such acts of kindness on their relationships. The additional objective and discussion we added to the start of each classwide session is in Figure 7.2.

Student–Student Relationships

The goals of the initial meeting between the practitioner and the class include establish a supportive environment, set clear behavioral expectations, identify commonalities among the students, and instill teamwork. The practitioners introduce themselves, with a focus on their role at the school and availability to support the students. For instance, the school psycholo-

---

A. Group Discussion: Strengthening Classroom Relationships	
To reinforce prior discussions of ties between positive social relationships and happiness, revisit positive student–teacher and student–student relationships.	
Teacher Support	• Before the session, check in with the teacher regarding words and actions he or she used in the past week to convey support to children. Inquire: 　1. What did you do or say to show support/care to your students? 　2. How did students respond to intentional displays of teacher support and care? 　3. Which strategies appeared effective in conveying support? 　4. What differences did you notice in classroom climate or relationships with specific students after such communications of care and support?
Classmate Support and Care	• Begin the session with directing the students' attention to positive qualities and actions displayed by their classmates and teachers. *Earlier, we discussed how working together cooperatively and treating each other kindly makes people feel happier. Tell us about some times that, since our last meeting, you've seen your classmates be particularly nice to you or another student, or times you've gone out of your way to help or support a classmate.* • Reinforce student sharing. *Ms. Smith, thinking over the past week, when have you noticed your students treated each other particularly nicely, or worked together cooperatively?* • Ask students to recall how they felt during that event/time. 　○ *Happier?* 　○ *Like schoolwork was more enjoyable?* • Prompt the students to reflect on instances of positive student–teacher relationships and teacher support. *Happy children also feel close to adults at school. What nice or supportive things have you noticed your teacher(s) do or say?* *Other kind behaviors or actions from other people at the school?*

FIGURE 7.2. Supplemental procedure for classwide application of the core Well-Being Promotion Program.

gist and trainees who worked with Ms. Smith's classroom explained that students could expect to work with them on Friday afternoons after lunch, and reminded them where they could locate the school psychologist's office on the school campus. A behavior management system should be implemented that is familiar to students (e.g., in line with the school's positive behavioral interventions and supports) and matched to the level of additional structure needed to ensure students' focus on the interventionist. Educators throughout Ms. Smith's school often referred to the following prompts for each activity: Conversation level? Help-seeking method? Activity/assignment? Movement level? Participation method? Success = adhering to those five guidelines (CHAMPS; Sprick, 2009). Therefore, students readily understood they would earn rewards (stickers, candy) for complying with the behavioral expectations (CHAMPS) communicated at the start of each session.

Once these ground rules are in place, the focus of the session turns to strengthening students' bonds with one another. This process begins with an activity intended to encourage students to recognize and reflect on their similarities and shared connections with classmates. In this icebreaker, students are instructed to stand side by side in a line and take a step forward if they can answer "yes" to a situation. The situations start out mild (e.g., "Have at least one brother or sister?") and gradually progress to more sensitive topics that have to do with times when students may feel alone and not realize the commonality of stressors (e.g., "Have ever been picked on or teased?"). Next, students participate in a team-building activity—for instance, figuring out how to work collaboratively in order to complete an art project. In Creative Coloring (Jones, 1998), students come to understand the challenges and benefits to working as a team, and ultimately gain a supervised experience in cooperative play. Small groups of students are given a single picture to color. Each student is given a single crayon; no sharing or trading colors is allowed. After the children cooperate to color the picture, the practitioner facilitates a discussion with the small group or whole class, and encourages the students to reflect on their experiences in working with and supporting their classmates. The practitioner makes clear the relationship between students' happiness and the strength of their relationships with people in their lives. This discussion leads to an introduction to the purpose of the Well-Being Promotion Program.

In later sessions, students' peer relationships are targeted through follow-up discussions of classmate support and care. As shown in Figure 7.2, at the beginning of a session, the practitioner asks the students to share aloud acts of kindness displayed by classmates or by themselves during deliberate attempts to support classmates. The teacher also comments on recent observations of kindness and other positive social behaviors in the classroom. Students are prompted to reflect on the impact of kind interactions on their happiness and relationships.

Preliminary Support for Intervention Efficacy

Ms. Smith's students recompleted the SLSS and MSLSS, as well as the PANAS-C, after the intervention concluded and 2 months later. As reported in Suldo, Hearon, Bander, and colleagues (2015), the children experienced statistically significant and clinically meaningful lasting gains in multiple indicators of subjective well-being, particularly positive affect and satisfaction with self (effect size as estimated by Cohen's $d = 0.52$ and 0.40, respectively, at intervention conclusion). At postintervention, medium-size effects were also reflected in students' growth in global life satisfaction ($d = 0.40$), as well as satisfaction in the domains of living environment

(d = 0.52) and friends (d = 0.43). At the follow-up assessment, moderate- to large-size effects became apparent in ratings of satisfaction with school (d = 0.68) and family (d = 0.44) as compared with ratings at postintervention. In contrast to these improvements in students' subjective well-being, students' behavioral engagement at school in terms of attendance and frequency of office disciplinary referrals did not change. This initial application by school psychologists partnering with a classroom teacher provides evidence of promise that elementary school children can benefit from participation in universal positive psychology interventions that target internal assets (gratitude, kindness, and signature strengths) and environmental resources (student–teacher and peer relationships). The improvements in students' happiness were shared with Ms. Smith and her school administration, through graphed comparisons of average scores as depicted in Figure 7.3.

Modified Version with Less Direct Involvement of Teachers

Encouraged by such improvements in students' subjective well-being, the partnering school chose to implement this multicomponent intervention the following school year but with a different service delivery modality. Rather than work with entire classrooms during the academic day, the students in grades 3–5 who began the school year with room for growth in life satisfaction (as indicated by average scores on the BMSLSS ≤ 6.0 on the 1–7 metric) were targeted for participation in small groups that were held during students' lunch periods (Suldo, Hearon, Dickinson, et al., 2015). The 29 children who took part received the same multicomponent positive psychology intervention described above and in Suldo, Hearon, Bander, and colleagues (2015), with the exception of two primary changes: (1) the addition of two sessions at the beginning of the intervention to permit an individualized multidimensional assessment of a specific child's life satisfaction level and determinants (as described in Chapter 6); and (2) change in teacher's expected involvement from a co-interventionist who was present during sessions, to an informed consultant who communicated with the school mental health provider before or after

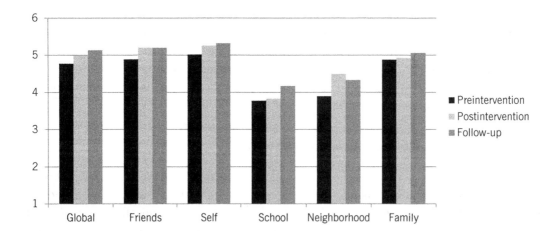

FIGURE 7.3. Comparison of preintervention, postintervention, and follow-up life satisfaction of Ms. Smith's students (January, April, and June 2014). Score range: 1 (*very dissatisfied*) to 6 (*very satisfied*).

the small-group sessions. Teachers of participating students were given the choice of meeting with the practitioner in person at mutually convenient times, and/or receiving written summaries of the activities the students were completing in group, primarily through e-mail. Teachers' full schedules limited opportunities for in-person meetings to discuss what their students were learning in the group. However, they were interested in brief written summaries that shared the content discussed during a given session and suggested ways that teachers could promote practice and generalization of content.

The online supplement to this book includes these one-page handouts ("notes for teachers") ready for distribution to teachers of students who take part in the elementary school version of the Well-Being Promotion Program described in Chapters 5 and 6. These handouts may facilitate teachers' connections with the student-focused positive psychology interventions. The Appendix also includes handouts to accompany the teacher- and peer-relationship-strengthening components described within this chapter. Of note, the session on building strong student–teacher relationships described in this chapter is optimally delivered through an in-person meeting with the teacher to permit a dialogue about strategies for communicating social support that are most authentic to the specific teacher, including behaviors already in the teacher's repertoire. The handouts to accompany this session can serve as either permanent products to be referenced during that meeting, or if needed, can serve as an alternative means for communicating the session content in the event the teacher is unable to meet in person. The weekly handouts can be provided to the teacher via e-mail, in person when students are returned to class, or left in the teacher's mailbox at school. All strategies enable teachers to review the information on their own time and at their own pace.

Promising outcomes were yielded from the pilot of the Well-Being Promotion Program when implemented with small groups of students with teachers as informed consultants. The elementary school children twice completed the SLSS and MSLSS to indicate life satisfaction at the beginning and end of the intervention period. A repeated measures analysis of scores showed that, on average, the 29 children who completed the intervention experienced statistically significant ($p \leq .05$; two-tailed) increases in global life satisfaction, as well as significant gains in satisfaction with their friends and family, with a trend in the data for an increase in school satisfaction ($p = .10$). Effect sizes were medium in magnitude for global life satisfaction ($d = 0.51$) and satisfaction with friends ($d = 0.52$) and family ($d = 0.42$), and small for school ($d = 0.24$). These immediate effects of the intervention are comparable in magnitude to those obtained in the classwide implementation version with different students at the same school.

SUMMARY

This chapter has described multiple intervention programs yielded from design and development research undertaken to promote students' subjective well-being through applications of pertinent theory and research (correlates of youth happiness). These classwide, small-group, and teacher-focused positive psychology interventions have proven feasible for in-school implementation, and provided evidence of promise that the intended outcome—improved subjective well-being—follows program participation. Studies of impact are the logical next step in the evaluation of the efficacy of these interventions.

CHAPTER 8

Family-Focused Strategies for Promoting Youth Happiness

with Rachel Roth

Features of the family context prove among the most robust determinants of subjective well-being, for children and adolescents in any culture (e.g., Schwarz et al., 2012). As summarized in Chapters 3 and 4, happy children have strong relationships with their parents; perceive their parents to express warmth, care, and support; and have parents who are happier themselves. Thus, the primary "power" to increase youth happiness to the upper end of one's set range may lie in reaching out to people beyond the relative convenience of the school setting.

This chapter focuses on (1) interventions directed toward the well-being of parents; and (2) parent-focused components in interventions to improve children's mental health, in terms of reducing psychopathology or increasing subjective well-being. We also recap the parenting practices tied to increased child happiness, and provide reference to psychoeducational materials for parents that describe how to increase authoritative parenting and family communication practices that are the hallmarks of strong parent–child relationships. Given the ties between parents' and children's subjective well-being, we describe in detail innovations in research and development efforts that have yielded promising ways to apply positive psychology principles to increase the well-being of parents. After summarizing the literature on the value added of parent involvement in youth mental health care, we present a feasible method for involving parents in student-focused positive psychology interventions, specifically the Well-Being Promotion Program discussed in Chapter 5. The parent component in our approach (Roth et al., 2016) is limited to including parents in the role of informed consultant, specifically so that they are kept abreast of the student-focused intervention strategies in a manner similar to that which

---

Rachel Roth, PhD, is a Postdoctoral Fellow at Boston Children's Hospital, and a 2015 graduate of the School Psychology Program at the University of South Florida.

we described for teachers in Chapter 7, with the goal of reinforcing and generalizing positive psychology strategies learned at school to the home. We selected a minimally intensive strategy in line with the accumulating research that paints an underwhelming benefit of extensive parent components in psychological interventions to improve mental health through reductions of internalizing problems, such as anxiety and depression. Extensive parent involvement in interventions to address disruptive behavior disorders is generally well supported, but youth subjective well-being tends to correlate more strongly with internalizing than externalizing symptoms (Bartels, Cacioppo, van Beijsterveldt, & Boomsma, 2013).

THE IMPORTANCE OF PARENTS' WELL-BEING

"If mama ain't happy, ain't nobody happy," turns out to be sage advice backed by extensive research on interfamilial transmission of mental health, for better or worse. However, this popular saying should be complemented by similar attention to fathers' happiness. Large-scale studies have established that the offspring of mothers and fathers who have mental health problems—including forms of anxiety, depression, conduct disturbance, and substance abuse—have a greater likelihood of mood, anxiety, substance, and behavior disorders themselves (McLaughlin et al., 2012). Parental emotional distress and stress also predicts diminished life satisfaction among their adolescents, with fathers' emotional distress being a particularly strong determinant (Powdthavee & Vignoles, 2008). As summarized in Chapter 4, abundant evidence also supports that happier children have happier parents, as indicated by significant associations between parents' and children's life satisfaction (e.g., Hoy, Suldo, & Raffaele Mendez, 2013), with mothers' life satisfaction being a particularly strong determinant among adult offspring (Headey et al., 2014). These ties between parents' and children's well-being are in line with the known genetic set point determinant of happiness. Above and beyond the genetic similarities that often manifest in shared personality features, environmental features attributable to parents influence children's happiness. Specifically, parents transmit values (e.g., about the importance of family, community, and material success) and behavioral choices (e.g., about work hours, social engagement, and exercise) to their children, which influence the purposeful actions that further relate to happiness (Headey et al., 2014). Of note, reciprocal effects have been observed, such that children's well-being also shapes their family experiences. For example, children with high life satisfaction have less emotionally distressed fathers a year later (Powdthavee & Vignoles, 2008), and life satisfaction of adult offspring continues to exert significant effects on parents' life satisfaction long after the child has left the family home (Headey et al., 2014). In fact, Saha, Huebner, Suldo, and Valois (2010) found evidence that adolescents' life satisfaction predicts increases in supporting parenting practices a year later, as opposed to authoritative parenting predicting improvements in youth life satisfaction. Nevertheless, modern-day parenting involves a flurry of activity. Practitioners' success in promoting students' happiness through positive psychology interventions like the Well-Being Promotion Program depends in part on students' success with practicing the exercises between meetings. To maximize such at-home applications as well as capitalize on the primary influences on children's mental health, consideration of parents' well-being and their inclusion in student-focused interventions simply makes sense.

POSITIVE PSYCHOLOGY INTERVENTIONS FOCUSED ON PARENT WELL-BEING

Promoting parent well-being is crucial to ensuring an optimal home environment for students. Practitioners may indirectly improve students' happiness by directing parents to the growing number of positive psychology interventions associated with lasting improvements in adults' happiness, as referenced in Chapter 4 (see Sin & Lyubomirsky, 2009, for a review). Adults with more personal motivation to seek happiness and sustain effort on the purposeful activities that lead to improved happiness tend to see greater impact from the exercises (Layous & Lyubomirsky, 2014). Perhaps learning how their happiness is tied to their children's happiness would raise parents' motivation to participate with gusto in positive psychology interventions.

There is no reason to suspect that parents would be less receptive than nonparents to any positive psychology intervention that has proven efficacious in adult samples. However, recent advances in positive psychology involve developing and testing applications geared specifically toward supporting parents. Whereas most psychological interventions developed for parents have focused on instruction in how to effectively manage children's behavior, positive psychology interventions have promise in facilitating parent well-being. Such innovations in intervention development, described below, include (1) combining approaches intended to increase parents' positive emotions, most commonly through mindfulness, with established behavior management approaches; and (2) advancing interventions for parents of children with special needs, such as disabilities or chronic illness, who may be in particular need of mental health support given the increased stressors and physical demands associated with caregiving. Although research on applying positive psychology to improve parent well-being is in the early stages, findings to date provide evidence of promise with regard to the targets described next.

Mindfulness

Increased mindfulness is posited to help parents focus on the present and become attuned to their child's emotions, reduce overly negative reactions to challenging child behaviors, and help parents to thoughtfully select more desirable methods of communicating with their children. Consequently, mindful parenting may positively influence the parent–child relationship, enhancing positive outcomes in youth. This rationale for positive results of mindfulness-focused interventions has been evaluated at a universal level and as a targeted intervention for parents with heightened stress. As a universal preventative intervention for families of middle school students, Coatsworth and colleagues (2015) aimed to enhance outcomes from evidence-based parent training programs by adding a mindfulness component. In the Mindfulness-Enhanced Strengthening Families Program (MSFP), the core program (seven 2-hour group sessions) was adapted to teach the principles of mindful parenting (e.g., listen attentively during each parent–child communication, be less judgmental) and affective education, practice deep-breathing exercises to direct attention to one's current experience briefly before and after each session, and teach loving-kindness reflections to be further practiced at home. In comparison to a bibliotherapy control group, at postintervention and 1-year follow-up both versions of the behavioral parent training program (with and without mindfulness) showed positive effects on various indicators of mothers' mindful parenting and parent–child relationship quality. For mothers and fathers, the added benefit of the mindfulness component was apparent in greater monitoring of youth behavior (a key feature of effective behavioral management). For fathers, MSFP was also tied to significantly greater improvement in mindful parenting, including compassion, active listening, and emotional awareness of youth. Although there were no unique effects of the mindfulness component on parent well-being, this study provides support that fathers in particular experience more mindful interpersonal interactions and more supportive relationships with their adolescent after direct instruction such as in MSFP, and that mindfulness training may enhance both parents' monitoring of youth.

As a targeted intervention, mindfulness practices have been conceptualized as a promising method for supporting the mental health of parents who experience the greater caregiving demands common to parenting a child with a disability or an infant. Benn and colleagues (2012) randomly assigned parents of children who were receiving special education services (primary disabilities: autism, ADHD/learning disability, or cognitive or health impairment) to an intensive 5-week group mindfulness intervention (twice weekly 2.5-hour sessions plus 2 full days, content focused on instruction and practice of mindfulness exercises; additional content on forgiveness, kindness, and compassion) or a wait-list control group. Parents who participated in the intervention experienced significant gains in acquisition of mindfulness skills such as being more present and less judgmental, which translated to immediate or later improvements in eudaimonic well-being and compassion, as well as reductions in stress and internalizing symptoms (anxiety, depression). In spite of improvements in mental health, no changes were detected in parenting self-efficacy or parent–child relationship quality. The sample was limited to 25 parents; different results may be obtained with larger samples. In an 8-week intervention (weekly 2-hour group sessions) for parents of children with autism, larger effects on parental stress and general health (both somatic and emotional symptoms) were associated with parents who received group mindfulness training as compared with parents in an alternate well-established intervention: group behavioral parent training (Ferraioli & Harris, 2013). This study was limited by small sample size (15 parents randomly assigned to either condition), but the large effect sizes yielded provide initial support for the efficacy of an approach to cultivating mindfulness skills (e.g., observing, acceptance, staying present) to support parents' mental health.

Positive outcomes were also yielded from an 8-week intervention targeting mindfulness for parents of infants (Perez-Blasco, Viguer, & Rodrigo, 2013). Compared with mothers randomly assigned to a no-treatment control group, this intervention yielded positive effects on self-compassion, mindfulness skills, and parenting self-efficacy beliefs, as well as significant reductions in internalizing forms of psychopathology. Likely because the study was underpowered ($n = 26$), the trend toward increased life satisfaction was not significant. Within a larger sample ($n = 86$) of parents referred for mental health care due to a range of problems (e.g., own or child's psychopathology, parent–child conflict), an 8-week mindful parenting program (weekly 3-hour group sessions) had positive effects on parent and child mental health (Bögels, Hellemans, van Deursen, Römer, & van der Meulen, 2014). Children of parents in the intervention incurred reductions in internalizing and externalizing symptoms. Parents also experienced declines in psychopathology, reduced parental stress, and improved parenting practices. This growing body of literature supports mindfulness interventions as an evidence-based way to improve parent well-being and other correlates of youth subjective well-being.

Gratitude

Harmony between parents is crucial to youth well-being. For instance, an observational study found that stress in the family explained 37% of the variance in differences in early adolescents' life satisfaction, with the chronic stressor of interparental conflict exerting the strongest (negative) influence (Chappel et al., 2014). Promising strategies for improving relationships between parents involve applying positive psychology principles of increasing positive emotions that may broaden and build social relationships. In one test of this approach, Rye and colleagues (2012) developed ways to foster positive emotions about the past between divorced parents who still need to effectively co-parent their children. These researchers worked with 99 parents who had either divorced or separated on average 3 years ago. Nearly half of the participants were receiving professional help for high levels of perceived harm on behalf of their ex-spouse. In a 6-hour workshop, parents learned the negative effects of anger and conflict on themselves and their children, cognitive-behavioral strategies to increase more pleasant feelings and empathy, positive effects of forgiveness on mental health, and strategies for increasing forgiveness. Prior to the intervention, parents who had higher levels of forgiveness (as a general trait, as well as an ability to recall the positive features of an ex-spouse) also reported greater co-parenting (more cooperation and direct communication between parents, less conflict) and fewer depressive symptoms, suggesting that increasing forgiveness may have a positive impact on harmonious parenting and parent well-being. Furthermore, higher gratitude co-occurred with higher forgiveness of one's ex-spouse, suggesting that increasing gratitude may be one way to facilitate other positive reinterpretations of the past and thereby improve parent outcomes. After completing the workshop, parents who were assigned a supplemental gratitude journaling exercise (daily for 10 weeks) experienced significantly greater growth in forgiveness (both toward their ex-spouse and as a general disposition) as compared with parents not assigned to the follow-up gratitude exercises but instead asked to journal about daily events. This finding suggests that focusing attention on positive aspects of one's life via gratitude journaling helps cultivate more positive emotions through forgiveness. There was also a trend toward improved parent–child relationships among parents who completed the gratitude journaling. No differences between intervention groups were seen on indicators of parent mental health or co-parenting after the writing portion of the program concluded, suggesting either positive impacts on well-being may appear later (plausible given the challenge of altering custody arrangements and making other collaborative changes), or that a more intense dosage of positive psychology interventions may be needed to alter relationships and well-being after a major stressor like divorce.

Multitarget Intervention

To provide support and foster well-being among parents of children with cerebral palsy, Fung and colleagues (2011) prioritized feasibility and attention to the positive when creating a group intervention that consisted of four weekly sessions and a booster session 1 month later. In-session time focused on the identification of character strengths in parents and their children, followed by the creation of plans to increase use of the children's signature strengths in daily life and to solve family problems. Between sessions, parents completed exercises targeting gratitude, including "counting blessings" and a gratitude visit. After the intervention concluded and at 1-month follow-up, parents reported significant increases in hope and decreases in parenting stress. While the group was in session, parents also gained in social support and reduced depressive symptoms; those effects were smaller at follow-up. Parents' weekly ratings of life satisfaction during the intervention period also showed an increasing trend. Although this pilot was limited to 12 parents in Hong Kong, these improvements in positive and negative indicators of mental health among a subgroup of parents with extensive caregiving demands suggests that a brief strengths-based program may be a promising alternative to lengthier stress management programs.

SALIENCE OF PARENT–CHILD RELATIONSHIPS TO CHILDREN'S WELL-BEING

Across numerous samples of children and adolescents, our research over the years has consistently confirmed that the happiest children perceive close, supportive relationships with their mothers and fathers, whom they report parent from an authoritative style. Positive parent–child relationships exert promotive and protective effects on youth subjective well-being. As one example of the effect of close, supportive relationships, in a study of 500 high school students we found that the adolescents who reported their parents often provided emotional support, practical assistance, and positive feedback also reported the greatest subjective well-being (Hoy, Thalji, Frey, Kuzia, & Suldo, 2012). When social support from parents, classmates, and teachers was considered together, parent support had the strongest unique influence by far, accounting for 17% of the variance in students' subjective well-being (vs. 2% for classmate support). Furthermore, high levels of parent support protected students' happiness in the face of peer victimization. In contrast, for students with medium and low levels of parent support, increased peer victimization co-occurred with lower happiness. This buffer effect, depicted in Figure 8.1, demonstrates the importance of positive parent–child relationships to youth subjective well-being, above and beyond the important main effect that is present regardless of social experiences.

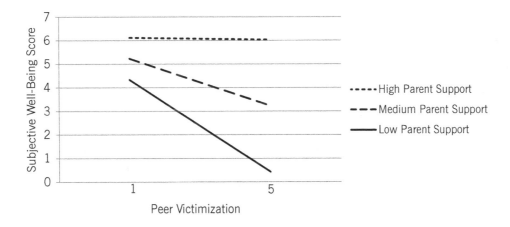

FIGURE 8.1. Parent support as a protective factor in the association between peer victimization and adolescent subjective well-being.

Support is a key feature of authoritative parenting, in which high levels of such expressed warmth and responsiveness are coupled with demandingness and monitoring of the youth's whereabouts, all while permitting the youth with opportunities to make age-appropriate decisions. The robust associations between family functioning and youth subjective well-being provide a strong rationale for targeting parents as a logical partner to cultivate children's subjective well-being, either by implementing evidence-based strategies to improve parent–child relationships (most commonly through behavioral parent training) or through including parents in the youth-focused interventions that stem from the positive psychology literature (discussed in the next section). A full discussion of universal and targeted behavioral strategies for increasing these authoritative parenting practices is beyond the scope of this chapter, but is provided in Suldo and Fefer (2013). For self-study, practitioners can refer parents to reputable and user-friendly books for general readers. Some of our favorites are *The Ten Basic Principles of Good Parenting* (Steinberg, 2004) as well as *Parents and Adolescents Living Together. Part 1: The Basics* (Patterson & Forgatch, 2005) and *Part 2: Family Problem Solving* (Forgatch & Patterson, 2005). Written by the lead researchers themselves, these books translate decades of studies that have pin-pointed positive parenting practices into practical guidance for how to increase authoritative parenting and family communication, key family correlates of youth subjective well-being.

INCLUDING PARENTS IN PSYCHOLOGICAL INTERVENTIONS

Given the salience of family functioning and parenting practices to youth mental health, it would seem logical that including parents in youth-focused interventions would cause a stronger impact on the target (reduced psychopathology, increased subjective well-being) than child-only modalities, such as individual or group counseling. To date, no published research has directly compared the impact of positive psychology interventions for youth with and without parent components. Some insight into the promise of including parents in any psychological intervention can be gleaned from the literature pertinent to prevention and treatment of youth psychopathology. We focused on interventions for anxiety and depression, because although youth subjective well-being is inversely related to both internalizing and externalizing symptoms of psychopathology, the larger association is with internalizing in part due to shared genetic influences (Bartels et al., 2013).

In a meta-analysis of the effectiveness of psychological interventions for youth anxiety, Reynolds, Wilson, Austin, and Hooper (2012) identified 55 relevant randomized controlled trials. They classified parent involvement into four levels: *extensive* (parents routinely attended most or all treatment sessions, or separate parent-only sessions ran parallel to child-focused sessions), *some* (parents involved in selected but not most sessions, or separate parent-only sessions that were fewer in number than the child-focused sessions), *minimal* (parents part of a few sessions, such as for psychoeducation only, or could participate in a short part of their child-focused session to share information with the therapist), or *none* (no mention of parents in youth-focused treatment). The number of studies within each of the four categories ranged from 11 for the minimal and some levels to 20 for none. The effect size of psychotherapy was medium within each category, suggesting that little was to be gained from including parents in treatment of their children's anxiety. Although differences were small, the largest effect size

(0.69) was associated with minimal levels of involvement; the effect size of interventions with no parent involvement was 0.57, with the more intensive levels in the middle (0.65 for some, 0.63 for extensive). Further research suggests that the nature of the parent activities during involvement may influence the maintenance of intervention gains (Manassis et al., 2014). Interventions with extensive parent involvement in which parents learn evidence-based cognitive-behavioral strategies (e.g., contingency management) are associated with continued improvement over time in terms of reduced youth anxiety, whereas youth in interventions with either minimal or some parent involvement or extensive parent involvement that focused less on managing the child's anxious behavior (instead, focus was on parental anxiety, parent–child communication, or other aspects of parent/family functioning) merely maintain gains across time. In an analogous manner, after the active ingredients of positive psychology interventions are well established, extensive parent components that mirror key youth activities may prove quite impactful.

Some interventions developed to treat youth mood disorders that included a parent component have produced positive results. For example, in time-limited treatment of child bipolar disorder, child- and family-focused cognitive-behavioral therapy (CFF-CBT) outperformed psychotherapy as usual in a randomized controlled trial (West et al., 2014). In CFF-CBT, parents were included in eight of the 12 sessions (including two sessions without the child present) and learned how to coach their children to use cognitive techniques taught in the child-focused sessions. Relative to the comparison group, children randomly assigned to CFF-CBT showed greater reductions in mania and depression at postintervention and 6-month follow-up. In discussing directions for future research in adolescent research, Curry (2014) wonders if increasing parent involvement in well-established treatments (e.g., cognitive-behavioral therapy, interpersonal therapy) or newer therapies would improve youth outcomes. He summarizes that the early evaluations of cognitive-behavioral therapy did not indicate superiority of conditions with parallel parent groups, and that other promising approaches like attachment-based family therapy had not yet been compared against a primarily individual treatment.

Indeed, in an evaluation of the Penn Resiliency Program, Gillham and colleagues (2012) randomly assigned over 400 middle school students (many with elevated levels of depression at baseline) to three conditions: after-school participation in the Penn Resiliency Program either with or without a parent component, or no treatment control. The parent component was relatively extensive; in up to seven 90-minute meetings, groups of parents learned the same cognitive restructuring and assertiveness skills their children were taught, including how to apply the skills in their own lives and support their children's use of the skills. Comparative analyses of the postintervention and 6-month follow-up data indicated no added benefit of the parent component. Instead, particularly for students who began the study with moderate to high levels of hopelessness, participation in either version of the Penn Resiliency Program was associated with reduced symptoms of depression and anxiety, as well as increased use of adaptive coping strategies. Furthermore, no dose effects were detected, indicating improved youth outcomes (reduced anxiety or depression) were not reserved for youth whose parents attended more of the parent sessions. In sum, there is not overwhelming evidence on the side of including parent components in the prevention and treatment of depression.

The effect of including parents in interventions intended to foster subjective well-being is even less studied. A hope-focused positive psychology intervention with minimal parent involvement (single 1-hour psychoeducational session for parents) was associated with significant and lasting gains in middle school students' hope and life satisfaction, relative to peers in a no-treatment control condition (Marques et al., 2011). In contrast, a pilot of a classwide strengths-focused curriculum that included a minimal parent component also psychoeducational in nature was not associated with significant gains in subjective well-being, although improvements in youth externalizing symptoms were noted (Rashid et al., 2013). Next, we describe our recent development of a parent component for middle school students taking part in a multitarget positive psychology intervention. Parents were involved in a manner akin to Marques and colleagues (2011), and the student outcomes were quite promising.

Application of a Multitarget Positive Psychology Intervention with a Parent Component

We modified the core well-being program described in Chapter 5 to include a minimal parent component, focused primarily on sharing information regarding positive psychology and targets/exercises in the weekly student-focused sessions (Roth et al., 2016). In total, the parent component entailed a 1-hour psychoeducational session at the onset of the student-focused component, and regular written correspondence to keep parents abreast of strategies their children learned in each group session with ideas for how to reinforce activities at home. One new parent psychoeducational session was developed, and the protocol for this supplemental session is presented in the Appendix. We also developed brief written summaries that specified the content discussed during each student-focused session, and suggested ways that parents could promote practice of content at home. The online supplement to this book includes these one-page handouts ("Notes for Parents") ready for distribution to parents of students who take part in the core program. In the 2 months after the core intervention with the parent component, we also provide monthly follow-up sessions for students (described in Chapter 5).

The goals of the parent information session are to establish rapport, introduce key concepts within positive psychology, demonstrate an example of a positive intervention, and overview the focus of sessions in the core program. The meeting is intended to occur at a time that the parent does not have responsibility for supervising his or her children, so that the parent's attention can be focused on the discussion with the practitioner. For evening sessions, consider making child care available.

The general introduction to the purpose and methods in the positive psychology intervention can be facilitated with reference to a handout (see "Overview of Positive Psychology and Program Activities" in the Appendix). We have found it useful to work from a brief PowerPoint presentation that shares key terms within positive psychology, how we conceptualized students' well-being, the benefits of high subjective well-being for youth and parents, and the specific constructs targeted in the core program (e.g., gratitude, acts of kindness, hope, optimism, character strengths). Takeaway points gleaned from this and earlier chapters in this book can be included in this presentation. To illustrate positive psychology interventions, we lead the parents through a savoring activity. The practitioner underscores that the purpose of the student intervention is to raise the child's current happiness level, and clarifies any misconceptions about the intervention identification process, such as that children were asked to participate because they have mental health *problems*. Parents learn that they will receive regular updates on the group activities from the practitioner. Each handout provides (1) an overview of the lesson covered that week in the child's well-being promotion session, (2) a description of the home-work task(s) assigned to the child that corresponds to the content covered in session, and (3) suggestions for parents to apply the intervention strategies in their own lives or as a family unit. The practitioner urges parents to follow the suggestions on these brief summary sheets in order to reinforce at home the strategies the child learned at school, and enhance their own well-being by completing the activities in parallel with their child. Ideally, the handout that corresponds to a given session should be sent to parents the same day the student participates in that session. The handout can be delivered in hard copy to the parent via the student (we recommend sealing it in an envelope addressed to the parent) or sent directly to the parent, such as in the form of a file attached to an e-mail from the practitioner.

Preliminary Support for Intervention Feasibility

We assessed the feasibility of the parent component through attendance, weekly monitoring of students' discussion of session content with parents (per recommendations in parent handouts), and program satisfaction, as reported in Roth and colleagues (2016). We experienced some challenges with getting parents to come to school for the information session. We offered multiple opportunities at different times of the day and evening, and were eventually successful in holding this 60-minute meeting with parents of 14 of the 21 students in the intervention condition. All parents presumably received the e-mailed handouts following student sessions; although we did not request a "read message" receipt, no e-mails bounced back. At the start of each group session, we privately asked students how much they discussed the session content or exercises from the session prior with parents. We coded students' reports from *none* to *some* to *a lot/ detailed*. Across responses over the 10 opportunities (after the first nine sessions in the core program and the first booster session), students' average level of weekly parental involvement in program-related activities corresponded to between *some* and *detailed*. No student indicated "none" for more than 5 weeks, suggesting that the e-mailed handouts reached the parents as intended.

Student attendance was exceptional; all participated in 100% of core sessions, either at the regularly scheduled time or during a make-up session offered later in the week. After the final session in the core program, youth participants expressed considerable satisfaction with the intervention. When completing open-ended questions about what they learned and their favorite aspects of the intervention, students noted learning how to improve their views of the past, present, and future, and mentioned specific exercises they liked the most, such as a gratitude visit, and aspects of peer support afforded by the group nature of the intervention. In completing this feedback form, no students spontaneously mentioned any aspect of the parent component or home-based applications of the program. We did not gather parallel intervention acceptability data systemically from parents, who had not interacted with us in person since the first week. However, several parents independently reached out (primarily via reply e-mails) at various points and reported noticeable gains in their child's happiness or expressed appreciation for being kept in the loop regarding activities that transpired during the student-focused sessions.

Preliminary Support for Intervention Efficacy

We examined the effects of this multicomponent positive psychology intervention on each aspect of subjective well-being (i.e., positive and negative affect, life satisfaction) and on internalizing and externalizing forms of psychopathology. The students in the intervention condition ($n = 21$) and their peers who had been randomly assigned to the wait-list control ($n = 21$) completed the SLSS, PANAS-C, and the Brief Problem Monitor—Youth of the ASEBA at four time points: baseline, postintervention, and approximately 1 and 2 months later. As reported in Roth and colleagues (2016), after completion of the core intervention with the parent component, the students experienced significant and clinically meaningful gains in all indicators of subjective well-being, as well as a trend for reductions in internalizing and externalizing symptoms of psychopathology relative to the control group. Throughout the follow-up period, gains in positive affect were maintained with a sustained large effect size. In general, this version of the Well-Being Promotion Program with a parent component exerted a stronger effect on more indicators of mental health than a prior implementation without the parent component (Suldo, Savage, et al., 2014).

The feasibility and efficacy findings described here provide support for this multicomponent, multitarget positive psychology intervention as a promising school-based intervention associated with long-lasting improvements in early adolescents' positive affect, a primary indicator of subjective well-being. Logical next steps in intervention evaluation should involve efficacy studies with larger numbers of youth, to be randomly assigned to experimental groups with and without the parent component. Pending sufficient support for added utility of the parent component, it would help to know which element (e.g., attendance at parent information session, weekly home-based parental involvement in student homework activities, parents' own use of the positive psychology intervention) drives effects on outcomes and are thus of the most critical importance.

PART IV

PROFESSIONAL CONSIDERATIONS IN PROMOTING HAPPINESS ACROSS CULTURES AND SYSTEMS

CHAPTER 9

Cross-Cultural and International Considerations

with Gary Yu Hin Lam

Practitioners interested in promoting youth happiness in line with the intervention strategies described in Chapters 5–8 should keep in mind that this work stemmed from, and has been tested mostly with, Western samples. Prior to implementation in countries other than the United States, or even applications with youth in minority cultural groups, practitioners should consider how to adapt the assessment and intervention procedures in a manner that is appropriate for the intended population. While it would take a separate book to create general recommendations for diverse cultural groups, this chapter draws attention to some of the ways that cultures can differ in terms of how happiness is conceptualized, measured, determined, and fostered. We begin by suggesting that happiness may be viewed differently in cultures with different worldviews and values (e.g., individualist vs. collectivist cultures). Out of necessity, this discussion is based on research and theory pertinent to adults given the focus of the available literature.

We also discuss the extent to which determinants of happiness may vary across children from different cultures. Cross-national research on youth subjective well-being is scant but growing, as evidenced in a 2015 special issue of *Child Indicators Research* titled "Child Subjective Well-Being: Early Findings from the Children's Worlds Project" (Vol. 8, No. 1). The opening editorial of this special issue introduces the Children's Worlds: International Survey of Children's Well-Being (ISCWeB). The ISCWeB is a new worldwide research project devoted to monitoring, understanding, and comparing the subjective well-being of children (ages 8, 10, and 12), with the intent that such data will yield implications for local, national, and international policy (Dinisman, Fernandes, & Main, 2015). That special issue contains findings from the first wave of data collection (with 34,000 children from 14 countries) using the international survey

---

Gary Yu Hin Lam, MA, is a doctoral student in the School Psychology Program at the University of South Florida.

of subjective well-being that had been in development since 2009. We suspect that the tentative discussions contained in this chapter, which were informed by previously conducted studies with youth on a smaller scale; initial knowledge gleaned from the ISCWeB; and findings from research with adults, will be able to be refined and strengthened following advances in the literature sure to be made possible through the ISCWeB project.

After a discussion of cultural fit in clinical assessment and intervention, we review examples of positive psychology interventions evaluated in different nations outside the United States. We conclude by considering the cross-cultural applicability of the specific targets within our Well-Being Promotion Program, and note an alternative intervention for consideration by interventionists interested in a program with theoretical roots in the eudemonic tradition of well-being. Further research is needed to determine if positive psychology interventions that diverge in underlying theory and choice of targets indeed differentially impact indicators of hedonic versus eudemonic well-being.

CULTURAL CONSIDERATIONS IN DEFINING HAPPINESS

The literature cited throughout this book, particularly in Chapter 3, shares the growing knowledge base of correlates of subjective well-being as indicated by emotional indicators (e.g., feelings of happiness and contentment) that are aligned with the hedonic conceptualization of well-being. In general, more attention has been afforded to hedonic aspects of well-being in Western cultures. Since indicators of subjective well-being have been used more often in research, more is currently known about what predicts feeling good. The Well-Being Promotion Program that is described in greatest detail in this book was developed with the explicit goal to increase students' subjective well-being, in line with the hedonic tradition of well-being. As described in Chapter 1, hedonic elements of well-being pertain to one's current emotional state, as indicated by one's positive emotions and present appraisals of life quality. The goal of increasing children's personal happiness has been well received by the parents, teachers, and youth with whom we have worked. When questions regarding desirable outcomes have arisen, they mostly involve "To what extent does the program also impact children's mental distress (e.g., make children less depressed or anxious) or academic performance (e.g., make them more on-task in the classroom or earn better grades)?" Anecdotally, we have not encountered resistance around the idea that sufficient impact on well-being would be reflected in helping students to feel good. This may reflect the individualistic nature of American culture, and the emphasis on personal choice and achievement (even in terms of achieving high levels of positive emotions).

However, the focus of well-being research, even in Western cultures, is moving from an exclusive focus on subjective well-being to the PERMA model (see Chapter 1) that recognizes aspects of hedonic *and* eudemonic well-being. Eudemonic elements of well-being pertain to leading a virtuous and meaningful life, which includes self-actualization in part to contribute fully to society. Seligman's (2011) recent conceptualization is aligned with other American scholars' highly regarded views of well-being that emphasize eudemonic aspects, such as Corey Keyes and Carol Ryff's attention to *psychological* well-being as manifested in environmental mastery, positive relations with others, and personal growth (Ryff & Keyes, 1995), and *social* well-being as manifested in social contribution and social integration (Keyes, 2006).

Although "What is well-being?" remains debatable within the United States, the focus on self-fulfillment and striving toward personal happiness is obvious in mainstream American culture. In contrast, people in a more collectivistic society such as Chinese clearly prioritize eudemonic well-being and are more sensitive to the well-being of others. Ho, Duan, and Tang (2014) summarized that pursuit of personal happiness in collectivist cultures involves consideration of social norms and the well-being of significant others. In collectivist and possibly even some European cultures, personal choice may be less important than belonging to a group, thus enhancing well-being is usually considered in a social context as much as it is viewed as an individual effort (D. Quinlan, personal communication, May 14, 2015). In a particularly eloquent description of the differences between Eastern and Western cultures that are relevant to well-being, Ryff and colleagues (2014) underscore that for the former, well-being is more "relational, intersubjective, and collective in scope" (p. 2), which contrasts the personal and individual emphasis in the latter. Because this need to consider the happiness of significant others is so fundamental to understanding a Chinese individual's happiness, Ho and Cheung (2007) felt compelled to expand the most popular measure of adults' life satisfaction: Diener and colleagues' (1985) Satisfaction with Life Scale. Developed in the United States, the Satisfaction with Life Scale includes five items like "So far I have gotten the important things I want in life" and "I am satisfied with life." Ho and Cheung's version includes five additional other-oriented items, such as "The conditions of my family members' lives are excellent" and "So far I believe my family members have gotten the important things they want in life." The resulting measure that includes intrapersonal and interpersonal dimensions of life satisfaction is deemed more appropriate for Chinese populations.

Another way that cultures may differ is in terms of the perceived optimal level of happiness. In Western societies, the general notion is that the higher the subjective well-being, the better. Research with samples in the United States and the United Kingdom support that very happy people are not pathological, but rather adults (Diener & Seligman, 2002) and youth (Proctor, Linley, & Maltby, 2010; Suldo & Huebner, 2006) with the highest levels of life satisfaction are the highest-functioning individuals. But is very high subjective well-being the appropriate goal, or even the most adaptive status, across cultures? Joshanloo and Weijers (2014) describe how for many non-Western cultures, personal happiness is not the primary value, often due to the aforementioned emphasis on social harmony. They also describe that an "aversion to happiness" phenomenon exists within some individuals and cultures for additional reasons, including fearing that feeling or expressing happiness may (1) leave one more vulnerable to negative events; (2) infer one is a morally, spiritually, or intellectually deficient individual; (3) invoke feelings of jealousy, suspicion, or resentfulness from others; and (4) bring adverse effects to oneself and close others. Ryff and colleagues (2014) note that in Japan, achieving balance and moderation is preferable to maximizing personal happiness. Whereas Americans tend to describe themselves in highly positive terms, Japanese invoke more self-critical statements that reflect greater compassion and sensitivity to others as part of well-being. Among Westerners, positive emotions and negative emotions are strongly inversely correlated, suggesting that inducing positive emotions is likely to reduce the concurrent experience of negative emotions. In contrast, East Asians appear more prone to experience both positive and negative emotions at a similar frequency, termed a "dialectical" emotional style. A moderate dialectical style, which is characterized by balance in positive and negative emotions (as compared with the mostly positive nondialectical style that is more common to adults in the United States), is linked to health advantages among Japanese adults (Miyamoto & Ryff, 2011).

Another distinguishing feature of Eastern traditions is a view that happiness is transient. Kan, Karasawa, and Kitayama (2009) summarize that in

> Eastern traditions happiness is regarded as something that is noted and appreciated, but never to be reified because it is fluid, incomprehensible, and transitory. Experience of happiness comes with a feeling of gratitude for a life that affords the momentary glimpse of happiness. (p. 303)

In cases in which happiness is viewed as fleeting, it may not make sense to take as serious activities intended to systematically increase one's level of well-being.

In light of such findings, practitioners may want to consider the ultimate indicator of subjective well-being "success" when working with youth from Eastern cultures, as well as how to harness motivation to pursue subjective emotional well-being if that is indeed the program goal. Whereas achievement-oriented youth raised in Western cultures may quickly warm to the idea of increasing personal happiness, relationally oriented youth may be more drawn to happiness that is embedded in social connections.

CULTURAL CONSIDERATIONS IN ASSESSMENT OF SUBJECTIVE WELL-BEING

As described in Chapter 2, promoting students' happiness often involves measuring it, whether in a universal manner (e.g., for purposes of research, identification of students in possible need of supplemental services, or to understand and track the well-being of youth in a given school or community) or with targeted students (e.g., to assess response to positive psychology interventions). The measures described in Chapter 2 were developed in the United States. Does measuring life satisfaction in another context simply involve translation to the native language? Gilman and colleagues' (2008) analysis of the MSLSS, which has been translated to many different languages, suggested that neither general nor domain-specific mean scores yielded from this instrument are equivalent across countries. Rather, adolescents from Western, more individualistic societies (specifically, Ireland and the United States) reported higher levels of self-satisfaction as compared with adolescents from collectivist countries (specifically, China and South Korea). In contrast, Chinese youth reported significantly higher levels of satisfaction with school and family (South Korean youth reported the lowest means in these two areas and in terms of the total/general life satisfaction score). A comparison of response styles indicated that youth from individualistic countries were more prone to extreme responding (reflected in choosing response options at the farthest end of the metric) and response acquiescence (reflected in agreement with items regardless of content), particularly when responding to items about friends, as compared with adolescents from collectivistic nations.

More recent studies with youth in different countries have arrived at similar conclusions with different measures. For instance, cross-country administration of the BMSLSS and other measures of item-specific satisfaction that originated overseas (e.g., Australia, Spain) concluded that a core set of 14 satisfaction items explained the latent life satisfaction construct well among the adolescents sampled from all three participating countries: Chile, Spain, and Brazil (Casas et al., 2015). These items tapped satisfaction with relationships, living environment, physical health, and religion, among others. However, Casas and colleagues (2015) cautioned against comparing average life satisfaction scores across countries, citing cultural differences in response styles. In a larger-scale study of the same topic, this time with 16,000 adolescents in 11 countries (Algeria, Brazil, Chile, England, Israel, Romania, South Africa, South Korea, Spain, Uganda, the United States) during a pilot wave of the ISCWeB, Casas and Rees (2015) again concluded that although it is defensible to make cross-national comparisons of associations among life satisfaction items and presumed correlates, it is generally not appropriate to compare mean levels of life satisfaction as derived from the measures. Why not? Casas and Rees noted that comparing levels of life satisfaction across countries is complicated by the reality that children in different cultures differ in (1) understanding concepts, such as happiness; (2) response styles, such as extreme responding; and (3) familiarity with the experience of completing surveys about their opinions or beliefs. Furthermore, some words in the life satisfaction scales simply do not have a clear one-to-one correspondence with a similar word in another language to represent the same underlying subjective well-being construct. If one would truly want to make a cross-national comparison of mean scores, one way to mitigate such problems of cultural biases and barriers is to triangulate the analyses of mean scores with responses from multiple types of questions (evaluative, satifaction) and compare mean scores with external data sources, such as other objective indices of social, institutional, and economic conditions (Rees & Dinisman, 2015).

Informed by the adult literature on cultural differences in defining well-being, when assessing children's well-being cross-culturally, we have to be equally careful in conceptualizing what life satisfaction or happiness actually means to children from different cultures around the world. Recent exploratory research with children in Nepal indicated research limitations that come from using an instrument with questions grounded in a Western-oriented concept of what constitutes a "good childhood" (Wilmes & Andresen, 2015). For instance, survey items about use of leisure time reflected Western ideas of how children spend their time, and ignored that in Nepal, employment and time spent with family play important roles in children's everyday life. Nevertheless, the study found that, in general, children in both Nepal and Germany were satisfied with their lives, as well as yielded important implications about the relevance of self-determination to children in both countries. Not only do we have to ask how much of a difference children from various cultural backgrounds experience happiness, but we also need to recruit children's own perspective and give voice to them in order to understand what construes their perception of a happy, satisfied life.

INTERNATIONAL AND CULTURAL CONSIDERATIONS IN DETERMINANTS OF SUBJECTIVE WELL-BEING

The rapidly growing body of literature on predictors of subjective well-being, particularly life satisfaction and satisfaction with specific domains, such as school, now includes youth from multiple continents. A recent review of correlates of *school* satisfaction indicated remarkable similarity in the predictors of school satisfaction across adolescents from different countries, likely due to strivings for independence common to virtually all teenagers, even those in more collectivistic cultures; mean differences in school satisfaction were conceptualized as reflecting mean differences in the extent to which cultures provide opportunities for adolescents to experience relatedness, autonomy, and competence (Suldo, Bateman, & Gelley, 2014). Accordingly, the primary correlates (also referred to as determinants) of subjective well-being that are presented in Chapter 3 are, in general, robust across studies with different samples from different countries. Thus, what makes children happy seems to be relatively stable, and reflects the environmental and internal features summarized in Chapter 3. For example, a synthesis of studies that examined associations between parent–child relationships and student subjective well-being concluded that a steady supply of parental emotional support and respect predicts greater happiness for youth from any sample in any locale; in a similar manner, across cultures a child who perceives harsh, punishment-oriented parenting practices and parent–child conflict is at high risk for low subjective well-being (Suldo & Fefer, 2013). This conclusion is illustrated by a study of 1,034 early adolescents (ages 10–14) from 11 cultures that evaluated the relationships between children's life satisfaction and their peer and parent relationships, while considering average levels of family values in a given culture (e.g., family vs. individualistic orientation; Schwarz et al., 2012). Results of multilevel modeling indicated that whereas the strength of the association between peer acceptance and life satisfaction was weaker within cultures that placed greater importance on family values, admiration from parents yielded strong, positive associations with life satisfaction across cultural groups and a positive trend between intimacy with parents and life satisfaction was noted across cultures, leading the researchers to conclude that "parental warmth and acceptance are important for early adolescents relatively independent of the respective cultural values" (Schwarz et al., p. 72).

Perhaps the strongest evidence of cross-cultural similarity and applicability of correlates comes from findings from the first wave of the ISCWeB. In a sample of over 12,000 12-year-olds from 11 countries, Lee and Yoo (2015) reported that variability in children's well-being was significantly tied to their country of origin, suggesting that country-specific cultural and contextual factors explain a reliable amount of the between-child differences in well-being. However, after accounting for these country-specific effects, a common set of environmental factors emerged as unique and strong predictors of youth subjective well-being. Results of regression analyses indicated that whereas a child's country of residence explained about 5% of the variance in subjective well-being, 55% of the variance was explained by factors pertinent to family (e.g., time spent together, home safety, family structure), school climate (e.g., peer social support, school safety, peer victimization), and community (e.g., neighborhood safety, areas to play). Lee and Yoo summarized that

> . . . GDP and inequality are not significant factors predicting children's subjective well-being. Rather it is the nature of children's relationships with immediate surrounding environments, such as frequency of family activities, frequency of peer activities, and neighborhood safety, [that] are most consistently related to the levels of children's subjective wellbeing across the nations. (p. 151)

A notable caveat in the apparent universality of correlates pertains to the relative economic strain that is placed on a given subgroup, as determinants that may best be considered basic needs become more pronounced and influential among disadvantaged groups. Case in point, initial findings from the ISCWeB indicate that personal access to material resources (i.e., computer, phone, Internet, and clothes in good condition) is particularly relevant to the subjective well-being of children in countries that on average have severe resource deprivation, such as Uganda and Algeria (Sarriera et al., 2015).

INTERNATIONAL AND CULTURAL CONSIDERATIONS IN POSITIVE INTERVENTION STRATEGIES

Chapter 5 of this book presents a set of intervention strategies for use in promoting youth happiness. The multitarget positive psychology program has been evaluated only in the context of American students, although other multitarget interventions often with overlapping strategies have been advanced in other countries. Our use with the positive psychology intervention protocols presented in the Appendix has been limited to youth in Florida. These students have been from a variety of socioeconomic backgrounds, attending schools that serve rather transient and poor families to schools that are considerably resourced and suburban. The students who have taken part in our trials have reflected the considerable ethnic and cultural diversity of the Tampa area. However, we have no direct knowledge of how the intervention strategies would "work" in populations outside of Florida. When we turned to the literature to examine the cultural appropriateness of other positive psychology interventions or programs, we were surprised by the scarcity of research that has investigated how different strategies do or do not work for adults or youth in different cultures. Rarely could we locate discussion of how researchers or practitioners had adapted certain elements of positive psychology interventions to fit the local culture. Nevertheless, best practices in clinical interventions generally involve considering the cultural fit of a given approach or strategy.

Cultural Fit

It is argued that people's subjective well-being may be related to the fit between one's individual culture at a personal level and the culture in the broader societal level in which a person situates. Lu (2006) investigated the effects of "cultural fit" between personal values (in terms of independence and interdependence at the self-concept level) and cultural beliefs (perception of how other people in the dominant society believe in exercising active control and maintaining social harmony) in relation to subjective well-being. Preliminary evidence supported higher subjective well-being among Chinese college students (in Taiwan and mainland China) who perceived less discrepancy between the individual's values and beliefs and the values and beliefs endorsed by the people in the society. In analyzing the different cultural-fit patterns, it was found that students who endorsed an independent self-concept but perceived the societal beliefs as relatively interdependent were better off in subjective well-being than those with interdependent self but expected the society to be independent. Relating the cultural-fit proposition in the context of positive psychology interventions, practitioners have to actively consider interpreting individuals' responses to the interventions and program effectiveness by (1) incorporating information about the broader contexts and cultures, and (2) conceptualizing "culture" at multiple levels (i.e., personal values in self and common beliefs in society) and analyzing the interactions between different levels. Related to this, McNulty and Fincham (2012) also cautioned the field of positive psychology to examine the contextual factors (both interpersonal and intrapersonal contexts) as to how the psychological traits and processes associated with positive psychology contribute to people's well-being.

Ho and colleagues (2014) discussed the combination of emic and etic approaches (see also Leong, Leung, & Cheung, 2010) in addressing cross-cultural issues in positive psychology, in particular instrument development. This approach involves employing both insider and outsider perspectives and taking into consideration the cultural views and understandings when adapting specific positive psychology constructs to a particular culture. When adapting a measure developed in another culture, it is suggested that we first identify the universal (etic) items that are compatible across local and foreign contexts. We then can add items with concepts relevant to local culture (emic) to the etic items. Through this way, we can produce measures with high ecological validity that are potentially cross-culturally comparable. This approach was exemplified in the aforementioned development of the Expanded Satisfaction with Life Scale (Ho & Cheung, 2007).

The VIA Classification System was created with cross-national applicability in mind. Using the combined etic–emic approach, Ho and Cheung (2007) modified the original 240-item VIA-IS questionnaire into the 96-item Chinese Virtues Questionnaire that reflects the three virtues of relationships, vitality, and conscientiousness (Duan et al., 2012). In the process of cross-cultural adaptation, some items in the original assessment were deemed incompatible with the cultural contexts in mainland China. Removal of these items was determined based on the following reasons identified through cognitive interviewing with local Chinese people: (1) the behavior deviates from Chinese social norms (e.g., "I always speak up in protest when I hear someone say mean things"), (2) the behavior carries religious connotation that might elicit different interpretations for Chinese people (e.g., "At least once a day, I stop and count my blessings"), and (3) the virtue is represented by a different set of behaviors (e.g., "I stick with whatever I decide to do" does not capture what perseverance looks like in Chinese culture).

Beyond such item-level considerations, issues of construct validity are important when considering if and how to use the VIA Classification System and corresponding survey. The ambition to create a core set of strengths that reflect values across cultures and societies is admirable, but this inherently implies that a particular trait that may be quite useful in a given faction of society is less important if it is irrelevant in the majority culture or in other societies. Instead, some traits may merit attention and cultivation because they reflect behaviors and values that are quite adaptive for a particular subgroup even if they are less applicable across society. This may be particularly salient when supporting youth who may already feel disenfranchised, such as individuals from a lower socioeconomic or social class, ethnic minorities who continue to experience discrimination, immigrants who struggle with acculturation, or a historically mistreated group such as indigenous people who have been displaced or colonized. When working with such populations who may be (rightfully) sensitive to feeling less valued, practitioners should consider viewing the VIA framework as a starting point for identifying character strengths, with the 24 strengths to be supplemented by the traits and actions that the youth and family proclaim to be features valued in their community. In sum, practitioners are urged to view the VIA framework as one option (albeit the most studied one) for categorizing strengths, and remain flexible for what they deem a "strength of character" such that strengths unique to a given group are valued in their own right, either as a supplement to the VIA framework or as a complete alternative through taking a community-specific approach to allowing traits that are strengths in that context to be recognized and valued.

Efficacy of Positive Psychology Interventions Around the Globe

The growing literature on positive psychology interventions in youth includes many examples of studies completed outside of North America. These interventions have targeted hope in after-school meetings with small groups of youth in Portugal (Marques et al., 2011) and character strengths via classwide application in England and New Zealand (Proctor et al., 2011; Quinlan, Swain, et al., 2015). Other examples include coaching interventions that target strengths and hope in Australia (Green et al., 2007; Madden et al., 2011), and a multicomponent, multitarget schoolwide intervention in Israel (Shoshani & Steinmetz, 2014).

Other international efforts have entailed modified applications of interventions that originated in the United States. In reviewing the literature on positive psychology interventions in the educational context in countries other than the United States, we were struck by the minimal explication within a published journal article about the way(s) a given exercise developed in America was modified to be appropriate for use in a different country. Authors often describe how they translated outcome measures to the language native to the participants, but aside from discussing translation issues as a routine practice, there were few mentions of how intervention procedures may have been adapted to be more culturally appropriate. Part of that may have to do with length restrictions set by publishers. When cultural adaptations are referenced, they range from rather minimal to extensive. A minimal-level adaptation would likely involve work with other Western cultures. For example, Challen, Machin, and Gillham (2014) implemented the Penn Resiliency Program on a large scale in 16 schools in the United Kingdom. They termed their adapted version the UK Resilience Programme (UKRP) and noted it contains "minor changes in examples and adaptations made for vocabulary" (p. 77). These modifications included a translation of the curriculum from American English to British English, a process in which local educational officials as well as a British children's author reviewed the materials and suggested changes (Challen, Noden, West, & Machin, 2010). Then, references to American culture were changed as long as the modification did not require changes in artwork, which resulted in materials that were deemed more appropriate for the United Kingdom but "still had an American feel" (p. 10). After a year of implementation, the group noted that further changes were needed to address lingering issues of cultural fit as well as teaching style (i.e., overly didactic for students, some of whom struggled with the program content and materials).

More extensive revisions may be expected when adapting interventions from Western to Eastern cultures. For instance, Chan (2010, 2011, 2013) described modifying gratitude journaling to be appropriate for the school teachers in Hong Kong. Chan (2010) adapted the "Three Good Things" gratitude intervention to be appropriate for the cultural background of Chinese school teachers, specifically by using three Naikan-meditation-like questions (i.e., "What did I receive?" "What did I give?" and "What more could I do?") to mirror Confucian teaching of "daily self-reflection on three things (*wu ri san xing wu shen* [吾日三省吾身])." Analyses of subgroups of teachers with high and low dispositional gratitude at baseline showed differential responses to the intervention, which led to the hypothesis that the questions might elicit the feelings of both gratitude and indebtedness, the latter of which might offset the positive effects of the intervention (Chan, 2010). Accordingly, the intervention was further modified with an aim to enhance both gratitude and life meanings (Chan, 2011). In addition to the self-reflection activity, teachers were asked to meditate with the three questions and think about the meanings of the good things or events, what these things could tell about them, and why these things happened to them. More recently, Chan (2013) found that while gratitude is predictive of teachers' subjective well-being and positive affect, forgiveness is predictive of subjective well-being and negative affect. He postulated the possibility of integrating both character strengths of gratitude by counting interpersonal kindness/blessings, and forgiveness by counting interpersonal conflicts to enhance positive emotions as well as reduce negative emotions in a holistic manner. These adaptations by Chan exemplified how existing culturally specific values and practices, Confucian teachings and Chinese cultural practice in this case, can complement the positive psychology intervention components developed in other cultures to formulate an effective intervention tailored to the local culture.

In another example, Lau and Hue (2011) adapted a mindfulness program derived from Eastern religious practices (Kabat-Zinn, 1990) that is popular in the United States for use with youth in Hong Kong. Minimal changes were made to the program curriculum and content prior to the 6-week trial. Effects of the intervention were modest; significant changes were observed on two indicators of mindfulness and psychological well-being (specifically in personal growth), but stress and the other five measured aspects of well-being did not improve. In discussing ways to improve outcomes, Lau and Hue noted "we can consider developing a curriculum for adolescents with modified means and local Chinese cultural elements" (p. 326). In sum, adapting any positive psychology intervention to be culturally appropriate is likely to be an iterative process, informed by feasibility data from the initial application (see Lam, Lau, Lo, & Woo, 2015, for an example).

Assumed Cross-Cultural Relevance of the Well-Being Promotion Program

We have no reason to believe any of the targets in the intervention we describe in Chapter 5 would be completely inappropriate for a particular group. This assertion is largely based on the fact that we found evidence of efficacy for interventions addressing each target in samples of adults from beyond North America. However, research on positive psychology interventions for youth in general is in its infancy, and our notion remains untested. Turning to studies with adults, some research has suggested that when applied to individuals from Eastern cultures, some specific targeted interventions have been less effective *or* required more changes. Regarding the former, Asian American adults (78% of whom were born in foreign Asian countries, predominantly China) experienced less gain in life satisfaction than Anglo Americans following interventions targeting gratitude and optimism (Boehm, Lyubomirsky, & Sheldon, 2011). However, there was tentative evidence that Asian Americans benefited more from gratitude than optimism intervention, potentially reflecting the relative importance of being grateful to people in life as compared with striving for personal optimism about the future. Enthusiasm for targeting gratitude may be tempered by findings from another study of young adults from Korea and the United States (Layous, Lee, Choi, & Lyubomirsky, 2013). Specifically, college students in the United States who wrote gratitude letters incurred gains in well-being, whereas college students in South Korea did not; in contrast, performing acts of kindness led to gains in well-being among participants in both countries.

Regarding the latter (i.e., required changes), a 6-week character strengths-based intervention was effective in producing short-term as well as long-term increases in life satisfaction in

Chinese college students in mainland China (Duan, Ho, Tang, Li, & Zhang, 2014). Despite its preliminary efficacy, the authors suggested a number of cultural considerations that could potentially benefit future intervention efforts in Chinese contexts: (1) consider interpersonal and intergroup factors in addition to the focus of individuals in traditional character strength interventions; (2) capitalize on and strengthen the virtue of vitality, a virtue uniquely identified in Chinese populations that is particularly predictive of life satisfaction (Duan et al., 2012); and (3) attend to both positive and negative aspects of satisfaction with life in accordance with the traditional conceptualizations of happiness and well-being in Eastern cultures.

As aforementioned, we developed the Well-Being Promotion Program to foster subjective *emotional* well-being, closely aligned with the hedonic tradition. As discussed earlier, some cultures may prioritize the striving for excellence and functioning well in life that are characteristics of the eudemonic tradition. Cultures with a strong preference for targeting the latter may find an alternate intervention, well-being therapy (Ruini et al., 2009), to be more appropriate. Well-being therapy, which originated in Italy, includes six 2-hour sessions that are intended for classwide delivery to middle school and high school students. The goals and activities within the first three sessions are comparable to traditional cognitive-behavioral programs that include affective education, detecting and evaluating automatic thoughts, and cognitive restructuring. The final three sessions contain content unique to positive psychology, and target (1) positive relationships and self-acceptance (through giving compliments), (2) autonomy and purpose in life (through developing and focusing on attainable goals for next year pertinent to social, athletic, academic, and leisure time), and (3) emotional well-being (through identifying and sharing [savoring] positive moments in life, both in the past and current). The nature of the activities has substantial overlap with our intervention, but with less explicit emphasis on character strengths and greater inclusion of content more common to clinical interventions intended to prevent and reduce emotional distress. In a randomized controlled trial, high school students who took part in weekly well-being therapy experienced growth in overall psychological well-being, in particular personal growth, as well as decreased anxious and somatic symptoms, in comparison with peers in an attention-placebo condition (Ruini et al., 2009). The researchers did not look for possible additional effects on indicators of subjective emotional well-being, so it is unknown if students also incurred changes in life satisfaction or positive affect. Similarly, the Well-Being Promotion Program described in Chapter 5 has not been evaluated in relation to psychological and social well-being, so possible impacts beyond emotional well-being are unknown. In sum, Ruini and colleagues' (2009) program might be an appealing option for practitioners interested in selecting a positive psychology intervention that is theoretically and empirically aligned with promoting the eudemonic aspects of well-being.

CHAPTER 10

Integrating Positive Psychology in a Multi-Tiered System of Support

with Natalie Romer

POSITIVE PSYCHOLOGY INTERVENTIONS WITHIN COMPREHENSIVE SCHOOL MENTAL HEALTH SERVICES

The positive psychology interventions described in this book are grounded in theory and research on how to foster subjective well-being, specifically life satisfaction and positive affect. Positive psychology interventions provide a planful way for practitioners to target positive indicators of mental health, including universal efforts to promote subjective well-being and, when low levels are detected, targeted activities to increase subjective well-being. As described in Chapter 1, *complete mental health* entails both high subjective well-being as well as minimal symptoms of mental illness (i.e., psychopathology). This conceptualization reflects the growing body of research on a dual-factor model of mental health that supports the distinctness of psychopathology and well-being among youth; the absence of psychopathology is correlated with but not equivalent to the presence of positive indicators of mental health (Suldo & Shaffer, 2008). Moreover, attending to students' subjective well-being matters in that the combination of high subjective well-being and low psychopathology is associated with the best outcomes. Students with complete mental health have superior social and physical health, and are the most academically successful on a range of indicators of academic enablers (behavioral and attitudinal engagement) and ultimate achievement as reflected in course grades and scores on high-stakes tests (Antaramian et al., 2010; Greenspoon & Saklofske, 2001; Suldo & Shaffer, 2008). Academic advantages associated with subjective well-being persist, as seen in better grades and attendance in later semesters and years, particularly among early adolescents (Lyons et al., 2013; Suldo et al., 2011). In addition to the predictive power of subjective well-being, psychopathology

Natalie Romer, PhD, is Assistant Professor in the Department of Child and Family Studies with the Florida Center for Inclusive Communities at the University of South Florida.

levels also cast independent effects on student success. For instance, high school students with elevated mental health problems are more likely to earn worse grades in courses, miss more school, and incur more ODRs than peers without mental health problems, even when subjective well-being is relatively intact (Suldo, Thalji-Raitano, et al., in press). As such, comprehensive approaches to promoting youth mental health involve providing interventions and supports that address targets that span across positive and negative indicators of mental health.

Schools have been the de facto setting in which services are provided to children and adolescents with mental health problems, and increasingly schools are focusing on promoting well-being and preventing problems among all youth. The strategies that are the foci of evidence-based interventions aim to facilitate the assets and protective factors that underlie subjective well-being, as well as reduce the risk factors that make mental health problems more likely to develop. Integrated models of school mental health that target multiple risk and protective factors have greater potential to produce better outcomes than a single program in isolation (Nelson et al., 2013). Accordingly, best practices in school mental health involve the adoption of programs and practices that support complete mental health, ensuring that all students have the competencies necessary for succeeding socially, emotionally, and academically. This chapter situates positive psychology interventions, in particular the Well-Being Promotion Program described in this book, within a multi-tiered framework of evidence-based school practices to support students' mental health that involves both the promotion of positive indicators of well-being and the prevention and reduction of negative indicators (i.e., symptoms of psychopathology). Figure 10.1 provides a summary of the range of indicators to be considered in the promotion of youth mental health, as well as common risk and resiliency factors that are targeted in order to effect change on those indicators. Resiliency factors include both promotive factors (i.e., internal and environmental assets that predict positive outcomes for virtually all youth, regardless of a person's level of risk) and protective factors (internal and environmental characteristics that serve as buffers, in that they predict positive outcomes especially in the face of risk factors; Masten et al., 2009).

We emphasize the importance of both promoting the factors within youth and their environments that co-occur with and predict better subjective well-being and social success, as well as preventing, reducing, and managing the risk factors within youth and their environments that cause and maintain mental health problems of an internalizing or externalizing nature. The preceding nine chapters of this book focused narrowly on the promotion of subjective well-being in part to fill a gap in dissemination of evidence-based strategies to which practitioners could turn for resources on promoting emotional well-being. In practice, it is important to consider how these positive psychology interventions can be strategically aligned with the myriad of programs and practices that have evolved from decades of empirical advances for preventing and treating mental health problems.

EDUCATIONAL FRAMEWORKS ALIGNED WITH FACILITATING POSITIVE STUDENT OUTCOMES

Educational practice and research has long been accused of emerging from separate silos, with surprisingly little communication and collaboration among youth-serving disciplines and systems. For instance, developmental psychologists have carried out sophisticated research studies that demonstrate the cascading effects of early mental health problems, such as disrup-

Youth Mental Health

Negative Indicators		Positive Indicators	
Internalizing problems, such as anxiety and depression	Disruptive behaviors, such as defiance, rule violations, and substance use	Life satisfaction and positive emotions, such as happiness	Strong social relationships
Cognitive errors, behavioral withdrawal	Risky/unsafe settings	Building blocks of well-being, such as gratitude, empathy, and persistence	Social skills
Trauma and other environmental stressors	Inconsistent rules and expectations across settings	Basic needs are met	Healthy interactions, such as high support and minimal bullying
Risk Factors		*Promotive and Protective Factors*	

FIGURE 10.1. Intervention targets for promoting complete mental health.

tive behaviors, on students' later social and academic challenges (Masten et al., 2005). Applied behavior analysis has informed and shares features with widely adopted interventions focused on academics (e.g., direct instruction; Watkins & Slocum, 2003) and social behavior (e.g., positive behavior support [PBS]; Carr et al., 2002). Child clinical psychologists have advanced manualized intervention protocols for therapists to use to reduce emotional distress (e.g., Weisz & Kazdin, 2010). School-based mental health proponents have demonstrated how to implement such interventions in schools with success (Mychailyszyn, Brodman, Read, & Kendall, 2012). At the same time, school psychologists and related disciplines have championed prevention frameworks for implementing interventions in such a way that the students most in need are identified fairly and that all students can access a continuum of evidence-based supports (Tilly, 2014). And as described throughout this book, positive psychologists have developed brief interventions to mimic the thoughts and behaviors of happy people, and modified the most promising strategies to be developmentally appropriate for youth. Despite the promising and growing evidence base for mental health promotion and intervention in schools (Durlak et al., 2011; Mychailyszyn et al., 2012), implementation of evidence-based practices within schools has historically been limited, often inconsistent, and unnecessarily fragmented in part due to insufficient collaboration between disciplines and youth-serving systems (Adelman & Taylor, 2009). Increasingly, research and policy have focused on the integration and systematic implementation of evidence-based interventions within multi-tiered implementation frameworks to facilitate the transfer of research to school practice.

Multi-Tiered System of Support

As schools adopt programs and practices that ensure all students succeed not only academically, but also socially and emotionally, multi-tiered system of support (MTSS) provide a framework for implementing a continuum of interventions that promote mental wellness and prosocial behavior for students to engage in learning while preventing the onset of behavioral, social, and emotional problems (Adelman & Taylor, 2009; Doll, Cummings, et al., 2014). Aligned with a growing body of research grounded in prevention and implementation science to increase the effectiveness of evidence-based practices in educational settings (Durlak & DuPre, 2008), schools have been adopting proactive approaches to intervention, rather than waiting for problems to begin to transpire. Multi-tiered prevention approaches include a continuum of evidence-based interventions for effectively and efficiently meeting the mental health needs of all students through systematic and coordinated services and practices (Doll, Cummings, et al., 2014; Weist, Lever, Bradshaw, & Owens, 2014). Aligned with a prevention-based approach, positive psychology interventions, as described throughout the previous chapters of this book, systematically build competence and capitalize on the protective processes within students and their environments to increase subjective well-being and other associated positive outcomes, as well as buffer against mental health problems (Nelson et al., 2013; Seligman & Csikszentmihalyi, 2000). Prevention-based approaches, such as MTSS being implemented across schools in the United States, have evolved over time from a public health perspective that conceptualized service delivery as a continuum of intervention ranging from health promotion to treatment as classified by primary, secondary, and tertiary prevention (Caplan, 1964).

A public health approach is often depicted as a triangle representing, in the case of schools, the entire student population (Doll, Cummings, et al., 2014). In a prototypical school, the bottom of the triangle represents the majority of students (about 80%) who will respond to Tier 1 (primary) interventions, with 15–20% of students in need of Tier 2 (secondary) interventions, and 1–5% of students in need of Tier 3 (tertiary) interventions. At Tier 1, interventions aim to prevent mental illness as well as promote complete mental health by teaching the social and emotional competencies that have been associated with resilience, and by creating positive learning environments that increase the likelihood that students practice prosocial and emotional skills and experience protective factors (e.g., positive peer and teacher relationships). At Tier 2, interventions aim to reduce risk factors and increase protective factors to prevent the onset of significant emotional and behavioral problems, which within a complete mental health approach would also include diminished subjective well-being. Thus, selected mental health interventions are typically aimed at a group of students at risk of developing social or emotional problems and who might benefit from similar interventions. Last, Tier 3 interventions target students who require individualized supports and often involve the delivery of coordinated services within the school and partnerships with outside community-based agencies. Proponents of multi-tiered approaches to mental health service delivery in schools emphasize that prevention requires that mental health standards are embedded throughout the school supporting all students through practices that emphasize positive aspects of development (Greenberg et al., 2003).

Research has identified evidence-based practices to support implementation of a continuum of supports within schools that prevent or minimize problems and promote prosocial behavior, mental wellness, and academic success (Durlak et al., 2011; Horner et al., 2009), yet the systems for supporting student needs, particularly mental health services, have in large part been fragmented and often fall short of embedding interventions into the day-to-day routines of the school context (Adelman & Taylor, 2009; Domitrovich et al., 2008). Barriers to embedding mental health supports into schools have included limited resources (personnel, time, logistical supplies), fragmented service delivery systems, competing priorities, and the stigma associated with accessing mental health supports (Suldo, Friedrich, & Michalowski, 2010). Moreover, while schools represent a common setting for students to access mental health supports, educators continue to report a lack of skills and training for identifying and implementing mental health interventions (Reinke, Stormont, Herman, Puri, & Goel, 2011). Multi-tiered approaches to mental health service delivery in schools provide a systematic and coordinated way for schools to identify, plan for, and implement a continuum of interventions based on data-based decisions and systems to support implementation, such as coaching and professional development (Doll, Cummings, et al., 2014; Eber et al., 2013). Many practitioners reading this book might be familiar with a positive behavioral interventions and supports (PBIS) framework, which is regarded as one of the most effectively scaled-up evidence-based practices with approximately 20,000 schools implementing PBIS the across the United States (Eber et al., 2013).

Positive Behavioral Interventions and Supports

PBIS is one example of a multi-tiered approach to achieve behavior change in schools. The goal of PBIS is to prevent behavior problems by implementing a three-tiered, public health framework and minimizing or neutralizing risk factors and enhancing protective factors (Sugai & Horner, 2006; Walker et al., 1996). A PBIS approach focuses on not only reducing problem behavior but also improving school climate by applying PBS (Carr et al., 2002) across multiple tiers to support all students. Commonalities between PBS and positive psychology have been eloquently articulated by Dunlap, Kincaid, and Jackson (2013) and include, for example, a shared emphasis on (1) contextual and ecological validity, (2) quality of life and happiness, (3) self-determination and the focus on the individual, and (4) not only reducing problems or symptoms but increasing well-being and teaching skills to achieve valued outcomes.

The PBIS implementation blueprint (Sugai et al., 2010) defines PBIS as "a framework or approach comprised of intervention practices and organizational systems for establishing the social culture, learning and teaching environment, and individual behavior supports needed to achieve social and academic success for all students" (p. 13). PBIS does not prescribe to a formal curriculum, but instead strives to alter the entire school environment through improved systems and procedures that build the capacity of educators to implement evidence-based practices, and, thereby, improve student behaviors. For example, educators and staff in PBIS schools use effective behavioral strategies to support all students by having a few clearly defined behavioral expectations that are posted throughout the school and explicitly taught throughout the school year. When students demonstrate behaviors that are aligned with these behavioral expectations, they are acknowledged by staff and positively reinforced (e.g., students receive public recognition or access tokens that can be exchanged for a valued item or activity). Behavioral practices such as these not only teach and provide motivation for students to use skills for meeting academic and behavioral expectations in school, but also improve social competency, student–teacher relationships, and create environments conducive to effective instruction and implementation of effective practices (McIntosh, Filter, Bennett, Ryan, & Sugai, 2010).

Consistent with a multi-tiered approach consisting of at least three tiers, within a PBIS framework it is expected that the majority of students (approximately 80%) will respond positively to Tier 1, 15–20% of students will need Tier 2 preventive interventions, and the remaining 1–5% will require intensive, Tier 3 supports and services. Core features of a PBIS framework include (1) prevention-focused continuum of supports, (2) data-based decision making, (3) regular universal screening and progress monitoring, (4) systems change through effective ongoing professional development and coaching, (5) team-based leadership, and (6) research-validated practices for improving behavior and learning (Eber et al., 2013; Horner, Sugai, & Anderson, 2010).

There is a growing evidence base supporting positive outcomes associated with PBIS implementation (Horner et al., 2010), including randomized control trials of PBIS implementation in elementary schools (Bradshaw, Mitchell, & Leaf, 2010; Horner et al., 2009). For example, PBIS implementation has been associated with increases in student academic achievement, on-task behavior, and students' social and emotional competencies (Algozzine & Algozzine, 2007; Nelson, Martella, & Marchand-Martella, 2002). Conversely, PBIS implementation has been associated with decreases in behavior problems, ODRs, and suspensions (Luiselli, Putnam, Handler, & Feinberg, 2005). Findings from observational and experimental studies indicate PBIS practices as an empirically supported means to facilitate a healthy school climate. For example, elementary school students in classes with greater features of PBIS in place (e.g., clearly defined behavioral expectations, teaching routines, clearly defined problem behaviors, frequent positive reinforcement of expected student behaviors, consistent consequences for problem behaviors, efficient transitions) reported greater perceptions of school climate on a majority of dimensions, including caring and helpful student–teacher relationships, order and discipline, and fairness (i.e., equal treatment of all students in a school), relative to students in classrooms whose teachers reported fewer PBIS classroom management features were in place (Mitchell & Bradshaw, 2013). Teachers with fewer classroom management strategies relied more on reactive and exclusionary discipline techniques, such as ODRs. Mitchell and Bradshaw (2013) found that teachers who referred more of their students to the office had students who reported significantly lower levels of order and discipline (i.e., perceived school as safe and under the teachers' control) than students of teachers with less frequent use of ODRs. Indeed, teacher ratings of their school's organizational health (especially positive relationships among teaching staff, student emphasis on academic achievement, and sufficient school resources) improved over the years that co-occurred with PBIS implementation (Bradshaw, Koth, Thornton, & Leaf, 2012). As such, in addition to the intended improvements in students' in-school behavior and reduced use of punitive strategies by educators, PBIS practices are associated with a positive school climate as indicated by teacher and student perceptions of safety, orderliness, and reduced bullying (McIntosh, Bennett, & Price, 2011).

As described in Chapter 3, students who report greater life satisfaction also tend to perform better academically, are more engaged in learning, and have more positive perceptions of school climate. More specifically, students who sense harmonious relationships at school (among classmates as well as between students and teachers) and view their school as generally orderly and safe in part because school rules are followed, report greater life satisfaction (Suldo, Thalji-Raitano, Hasemeyer, Gelley, & Hoy, 2013). As such, efforts to improve school climate, such as PBIS, may be considered universal strategies to promote students' emotional well-being. Although yet to be examined empirically, student subjective well-being may be another outcome that improves along with PBIS implementation (i.e., students in PBIS schools may be happier). However, promoting subjective well-being by targeting high-quality academic instruction and school climate alone may not be sufficient to cultivate the personal behaviors and thought patterns associated with subjective well-being and further buffer against mental health problems. The inclusion of positive psychology interventions, such as the ones described throughout this book, in a continuum of supports may not only enhance academic and behavioral outcomes but also increase the unique positive indicators of well-being that support complete mental health. Notably, a positive, well-managed learning environment also sets the stage for students to participate in positive psychology interventions. As such, universal PBIS practices not only provide a plausible means to improve subjective well-being through positive impacts on schooling experiences, but also enhance the likelihood that children can engage meaningfully with positive psychology strategies taught by practitioners and/or teachers in an academic setting more likely to feature on-task behavior.

BLENDING UNIVERSAL SUPPORTS

Recently, conceptual guidance specific to blending PBIS and school-based mental health supports has emerged (Eber et al., 2013). However, limited research is available on blending even the most predominant universal approaches, which are generally recognized as PBIS and SEL (Durlak et al., 2011). From an implementation standpoint this is unfortunate as adoption of different programs to address different problems can create system overload and thereby minimize sustainability, particularly if the programs are implemented in parallel without consideration for the complementary, conflicting, or redundant aspects of the programs. Cook and colleagues (2015) provide one of the few studies that describe the process and outcomes whereby elementary schools tested the implementation of an integrated SEL and PBIS approach. The researchers used a quasi-randomized control design to compare four classroom conditions: business as usual, PBIS alone, SEL alone, and a combination of PBIS and SEL. The classrooms that implemented either PBIS or SEL alone experienced significantly greater improvements in students' overall mental health functioning (as indicated by teacher-completed measures of internalizing and externalizing behavior problems) compared with business as usual. However, the largest improvement in student mental health was seen in classrooms that blended PBIS and SEL; the combination of PBIS and SEL resulted in significantly greater reductions in externalizing behaviors when compared with all three of the other conditions (Cook et al., 2015). Such studies make clear the value added of multiple universal programs that target different outcomes (in this case, internalizing and externalizing symptoms).

The dual-factor model of mental health establishes subjective well-being as correlated with but separable from mental health problems, such as internalizing and externalizing symptoms. In Cook and colleagues' (2015) experiment, the implementation of PBIS alone was not associated with improvements in internalizing forms of mental health problems. Instead, significant reductions in students' internalizing problems were apparent only in conditions that implemented SEL. Considering the alignment between intervention goals and intended outcomes, the particular impact on internalizing is not surprising given that SEL targets the thought and activity patterns that become risk factors for emotional distress. The SEL program implemented in this example provides direct instruction in adaptive styles of thinking and behaving (Merrell, Carrizales, Feuerborn, Gueldner, & Tran, 2007). In an analogous manner, positive impacts on the well-being component of mental health are most likely to come from those interventions that target the underlying promotive factors. Comprehensive blending of universal mental health supports may thus involve theoretically driven and evidence-based strategies for reducing internalizing and externalizing forms of psychopathology, as well as increasing subjective well-being.

In line with the quite recent development of positive psychology interventions, we lack data to share regarding the added benefit in student outcomes that may result from implementation with other universal strategies. More research is needed to investigate the possible benefits of integrating a positive psychology intervention (vs. SEL) with PBIS. These sorts of applications are needed to discern how selective positive psychology interventions for students with growth in subjective well-being (as described in Chapter 5) may benefit youth differently with and without foundational access to PBIS, and to examine the possible value of universal applications of positive psychology interventions to all students in a given classroom (as described in Chapter 7) who do or do not access PBIS. Although we are not aware of any studies investigating the blending or integration of positive psychology interventions and PBIS, given the complementary aims of these interventions and approaches described throughout this book of applications within a multi-tiered framework, schools may choose to consider integrating positive psychology interventions into their PBIS framework.

INTEGRATION OF POSITIVE PSYCHOLOGY INTERVENTIONS AND PBIS

We believe positive psychology interventions and PBIS are complementary approaches to intervention with the potential to more effectively support student well-being and associated competencies through systematic and coordinated programing. Both positive psychology interventions and PBIS focus on the prevention of problems that interfere with academic success and the promotion of positive skills and environments. At the same time, some foundational differences in the theoretical underpinnings of these approaches need to be acknowledged. With a firmly behavioral foundation, PBIS has generally focused on changing the environment (i.e., adult behavior) to more effectively teach and manage student behavior, whereas positive psychology interventions have focused on personal emotional growth associated with character strengths and virtues (e.g., gratitude, kindness, hope, and optimism). Despite these differences in conceptual and theoretical foundations, when implemented together, we would anticipate a positive reciprocal relationship in which features unique to each approach support one another. For example, PBIS practices have the potential to enhance implementation of positive psychology interventions through systematic teaching embedded into the curriculum and the use of positive reinforcement to promote acquisition, generalization, and maintenance of newly learned skills and behaviors. Similarly, well-managed classrooms that provide opportunities for practice and feedback may enhance program delivery of positive psychology interventions through increasing the likelihood that students can engage with the curricular material in a meaningful manner. Positive psychology interventions teach students strategies for promoting subjective well-being, thereby potentially increasing positive emotions and cognitions associated with prosocial behavior.

In light of PBIS providing a framework and foundation for implementing a range of programs and systems, a school's PBIS leadership team planning for the implementation of positive psychology interventions may:

- Develop a scope and sequence that links behavioral expectations and positive psychology intervention lessons (e.g., be kind).
- Create a professional development plan that ensures staff have access to training and ongoing coaching matched to their role in embedding positive psychology interventions within the continuum of supports.
- Prioritize the needed resources (time, materials, etc.) for effective implementation of positive psychology interventions.
- Include measures of subjective well-being and social–emotional outcomes to inform decision making and action planning.

Throughout this book, there have been illustrations of positive psychology practices and tools that are particularly aligned with the core features of an MTSS framework, such as PBIS. We highlight these examples of alignment next, to provide guidance to leadership teams that desire to integrate positive psychology interventions into their intervention continuum.

ILLUSTRATIONS OF POSITIVE PSYCHOLOGY PRACTICES WITHIN A MULTI-TIERED APPROACH

Three-Tiered Continuum of Supports

As introduced in Chapter 1, efforts to foster students' subjective well-being are consistent with a proactive, prevention-oriented approach to mental health services that focuses on building promotive factors. These internal and environmental assets may later serve protective functions in times of adversity, but are valued in and of themselves as the building blocks that underlie a flourishing level of emotional well-being. Specific strategies for enhancing these targets (e.g., gratitude, signature character strengths, hope, positive relationships) are described in great detail in the Appendix.

Tier 1

At the universal or primary level, educators can apply the strategies described in the Appendix with entire populations of students. Research summarized in Chapter 4 documents improvements in student mental health associated with schoolwide emphasis on multiple targets, including gratitude, optimism, character strengths, and strong relationships at home and school (Shoshani & Steinmetz, 2014). Schools can also choose to focus on a single target, such as kindness (Lawson et al., 2013) or character strengths (White & Waters, 2015).

Chapter 7 focuses on universal applications of positive psychology interventions at the class level. We describe in detail two promising classwide positive psychology programs that have been tested with promising results in elementary schools. One focuses on teaching students to recognize activity strengths and character strengths in themselves and others, and to use their character strengths to support meaningful goals (Quinlan, Swain, et al., 2015). The other program is a version of the Well-Being Promotion Program presented in Chapter 5 that was augmented with supplemental components targeting the larger classroom context through activities intended to strengthen classroom relationships (Suldo, Hearon, Bander, et al., 2015). These examples illustrate how positive psychology interventions not only provide an opportunity for all children to build internal assets that promote well-being, but also enhance social relationships through strengths spotting (i.e., noticing strengths in others), as well as directing kind acts and other supportive behaviors toward each other. The Appendix contains supplementary protocols intended to strengthen student–teacher and student–student relationships accordingly in order to enhance the emotional climate in a classroom.

Tier 2

At the selective or secondary level, practitioners can apply the strategies described in the Appendix to groups of students who have room for clinically meaningful growth in a given outcome or have a specific risk factor. We conceptualize the Well-Being Promotion Program as a selective-level intervention when offered to students identified through a universal screening of subjective well-being, such as with the BMSLSS (described in Chapter 2).

Chapter 5 focuses on implementation of the Well-Being Promotion Program as a selective support. The Well-Being Promotion Program entails 10 sessions of positive psychology interventions that target students' positive feelings about their past, present, and future through specific activities focused on gratitude, kindness, character strengths, optimistic thinking, and hope. To date, the primary modality for implementing this comprehensive, multitarget program has involved small groups of youth via 10 weekly meetings during a single class period (approximately 45 minutes). The complete manual for group leaders is presented in the Appendix. Chapter 5 concludes with a detailed example of implementation of the Well-Being Promotion Program with middle school students, including a description of the decision rules for identification of students in need of the intervention and progress monitoring. In the event that a small-group modality is not feasible or a student may benefit from a more individualized approach, Chapter 6 contains additional guidance for how practitioners may implement the Well-Being Promotion Program with an individual student. Chapter 6 also describes, in less detail, alternatives to our multitarget positive psychology intervention that may be applicable at the selective level. These other approaches include brief clinical interventions from a strengths-based approach, coaching using positive psychology principles, and positive psychotherapy.

Tier 3

Interventions at the indicated or tertiary level are reserved for the small number of students in need of intensive supports. At this level, positive psychology interventions are individualized, and the selected targets are often addressed by a practitioner working one on one with a given student. The students who would be appropriate for Tier 3 positive psychology interventions include those who did not respond to Tier 2 services (e.g., participation in the small-group Well-Being Promotion Program), as well as students who display concerning symptoms of mental health problems coupled with diminished subjective well-being and are either referred to the school mental health team for additional services or have already been identified with emotional/behavioral disabilities.

Chapter 6 focuses on the unique process of assessment, relationship building, and intervention/treatment planning that permits a practitioner to pursue the range of individualized intervention targets that are matched to level and type of student need in consideration of the complexity of a given student's mental health concerns. Regarding treatment planning, a practitioner may choose to provide the complete set of core positive psychology intervention protocols from the Well-Being Promotion Program, given that all strategies are appropriate for the intervention goal of increasing students' subjective well-being. However, the individualized nature of service delivery at this level of support permits the team to either select specific positive psychology intervention strategies that are consistent with a case conceptualization and/or blend these positive strategies into a comprehensive behavior support or intervention plan that may include other treatment approaches (e.g., behavioral parent training, trauma-focused cognitive-behavioral therapy) or individualized interventions in other areas (e.g., reading). Chapter 6 concludes with a case study of a high school student that details the integration of positive psychology interventions at this level of intensity.

Data-Based Decision Making

A key feature of MTSS is the use of data for decision making. Data are used not only to measure program effectiveness (i.e., outcomes) but are also analyzed for formative decision making followed by action planning. Thus, data must be directly pertinent to treatment outcomes and sensitive to changes. In the case of positive psychology interventions, this involves teams analyzing data on students' subjective well-being or promotive factors (assets or building blocks of well-being). Several examples of measures that teams might consider utilizing to inform their decision making when implementing positive psychology interventions within an MTSS are described throughout the book.

Chapter 2 describes psychometrically sound methods for measuring subjective well-being, particularly the cognitive component: life satisfaction, in school-based practice. Brief and full measures of global and multidimensional life satisfaction are described, specifically the SLSS (Huebner, 1991a, 1991b), the BMSLSS (Seligson et al., 2003), and the MSLSS (Huebner, 1994). Reproducible copies of these life satisfaction measures are provided in the Appendix. As brief measures of student life satisfaction, the SLSS and BMSLSS can be administered schoolwide to assess and monitor the collective health of the student population; as a screening instrument, the measures can be used to identify students appropriate for supplemental services (Chapter 5 contains an example of universal screening with the BMSLSS in this manner). Multiple chapters throughout this book illustrate ways the SLSS, BMSLSS, and MSLSS can and have been used to evaluate student response to participation in schoolwide (or classwide), small-group, and individual applications of the Well-Being Promotion Program. The case study in Chapter 5 also illustrates the process of collecting data on fidelity of program implementation. The Appendix includes a brief integrity checklist for each session in the Well-Being Promotion Program, for practitioners to complete to monitor the proportion of tasks described in the intervention protocol that are implemented in a given meeting. Such data on intervention fidelity are intended to be considered in tandem with student outcome data, particularly when considering next steps in the supports to be provided to a student whose life satisfaction remains low at postintervention. For example, in the event of low implementation fidelity, additional exposure to the intervention activities as intended (i.e., as implemented in the research trials that provided empirical support for the program) may be warranted.

Chapter 2 also describes the Social Emotional Health Survey (SEHS), developed to assess the positive psychological and social building blocks that predict subjective well-being. Chapter 2 describes schoolwide applications of the SEHS in a school mental health team's efforts to identify students most in need of supplemental supports in accordance with a dual-factor model of mental health (see also Dowdy et al., 2015). The importance of monitoring all students' assets comprehensively across a range of internal and environmental domains is backed by large-scale research that demonstrates that a larger number, and variety, of high-level assets predicts better emotional and behavioral health outcomes such as substance use and suicidality (Lenzi, Dougherty, Furlong, Sharkey, & Dowdy, 2015). Given the advantages associated with cumulative assets, universal applications of the SEHS include identifying students at risk for negative outcomes due to few assets, and promoting multiple assets (e.g., four assets from two or more domains) in all students. At the selective and indicated levels, the SEHS may be a useful tool for gathering additional data regarding specific students' psychosocial strengths for case conceptualization as well as progress monitoring; growth in SEHS scores would support response to intervention, whereas areas that remain low or decline would suggest targets most in need of subsequent supports. In sum, data from the SEHS may help guide the selection of positive psychology interventions applied at the Tier 2 and Tier 3 levels, and, as an outcome measure, supplement an indicator of subjective well-being (such as the SLSS) that would serve as the primary index of growth across time.

Professional Development and Coaching

A traditional model of mental health service delivery that relies on "pull-out" services provided by trained "experts" (e.g., mental health practitioners) is contraindicated in systems that prioritize student academic engaged time, have limited access to school-based mental health professionals, and take advantage of natural opportunities to build and generalize assets through strengthening relationships and teaching adaptive thought and behavior patterns (e.g., social–emotional competencies) in social settings such as the classroom, community, and family home. Accordingly, modern approaches to service delivery rely more on what have traditionally been referred to as consultative practices in which the "experts" support those individuals (e.g., teachers and parents) who interact with youth frequently and authentically.

Chapter 7 highlights ways to work with teachers in particular to either (1) increase their personal subjective well-being (relevant in part due to bidirectional relationships between teacher and student well-being), or (2) implement or reinforce positive psychology interventions with their students. Regarding the latter, Chapter 7 details an example of a classwide implementation in which a teacher served as co-interventionist. The intent of this rather resource-intense side-by-side implementation of a mental health practitioner with a teacher was intended to build the teacher's capacity to implement the intervention more independently with future classrooms of children. For instance, in the next school year, the teacher would implement alone with coaching support from the practitioner. Chapter 7 also presents a brief strengths-focused intervention intended to increase teachers' subjective well-being through increased use of signature character strengths in the classroom. This intervention serves the dual purpose of supporting teachers' well-being, and teaching them the vocabulary and activities that are involved in an evidence-based positive psychology intervention shown to cause enduring gains in happiness. Teachers who incur personal benefits from that character strengths intervention may be more likely to lead their students through the same process of identifying and using signature strengths.

Chapter 8 describes ways to support parents to either (1) increase their personal subjective well-being (relevant in part due to familial trends in well-being), or (2) reinforce positive psychology interventions that their children learn at school. The Appendix provides brief parent handouts that correspond to each session of the Well-Being Promotion Program. These handouts summarize what their child learned in a given meeting with a practitioner, and suggest follow-up activities the parents can do at home to facilitate practice of the positive psychology intervention.

Research-Validated Practices for Improving Student Outcomes

MTSS involve selection of evidence-based practices to support the needs of all students. Evidence-based approaches to improving students' subjective well-being can entail applying findings of studies that have discerned the potentially malleable factors within the environment (e.g., peers, family, and school) as well as within individuals (e.g., cognitions and activities) that are correlated with increased life satisfaction among children and adolescents. To that effect, Chapter 3 contains a summary of such correlates of youth subjective well-being. Practices to increase those factors associated with youth subjective well-being may logically contribute to elevations in subjective well-being, as we discussed in this chapter in the case of school climate.

Recent advances in the literature have lent more confidence in the positive outcomes that should follow implementation of positive psychology interventions, many of which were developed to target the promotive factors. Chapter 4 presents findings from the growing number of studies that support various single and multitarget positive psychology interventions as research-based practices for improving student subjective well-being. Because of the infancy of the study of positive psychology interventions with youth, the confidence in these strategies as "research validated" should be tempered; positive psychology interventions may be most accurately described as promising or perhaps probably efficacious, but not yet well established. More research is needed to ensure replication by independent research teams, as well as identify student demographic features (e.g., age level, cultural groups) that may moderate intervention effectiveness.

CONCLUSION

Mental health is increasingly viewed as a complete state of being, in which both negative indicators of problems and positive indicators of well-being matter. Comprehensive mental health services necessitate both the prevention and amelioration of internalizing and externalizing forms of psychopathology, and the promotion of subjective well-being (a scientific term for happiness). This book was developed to provide practical guidance for school mental health professionals who are interested in promoting children's subjective well-being through a continuum of supports that are student focused, as well as target the classroom and family contexts. The strategies described in the book are derived from a small but growing body of research on school-based positive psychology interventions. Those studies have found promising youth outcomes associated with universal, selective, and indicated interventions that target students' positive emotions, gratitude, hope and goal-directed thinking, optimism, use of character strengths, and positive relationships with friends, families, and educators.

When integrating positive psychology interventions or other evidence-based mental health interventions into a multi-tiered implementation framework such as PBIS, schools can systematically align interventions to enhance outcomes and maximize resources. Throughout this book, there have been illustrations of approaches that teams might consider when integrating positive psychology interventions into their MTSS framework. We encourage teams to consider how these positive psychology interventions can systematically be integrated into their current multi-tiered implementation framework to meet the complete mental health needs of their student population. Aligned with an emphasis on complete mental health, a multi-tiered framework provides schools with a systematic approach to teaching students skills and creating positive and effective learning environments to promote mental wellness, as well as social and academic success, and to prevent, reduce, and manage internalizing and/or externalizing problems.

Appendix

ADDITIONAL SESSION PROTOCOLS FOR APPLICATION WITH INDIVIDUAL STUDENTS (TO ACCOMPANY CHAPTER 6)

ADDITIONAL SESSION PROTOCOLS AND HANDOUTS FOR CLASSWIDE APPLICATION (TO ACCOMPANY CHAPTER 7)

ADDITIONAL SESSION PROTOCOL AND HANDOUTS FOR PARENT COMPONENT (TO ACCOMPANY CHAPTER 8)

INTERVENTION INTEGRITY CHECKLISTS (ONLINE SUPPLEMENT*)

---

*Purchasers of this book can download and print materials in the Online Supplement (see the box at the end of the table of contents).

Students' Life Satisfaction Scale (SLSS)

Student: _____   Date: _____

Teacher: _____

Instructions: We would like to know what thoughts about life you've had *during the past several weeks.* Think about how you spend each day and night, and then think about how your life has been during most of this time. Here are some questions that ask you to indicate your satisfaction with life. In answering each statement, circle a number from **1** to **6**, where **1** indicates you **strongly *dis*agree** with the statement and **6** indicates you **strongly agree** with the statement.

	Strongly disagree	Moderately disagree	Mildly disagree	Mildly agree	Moderately agree	Strongly agree
1. My life is going well.	1	2	3	4	5	6
2. My life is just right.	1	2	3	4	5	6
3. I would like to change many things in my life.*	1	2	3	4	5	6
4. I wish I had a different kind of life.*	1	2	3	4	5	6
5. I have a good life.	1	2	3	4	5	6
6. I have what I want in life.	1	2	3	4	5	6
7. My life is better than most kids'.	1	2	3	4	5	6

For Practitioner Use Only—Scoring Directions:

*Reverse-scored item (subtract student response from 7)

Global = (1 + 2 + 3 + 4 + 5 + 6 + 7) / 7

Multidimensional Students' Life Satisfaction Scale (MSLSS)

Student: _____ **Date:** _____

Teacher: _____

Instructions: We would like to know what thoughts about life you've had *during the past several weeks.* Think about how you spend each day and night, and then think about how your life has been during most of this time. Here are some questions that ask you to indicate your satisfaction with life. In answering each statement, circle a number from **1** to **6**, where **1** indicates you **strongly** *disagree* with the statement and **6** indicates you **strongly agree** with the statement.

	Strongly disagree	Moderately disagree	Mildly disagree	Mildly agree	Moderately agree	Strongly agree
1. My friends are nice to me.	1	2	3	4	5	6
2. I am fun to be around.	1	2	3	4	5	6
3. I feel bad at school.*	1	2	3	4	5	6
4. I have a bad time with my friends.*	1	2	3	4	5	6
5. There are lots of things I can do well.	1	2	3	4	5	6
6. I learn a lot at school.	1	2	3	4	5	6
7. I like spending time with my parents.	1	2	3	4	5	6
8. My family is better than most.	1	2	3	4	5	6
9. There are many things about school I don't like.*	1	2	3	4	5	6
10. I think I am good-looking.	1	2	3	4	5	6
11. My friends are great.	1	2	3	4	5	6
12. My friends will help me if I need it.	1	2	3	4	5	6
13. I wish I didn't have to go to school.*	1	2	3	4	5	6
14. I like myself.	1	2	3	4	5	6
15. There are lots of fun things to do where I live.	1	2	3	4	5	6
16. My friends treat me well.	1	2	3	4	5	6
17. Most people like me.	1	2	3	4	5	6
18. My family gets along well together.	1	2	3	4	5	6

(continued)

	Strongly disagree	Moderately disagree	Mildly disagree	Mildly agree	Moderately agree	Strongly agree
19. I look forward to going to school.	1	2	3	4	5	6
20. My parents treat me fairly.	1	2	3	4	5	6
21. I enjoy being at home with my family.	1	2	3	4	5	6
22. I like being in school.	1	2	3	4	5	6
23. My friends are mean to me.*	1	2	3	4	5	6
24. I wish I had different friends.*	1	2	3	4	5	6
25. School is interesting.	1	2	3	4	5	6
26. I enjoy school activities.	1	2	3	4	5	6
27. I wish I lived in a different house.*	1	2	3	4	5	6
28. Members of my family talk nicely to one another.	1	2	3	4	5	6
29. I have a lot of fun with my friends.	1	2	3	4	5	6
30. My parents and I do fun things together.	1	2	3	4	5	6
31. I like my neighborhood.	1	2	3	4	5	6
32. I wish I lived somewhere else.*	1	2	3	4	5	6
33. I am a nice person.	1	2	3	4	5	6
34. This town is filled with mean people.*	1	2	3	4	5	6
35. I like to try new things.	1	2	3	4	5	6
36. My family's house is nice.	1	2	3	4	5	6
37. I like my neighbors.	1	2	3	4	5	6
38. I have enough friends.	1	2	3	4	5	6
39. I wish there were different people in my neighborhood.*	1	2	3	4	5	6
40. I like where I live.	1	2	3	4	5	6

Student, please stop here, thank you!

(continued)

For Practitioner Use Only—Scoring Directions:

*Reverse-scored item (subtract student response from 7)

Friends = (1 + 4 + 11 + 12 + 16 + 23 + 24 + 29 + 38) / 9

Self = (2 + 5 + 10 + 14 + 17 + 33 + 35) / 7

School = (3 + 6 + 9 + 13 + 19 + 22 + 25 + 26) / 8

Family = (7 + 8 + 18 + 20 + 21 + 28 + 30) / 7

Living environment = (15 + 27 + 31 + 32 + 34 + 36 + 37 + 39 + 40) / 9

Brief Multidimensional Students' Life Satisfaction Scale (BMSLSS)

Student: _____   **Date:** _____

Teacher: _____

Instructions: We would like to know what thoughts about life you've had *during the past several weeks.* Think about how you spend each day and night, and then think about how your life has been during most of this time. Here are some questions that ask you to indicate your satisfaction with life. In answering each statement, circle a number from **1** to **7**, where **1** indicates you feel **terrible** about that area of life and **7** indicates you are **delighted** with that area of life.

	Terrible	Unhappy	Mostly dissatisfied	Mixed (about equally satisfied and dissatisfied)	Mostly satisfied	Pleased	Delighted
1. I would describe my satisfaction with my *family life* as:	1	2	3	4	5	6	7
2. I would describe my satisfaction with my *friendships* as:	1	2	3	4	5	6	7
3. I would describe my satisfaction with my *school experience* as:	1	2	3	4	5	6	7
4. I would describe my satisfaction with *myself* as:	1	2	3	4	5	6	7
5. I would describe my satisfaction with *where I live* as:	1	2	3	4	5	6	7
6. I would describe my satisfaction with my *overall life* as:	1	2	3	4	5	6	7

Social Emotional Health Survey—Secondary Version (SEHS-S)

Student: _____   **Date:** _____

Teacher: _____

Instructions: Please *circle* the number that corresponds to the response that indicates how true each of these statements is about you.

	Not at all true of me	A little true of me	Pretty much true of me	Very much true of me
1. I can work out my problems.	1	2	3	4
2. I can do most things if I try.	1	2	3	4
3. There are many things that I do well.	1	2	3	4
4. There is a purpose to my life.	1	2	3	4
5. I understand my moods and feelings.	1	2	3	4
6. I understand why I do what I do.	1	2	3	4
7. When I do not understand something, I ask the teacher again and again until I understand.	1	2	3	4
8. I try to answer all the questions asked in class.	1	2	3	4
9. When I try to solve a math problem, I will not stop until I find a final solution.	1	2	3	4
10. At my school there is a teacher or some other adult who always wants me to do my best.	1	2	3	4
11. At my school there is a teacher or some other adult who listens to me when I have something to say.	1	2	3	4
12. At my school there is a teacher or some other adult who believes that I will be a success.	1	2	3	4
13. My family members really help and support one another.	1	2	3	4
14. There is a feeling of togetherness in my family.	1	2	3	4
15. My family really gets along well with one another.	1	2	3	4
16. I have a friend my age who really cares about me.	1	2	3	4
17. I have a friend my age who talks with me about my problems.	1	2	3	4
18. I have a friend my age who helps me when I'm having a hard time.	1	2	3	4
19. I accept responsibility for my actions.	1	2	3	4
20. When I make a mistake I admit it.	1	2	3	4
21. I can deal with being told no.	1	2	3	4
22. I feel bad when someone gets his or her feelings hurt.	1	2	3	4

(continued)

	Not at all true of me	A little true of me	Pretty much true of me	Very much true of me
23. I try to understand what other people go through.	1	2	3	4
24. I try to understand how other people feel and think.	1	2	3	4
25. I can wait for what I want.	1	2	3	4
26. I don't bother others when they are busy.	1	2	3	4
27. I think before I act.	1	2	3	4
28. Each day I look forward to having a lot of fun.	1	2	3	4
29. I usually expect to have a good day.	1	2	3	4
30. Overall, I expect more good things to happen to me than bad things.	1	2	3	4

	Not at all	Very little	Somewhat	Quite a lot	Extremely
31. How much do you feel *energetic* right now?	1	2	3	4	5
32. How much do you feel *active* right now?	1	2	3	4	5
33. How much do you feel *lively* right now?	1	2	3	4	5
34. Since yesterday how much have you felt *grateful*?	1	2	3	4	5
35. Since yesterday how much have you felt *thankful*?	1	2	3	4	5
36. Since yesterday how much have you felt *appreciative*?	1	2	3	4	5

Student, please stop here, thank you!

(continued)

For Practitioner Use Only—Scoring Directions:

Belief in self = sum of items 1–9 [range = 9–36]

Belief in others = sum of items 10–18 [range = 9–36]

Emotional competence = sum of items 19–27 [range = 9–36]

Engaged living = sum of items 28–36 [range = 9–42]

Total covitality = sum of items 1–36 [range = 36–150]

*Low ≤ 85; low average = 86–106; high average = 107–127; high ≥ 128

Social Emotional Health Survey—Primary Version (SEHS-P)

Student: _____   **Date:** _____

Teacher: _____

Instructions: Please circle from **1** to **4**, where **1** is **almost never** and **4** is **very often**, how true each of the following statements is for you.

	Almost never	Sometimes	Often	Very often
1. I am lucky to go to school.	1	2	3	4
2. I am thankful that I get to learn new things at school.	1	2	3	4
3. We are lucky to have nice teachers at my school.	1	2	3	4
4. I feel thankful for my good friends at school.	1	2	3	4
5. When I have problems at school, I know they will get better in the future.	1	2	3	4
6. I expect good things to happen at my school.	1	2	3	4
7. Each week, I expect to feel happy in class.	1	2	3	4
8. I expect to have fun with my friends at school.	1	2	3	4
9. I get excited when I learn something new at school.	1	2	3	4
10. I get really excited about my school projects.	1	2	3	4
11. I wake up in the morning excited to go to school.	1	2	3	4
12. I get excited when I am doing my class assignments.	1	2	3	4
13. I finish all my class assignments.	1	2	3	4
14. When I get a bad (low) grade, I try even harder the next time.	1	2	3	4
15. I keep working until I get my schoolwork right.	1	2	3	4
16. I do my class assignments even when they are really hard for me.	1	2	3	4
17. I follow the classroom rules.	1	2	3	4
18. I follow the playground rules at recess and lunch/break times.	1	2	3	4
19. I listen when my teacher is talking.	1	2	3	4
20. I am nice to other students.	1	2	3	4

Session Protocols for Core Intervention Guide for School Mental Health Providers

INTRODUCTION TO THE WELL-BEING PROMOTION PROGRAM	Core Session 1: Student Group
Goals	• Establish a supportive group environment. • Increase awareness of subjective well-being. • Introduce students to the broad determinants of happiness.
Overview of Procedures	A. Get to Know You Activity: You at Your Best B. Group Discussion: Initial Definition and the Importance of Happiness C. Clarify Purpose of the Group D. Establish Group Norms E. Homework: You at Your Best
Materials	• *Binder* to hold documents provided and created throughout the program, to stay in the practitioner's possession for ready access at the beginning of each group session • *Folder* in which students can transport group homework assignments, to stay in the student's possession for ready access between group meetings • White board or easel • *What Determines Happiness?* figure • *What Determines Happiness?* handout • *Overview of Program Activities* handout • *Confidentiality* handout

Procedures Defined

A. Get to Know You Activity: You at Your Best

This activity provides an initial boost of happiness (Seligman et al., 2005). It is included here as an introductory exercise in part to enhance engagement and to amplify effects of later activities.

Set the Stage	*Before we talk about why we're all here in this group, I'd like to do an activity to help us get to know one another, in particular what we are each good at.*

Writing	• Provide students with a plain sheet of lined paper.
	• Ask them to write about a time when they were at their best.
	  o Doing something really well.
	  o Going above and beyond for someone else.
	  o Displaying a talent.
	  o Creating something.

Personal Reflection	• Once completed, ask them to take a few minutes to reflect on the story.
	  o Remember the feelings of that day.
	  o Identify the personal strengths they displayed in the story.
	  o Think about the time, effort, and creativity that comprised such an accomplishment.

(continued)

Shared Reflection	• Ask students to share their story with the group and one or two reflections.
	• Initiate reflections on each group member's story with identifications or reaffirmations of strengths displayed within the story.
	• Encourage group members to reflect on the positives in each other's stories.
	  o Something they admired or liked in the story.
	  o Strengths the presenter demonstrated in the story.
	  o A quality they share with the presenter.

Retain	• Make a photocopy of the "You at Your Best" stories. • File the copy of the story in a binder you will keep for future reference by you or the student, such as in the event the student forgets to bring his or her homework folder back to group the next session. • Place the original story in a folder the student will use to keep his or her homework assignments for, and notes from, the Well-Being Promotion Program group.

B. Group Discussion: Initial Definition and the Importance of Happiness

Set the Stage	*What do you think this group is all about?* • Once answers are received, state that the group is about happiness.
Introduction to Happiness	Pose these questions to the group and facilitate a brief discussion: • *When someone says he or she is "happy," what does he or she mean? What does "happiness" mean to you?* • *Why is being happy important? Why is happiness important to you?* • *What do you do to increase your own happiness?* No specific answers are necessary. Simply facilitate students' thoughts and discussions on these topics. Participate in the discussion as well with examples from your own life in order to develop a relationship with the group.

C. Clarify Purpose of the Group

This discussion will introduce students to the purpose of the group: to use our power to change our personal happiness to the upper bounds of our set point through building purposeful thoughts and activities that move us toward the upper part of our emotional range.

| Introduce the Determinants of Happiness Theory | • Share the *What Determines Happiness?* figure.
• Explain that happiness is determined by three things: our genetics, our life circumstances, and our purposeful activities. Example script:

Look at the What Determines Happiness? *figure. Scientists find happiness is made up of three things: a genetic or biological set point, purposeful activity, and life circumstances. Set point is the biggest cause of happiness and it is controlled by our genetics. We all have a range of ability to be happy based on what we're born with. Let's use the ruler and pretend that people can be happy on a scale of 1–6. Some people's ranges are naturally high, so even when they are at their lowest happy level, they may seem a lot happier than other people. In that case, their range could be 4–6. However, some people's ranges are lower, so they don't seem happy that often. They may have a range of 0–2. A person's set point is the level of happiness they usually have within their range. For example, a person could have a range of 3–5 but is usually at a 4 level of happiness. It is a good thing that genetics isn't the only thing that makes up happiness, or else we wouldn't be able to get any happier. Changes in life circumstances and purposeful ways of thinking and acting help us to move our level of happiness within our ranges. Circumstances are facts of life, such as the state you live in, your age,* |

(continued)

how much money you have, and the school you go to. These are things that we usually can't change or can't do so very easily. The key to increasing happiness within our ranges is purposeful activity—in other words, what you choose to do or think. Purposeful activity includes the things you do, the way you think, your attitudes, and your goals. Everyone has the opportunity to increase his or her level of happiness through purposeful activities and that's what we'll be talking about in the group. The purpose of this group is to increase your happiness by talking about good attitudes, feelings, thoughts, and activities from your past, present, and future. During our meetings, we'll learn how to make our purposeful activities (those things we choose to do and think about) more in line with activities seen in people who feel pretty happy with their lives. What questions do you have?

Check for Comprehension	• Distribute the *Overview of Program Activities* handout. • Ask students to complete the key for the figure (three determinants of happiness) and the first question regarding the focus of group meetings (answer: purposeful activities). • Reinforce effort; guide students to correct answers as needed.

D. Establish Group Norms

Provide clear expectations for appropriate behavior during meetings. Behavior should convey respect for classmates and maximize opportunities to engage with the activities and thereby increase personal happiness.

Set the Stage	• Discuss the logistics of group meetings. When, how often, and where students will meet with the group leader; how the group leader will coordinate this schedule with classroom teachers; use of hall passes, and so on. Example script: *We'll meet once each week, for the next 10 weeks, in this room, at this time— third period. No need to check in with your third-period teacher first; I'll e-mail her to confirm you were here today. When your second-period class is dismissed, stop by your locker to get your folder for our group, then come straight here.* • Revisit the *Overview of Program Activities* handout; complete questions 2–4. • File completed worksheet in students' folders for their future reference.
Confidentiality	• Pose these questions to the group and facilitate a brief discussion: ○ *Have you heard the word* confidentiality *before?* ○ *How would you define confidentiality for this group? (e.g., confidential = private or secret).* • Compile students' ideas into a confidentiality definition on the board. Make sure that it includes the following components: ○ Respect for others' privacy outside of group. ○ Times when the group leader will have to break confidentiality (e.g., danger to self, danger to others, student is in danger). ○ Any other concerns students express. • Distribute the *Confidentiality* handout. • Ask students to write the definition on the worksheet. • File the completed worksheet in students' folders for future reference.

(continued)

Develop Additional Group Rules for Behavior	• Develop a short list of group rules. These rules are intended to facilitate an atmosphere of trust and engagement. Rules for appropriate behavior in the group should also be consistent with existing school rules and behavioral expectations, such as those rules that are explicated in the school's PBIS program. • Record and post group rules for future reference.

E. Homework: You at Your Best

Set the Stage	• Discuss specific incentives that will be provided weekly for completion of group homework, such as school supplies, stickers, candy, tickets toward rewards used in the school's PBIS program, and so on.
Assign	• For each night this week, students should read their story and think about the strengths they demonstrated in the story. • Encourage students to add more details and length to the story. • They can share the story with family members or someone else if they like.
Looking Ahead	• A brief discussion in the next session will touch on student follow-through with homework and resulting feelings of happiness.

Session Protocols for Core Intervention Guide
for School Mental Health Providers

GRATITUDE JOURNALS	Core Session 2: Student Group

Goals	• Explore students' current levels of gratitude. • Define gratitude and how it can impact happiness. • Learn a method of using gratitude to focus on positive interpretations of past events.
Overview of Procedures	A. Review Homework: You at Your Best B. Group Discussion: Initial Definition and Importance of Gratitude C. Gratitude Journals D. Homework: Gratitude Journal on a Daily Basis
Materials	• Tangible rewards for homework completion (stickers, candy, pencils, etc.) • Blackboard, white board, or easel • Small squares of paper for students to note self-identified ratings • Notebook or journal with blank cover to be inserted in group folders • Pens, pencils, markers, or other colorful supplies to decorate journals

Procedures Defined

A. Review Homework Assignment: You at Your Best

Assignment Completion and Reward	• Ask students how often they read their "You at Your Best" stories. • Provide a small tangible reward (e.g., candy) for homework completion. • If students did not comply with the daily requirement, stress the importance of daily effort for changes in happiness to occur.
Reflection	• Ask students to share any new reflections that they had over the week when revisiting their "You at Your Best" story. • Ask students to share if they felt any difference in happiness since the last session.

B. Group Discussion: Initial Definition and Importance of Gratitude

Set the Stage	*What is gratitude?* • Facilitate a brief discussion on what students think constitutes gratitude. • Record students' responses on the board. Circle and discuss key terms, phrases, and or themes. Provide a common definition, such as: *You feel gratitude (thanks, appreciation, grateful) when you recognize that you received an intentional act of kindness from another person. More specifically, you feel gratitude after gaining a benefit that you view as valuable, that was provided intentionally and altruistically (not for ulterior motives), and occurred at some cost to the person who provided the benefit.*

(continued)

Rate Your Gratitude	*We are going to rate our own level of gratitude.*
	• Draw a number line from 0 to 10 on a white board.
	• Distribute small, blank pieces of paper.
	Think about how often you have felt grateful in the past few months. On a scale from 0 to 10 with 0 being never grateful, *5 being* sometimes grateful, *and 10 being* always grateful, *rate your gratitude.*
	• Ask students to write their ratings on a piece of paper and fold it over.
Shared Reflection	• In a round-robin fashion, ask each to student share his or her number and the reason he or she chose it.
Introduce Links between Gratitude and Happiness	• *Why may gratitude be important?*
	• *Why is it important or not important to have gratitude in your life?*
	• *Do you think being grateful can increase happiness? Why or why not?*
	o Discuss how *gratitude helps us focus our emotions on the positive parts of our pasts as related to school, friendships, and in family life.*
	o Provide a personal example of a time in which you have felt grateful and how that refocused your attention on a positive experience.

C. Gratitude Journals

Emmons and McCullough (2003) found that daily attention to grateful thoughts increased happiness. Gratitude journals are a method of focusing student thoughts on things, people, and events for which they are grateful. The intensity is high for the first week, in that students are asked to journal daily. This is in line with Emmons and McCullough's finding that higher intensity led to greater happiness gains. Later, journaling is suggested on a once-per-week basis.

Create a Gratitude Journal	• Provide each student with a plain-cover journal or notebook.
	• Ask students to use the writing/art materials to design a cover that shows something positive about their history.
	o Something they have done, was given to them, part of a family event, or any other kind of experience valued as positive.
	o Encourage them to draw a picture, write, or use a combination of writing and drawings/symbols.
Use the Gratitude Journal	• After the time to decorate the journals is over, explain their intended use.
	I want you to take 5 minutes, think about your day, and write down five things in your life that you are grateful for, including both small and large things, events, people, talents, or anything else you think of. Some examples may include generosity of my friends, my teacher giving me extra help, family dinner, your favorite band/singer, and so on. [Provide examples relevant to your students that you are aware of.]
	• Help students complete an initial entry in the group.
	o Give students about 5 minutes to list five things for which they are currently grateful.
	o Explain that a variety of responses is acceptable and expected.
Shared Reflection	• After the independent writing time is over, prompt each student to share one or two of their responses with the group.
	• In light of students' typically relatively low satisfaction with school, draw particular attention to things or people pertinent to school that students comment on in a positive manner.

(continued)

D. Homework: Gratitude Journal on a Daily Basis

Assign	*For each night this week, I want you to set aside 5 minutes before you go to sleep. At that time, think about your day and write down five things in your life that you are grateful for, just like we did here today in your journals. Remember that you can include events, people, talents, or anything else you think of, whether it is large or small. Also, you can repeat some things if they are really important to you. But also try to think of different ones as well.*
Looking Ahead	• Explain that students will never be asked to share all of their responses, but to become comfortable with sharing two to three of their recorded responses in the next group meeting. • Students should leave the meeting with the decorated notebooks added to their homework folder. • Remind students of the incentives they can receive contingent on homework completion and return of the gratitude journal.

Session Protocols for Core Intervention Guide for School Mental Health Providers

GRATITUDE VISITS	Core Session 3: Student Group

Goals	• Explore students' experiences with gratitude journals. • Make connections between grateful thoughts and positive feelings about the past. • Learn to incorporate actions/expressions of gratitude.
Overview of Procedures	A. Review Homework: Gratitude Journals B. Gratitude Visit C. Group Discussion: Positive Feelings about the Past D. Homework: Carry Out the Gratitude Visit
Materials	• Tangible rewards for homework completion (stickers, pencils, etc.) • Access to computer lab or letter stationery • Letter-size envelopes • *What Determines Happiness?* figure • *Gratitude Visit Planning Form* handout

Procedures Defined

A. Review Homework Assignment: Gratitude Journals

Assignment Completion and Reward	• Ask students how often they completed the gratitude journals. • Provide a small tangible reward (e.g., pencil, sticker) for homework completion. • If students did not journal regularly, stress the importance of daily effort for changes in happiness to occur.
Reflection	• Ask students to choose two to three things for which they recorded being grateful to share with the group. • Discuss the significance of gratitude for these things in terms of positive feelings about the past. • Ask students to share any changes in feelings of gratitude or happiness.

B. Gratitude Visit

Completion of a gratitude visit is associated with positive, enduring changes in happiness (Seligman et al., 2005). The activity below is adapted from that original research.

Set the Stage	*We all have people in our lives who have helped us in some way. This helping can be part of someone's job, like a teacher or parent, or help that someone gives without being required to. Even when people's kindness or help is provided as part of their job, the help can be important because of the way they did it or how it benefited us so much. Sometimes other people's kindness toward us goes unnoticed or unrecognized.*
Identify People to Whom We Are Grateful	• Provide some examples of people who were particularly kind or helpful to you during childhood who were never properly thanked. • Distribute the *Gratitude Visit Planning Form* • Ask students to write a list of people who had been especially kind to them but may not have been properly thanked.

(continued)

Plan a Gratitude Visit	• Help students identify someone from their list of people to whom they are grateful that they could feasibly meet in person to deliver such a letter. • Assist students in composing a one-page letter that describes the reason(s) why they are grateful to this person. o Secure access to computers in advance if students prefer to type. • Assist students in planning a day and time during which they will read the letter aloud to the person (complete the *Gratitude Visit Planning Form*) • Instruct students to read aloud the letter slowly with expression and eye contact during a face-to-face visit. • Ask students not to reveal the reason why they want to meet with the person; instead, simply make plans to spend time with the person.

C. Group Discussion: Positive Feelings about the Past

Introduce the Thoughts–Feelings Connection	• Discuss the connection between students' thoughts of the past and current affect. *How has gratitude—noticing, writing about, and talking about the good things in your life, and thinking about the people to whom you are thankful—refocused your thoughts and changed your feelings?*
Revisit the Determinants of Happiness Theory: Emphasis on Purposeful Activities	• Review the *What Determines Happiness?* figure and discuss how grateful thinking is a purposeful activity. Example script: *Doing things like gratitude journaling and visits refocuses thoughts on the positive parts of your past, which increases positive attitudes about your history and your life (brings you into the upper range of your set point [reference ruler]). Such activities can even help you feel more confident in your goals because you recognized people in your life who are there to help you.*

D. Homework: Carry Out the Gratitude Visit

Assignment 1	• Before the next group meeting, students should carry out the gratitude visit. • *Note:* In situations in which the student does not have the means to meet with someone to whom he or she is grateful, or cannot identify a person, ask the student to continue daily gratitude journals as done the previous week.
Assignment 2	• Ask all students to complete at least one gratitude journal entry at some point during the week before the next session.
Looking Ahead	• Students should leave the meeting with the completed *Gratitude Visit Planning Form* and the decorated notebooks in their homework folders. • Remind students of the incentives they can receive contingent on homework completion and return of the gratitude journal.

Session Protocols for Core Intervention Guide for School Mental Health Providers

ACTS OF KINDNESS	Core Session 4: Student Group
Goals	• Define kindness (i.e., a character strength), and how it can impact happiness. • Explore students' current frequency of kind acts. • Learn a method of using kindness to create a focus on positive interpretations of present events.
Overview of Procedures	A. Review Homework: Gratitude Visits and/or Gratitude Journals B. Group Discussion: Initial Definition and Importance of Kindness C. Student Estimations of Acts of Kindness D. Homework: Performing Acts of Kindness
Materials	• Tangible rewards for homework completion (stickers, pencils, etc.) • Blackboard, white board, or easel • *What Determines Happiness?* figure • *Performing Acts of Kindness Record Form* handout

Procedures Defined

A. Review Homework Assignment: Gratitude Visits and/or Gratitude Journals

Assignment Completion and Reward	• Ask students about their progress with carrying out the gratitude visit. • Ask students about their progress with completing one or more gratitude journal entry. • Provide a small tangible reward (e.g., candy) for homework completion. • If students did not complete the gratitude visit as assigned, problem solve barriers and create a plan for a visit this week. Stress the importance of continued effort between sessions for changes in happiness to occur.

Reflection	• Ask students to share their experiences during and after the gratitude visits.
	   o *How did the recipients of the visit respond?*
	   o *How did they and you feel following the visit?*
	 • For students who continued to complete gratitude journals, ask them to select and share one entry with the group.
	 • Ask students to share any changes in happiness since the last meeting.

B. Group Discussion: Initial Definition and Importance of Kindness

Acts of kindness provide a way to boost moods and make long-lasting changes in well-being through satisfying basic human needs of relatedness (Lyubomirsky, Sheldon, & Schkade, 2005). Kindness has been defined as a character strength, which causes and stems from happiness (Otake et al., 2006; Park, Peterson, & Seligman, 2004). The following discussion is based on this research.

(continued)

Set the Stage; Define Kindness as a Character Strength Related to Happiness	*What is kindness? What do you think of when someone is called a kind person? What specifically is that person doing?* • Facilitate a brief discussion on what students think constitutes kindness. • Record students' responses on the board. Circle and discuss key terms, phrases, and or themes. Provide a common definition, such as: *Acts of kindness are behaviors that benefit other people or make others happy, typically at the cost of your time and effort. When a person consistently performs these acts of kindness, we say he or she is kind, or he or she possesses the virtue of kindness. A virtue, also called strength of character, is a moral strength that people do by choice. We'll talk more about character strengths next week.*

Introduce Links between Kindness and Happiness	*Why may this particular character strength—kindness—be important?*
	  o *Why is it important to display kindness in your life?*
	  o *Do you think being kind can impact happiness? Why or why not?*
	• Discuss how *kindness helps us focus our emotions on the positive parts of our **present lives**, for example through:*
	  o Creating a positive view of others and the community.
	  o Increased cooperation.
	  o Awareness of your own good fortune.
	  o Seeing yourself as helpful.
	  o Increased confidence and optimism about being able to help others.
	  o Getting others to know and like us.
	  o Receipt of appreciation and gratitude.
	  o Others reciprocating kindness and friendship toward you.
	• Provide an example of a time when you have been kind to someone, and how that refocused your attention on a positive situation.

C. Student Estimations of Acts of Kindness

Otake and colleagues (2006) found that happiness could be increased through simply counting the acts of kindness that one performs over a week's time. The basis of that research is used in this preparatory exercise for the upcoming assignment to enact acts of kindness for homework.

Identify Acts of Kindness	• Facilitate a discussion of various acts of kindness performed by you, youth, and adults in students' lives, then the students themselves.
	• Begin by providing some examples of acts of kindness that you have performed recently, focusing mainly on the past week.
	  o Make sure that you provide a wide range of acts of kindness that are authentic to you but also relatable to the group.
	  o Give yourself a loose estimate of the amount of kind acts you perform in a week (e.g., three to five, four to six, or seven to 10).
	• Ask students to think about the people in their lives such as family, classmates, other friends, and teachers.
	  o Ask them to provide a few examples of kind acts they observed by these significant figures in their lives during the past week.
	  o Ask them to provide a weekly estimate of how often an identified person demonstrates such kind acts.

(continued)

Rate Your Kindness	*We are going to think about kind acts we have demonstrated, and estimate our own typical kind acts.* • Ask students to provide some examples of acts of kindness that they have performed in the past week. If it is too difficult for students to think of acts of kindness limited to this time frame, they can think back to the past 2 or 3 weeks. • Keep in mind that kindness was described as a moral virtue, and thus it can be interpreted as negative, perhaps even shameful, if a student shares he or she has low levels of kind acts. Facilitate a climate of openness and nonjudgmental attitudes. Example script: *People vary in the amount of kind acts they perform. This is not a reflection on the quality of their moral character. As will be examined in the next session, character strengths come in many forms. People are stronger than others in different areas.* • Distribute small, blank pieces of paper. • Ask students to give themselves a weekly estimate of personal kind acts; they can write this on the piece of paper and fold it over. • Explain that we are going to aim to increase this number in the coming week, through performing five acts of kindness on a single day.

D. Homework: Performing Acts of Kindness

Lyubomirsky, Tkach, and Sheldon (2004) found that people who performed five acts of kindness in 1 day, each week for 6 weeks, showed a significant increase in well-being. This week's homework assignment is based on that and subsequent research.

Assign	*I want you to pick a day this week to perform five acts of kindness. As we talked about, acts of kindness are behaviors that benefit other people or make others happy, typically at the cost of your time and effort. They can range from small acts, like giving a compliment or holding a door, to large acts like helping your dad wash his car.*
	• Help students brainstorm some ideas of the acts of kindness they might like to perform.
	  o Which can they do at school? [In the classroom? Before school or during lunch?]
	  o Which can they do at home?
	• Distribute the *Acts of Kindness Record Form* to jot down their plans as well as record additional kind acts after they have been performed.
	• Ask students to decide on a date to perform the acts.

Looking Ahead	• Explain students will never be asked to share all of their responses, but to become comfortable with sharing two to three of their acts of kindness and related feelings in the next group meeting. • Students should leave the meeting with the *Acts of Kindness Record Form* added to their homework folder. • Remind students of the incentives they can receive contingent on homework completion and return of the *Acts of Kindness Record Form.*

Session Protocols for Core Intervention Guide
for School Mental Health Providers

INTRODUCTION TO CHARACTER STRENGTHS	Core Session 5: Student Group

Goals	• Define character strengths and virtues, and how use of strengths can impact feelings of happiness in the present. • Explore students' perceived character strengths. • Reinforce acts of kindness.
Overview of Procedures	A. Review Homework: Performing Acts of Kindness B. Group Discussion: Character Strengths and Virtues C. Student Identification of Perceived Character Strengths D. Group Discussion: Positive Feelings in the Present E. Homework: Continue Performing Acts of Kindness
Materials	• Tangible rewards for homework completion (candy, stickers, etc.) • Blackboard, white board, or easel • Lined paper • *VIA Classification of 24 Character Strengths* handout • *Performing Acts of Kindness Record Form* handout

Procedures Defined

A. Review Homework Assignment: Performing Acts of Kindness

Assignment Completion and Reward	• Ask students about their progress with completing all five acts of kindness during the week. • Provide a small tangible reward (e.g., candy) for homework completion. • If students did not perform the acts of kindness as planned, problem solve barriers and explain that they will have another opportunity to do so this week. Stress the importance of continued effort between sessions for changes in happiness to occur.
Reflection	• Ask students to share two to three acts of kindness they carried out. • Discuss the significance of acts of kindness in terms of positive feelings about the present, ensuring that the acts performed benefited someone else at the cost of the student's time and/or effort. o *How did the people who benefited from your kind act(s) respond?* o *How did you feel following the kind act(s)?* • Inform students that their homework for this week will be to continue doing acts of kindness in the same manner.

B. Group Discussion: Character Strengths and Virtues

Park and colleagues (2004) defined character strengths as "traits that reflect thoughts, feelings, and behaviors" (p. 603). These strengths are identifiable but related and used voluntarily in differing degrees by individuals. Strengths are dispositions to act that require judgment and enable people to thrive. On this basis, lead the following discussion.

(continued)

Set the Stage; Distinguish Character Strength from Talent	*How would you define a character strength or virtue of a person?* • Encourage an active discussion of the meanings of these words. • Be sure to discuss that character strengths are moral strengths done by choice, which is different from talents: *Talents are qualities that you are born with but may be improved somewhat by purposeful actions (e.g., perfect pitch in your singing voice, rhythm in dance, running speed). However, character strengths are moral virtues that are built up and used by choice (honesty, kindness, fairness, creativity).* • Provide examples of your own talents versus moral strengths.
Introduce the VIA Classification System for Strengths	• Distribute the *VIA Classification of 24 Character Strengths* handout. • Interactively discuss the meanings of each of the 24 identified strengths. • With a round-robin method, ask each student to read aloud one of the character strength definitions and say what that means to him or her; ensure that students understand meanings by clarifying definitions as necessary. • Describe each virtue category before students read and discuss the strengths that comprise them. This will give the character strengths context and clarify that the broad virtue categories are more general, not character strengths in themselves. • Continue the round-robin to ensure each student has several turns to define and discuss character strengths.

C. Student Identification of Perceived Character Strengths

Strengths Spotting	• Retrieve students' completed "You at Your Best" activity (from leader binder or student folder) from the first group session. • Ask students to reread their stories to themselves. • Briefly summarize the "You at Your Best" story you shared earlier, and suggest some character strengths (consistent with the terminology used in the *VIA Classification of 24 Character Strengths* handout) of your own that you demonstrated in that story. • Ask students to identify which strengths listed on the *Classification of 24 Character Strengths* handout they personally demonstrated in the context of their "You at Your Best" stories. • Ask students to discuss strengths they have seen the other students in their group display in the context of the group meetings or elsewhere, such as in class or in another situation at school.
Identify Perceived Top Five Character Strengths	• Considering these strengths that students have noticed in themselves, or that their peers have recognized in them, ask students to identify what they believe are their top five strengths, as selected from the *VIA Classification of 24 Character Strengths* handout. ○ Ask each student to write down his or her own identified strengths on a piece of lined paper. ○ Ask students to share the strengths they chose for themselves and write them out on the white board. ○ Assist students to look at the strengths shared by different group members.

(continued)

185

D. Group Discussion: Positive Feelings in the Present	
Introduce the Actions–Feelings Connection	• Discuss the connection between how using character strengths may relate to feelings of happiness in the present (your day-to-day life): *When you are using your character strengths in everyday life, what are your thoughts and feelings typically like?* • Record students' ideas on the board. Add and discuss these ideas as needed: o Focus on current efforts; concentration. o Engaging in challenges that build on abilities and skills. o Absorption in a task where time flies by. o Creating and working on clear goals. o Immediate feedback from others and yourself. o Sense of self-control.
Revisit the Determinants of Happiness Theory: **Emphasis on Purposeful Activities**	• Review the *What Determines Happiness?* figure and discuss how good feelings resulting from use of character strengths are due to the choice and effort in using them; thus, enacting character strengths is another example of a purposeful activity tied to happiness. Provide an example: *A cashier undercharges you for your order. Although you think that the items are overpriced and you really want to keep the extra money, you tell the cashier that you owe more than he stated. (Or: You are walking behind a man at the mall. A 20-dollar bill falls to the ground. Although you have something you would like to buy and you really want to keep the extra money, you call out "Hey mister, you dropped some money" and run after him with the $20 you picked up). You feel good about yourself afterward because you chose to exercise your character strength of honesty.* • Ask students to pick one of the strengths they listed for themselves and explain to the group how it may take effort to use it. • Explain that the next few sessions will focus more on discovering and using top character strengths.
Prepare for Focus on Strengths	• Collect each student's list of self-identified strengths; store in your group binder for reference during the next session. • Explain that students will complete an online survey to identify their character strengths in the next session, and compare the strengths they chose for themselves with the survey results.

E. Homework: Continue Performing Acts of Kindness	
Assign	*Just like last week, I want you to pick a day this week to perform five acts of kindness. Remember, changes in happiness occur with repeated use of exercises such as performing acts of kindness.* • Distribute an *Acts of Kindness Record Form* to jot down their plans as well as to record additional kind acts after they have been performed. • Ask students to decide on a date to perform five acts of kindness. • Remind students that acts of kindness are small-to-large actions that benefit or make others happy, typically at the cost of their time and effort.
Looking Ahead	• Inform students that they will be asked to share two to three of their acts of kindness and related feelings in the next group meeting. • Students should leave the meeting with the *Acts of Kindness Record Form* added to their homework folder. • Remind students of the incentives they can receive contingent on homework completion and return of the *Acts of Kindness Record Form*.

Session Protocols for Core Intervention Guide
for School Mental Health Providers

ASSESSMENT OF SIGNATURE CHARACTER STRENGTHS	Core Session 6: Student Group

Goals	• Identify students' signature strengths through a survey that assesses multiple aspects of each strength. • Discuss students' individual signature character strengths. • Explore new ways to use one signature strength. • Develop individualized plan for new uses of one signature strength.
Overview of Procedures	A. Review Homework: Performing Acts of Kindness B. Survey Assessment of Character Strengths C. Discussion: Expected versus Survey-Identified Signature Strengths D. Homework: Use the First Signature Strength in a New Way
Materials	• Tangible rewards for homework completion (candy, stickers, etc.) • Blackboard, white board, or easel • Students' handwritten lists of self-identified strengths created in the previous session • Lined paper • Access to computer lab and the Internet • *VIA Classification of 24 Character Strengths* handout • *New Uses of My First Signature Strength* handout • *Performing Acts of Kindness Record Form* handout

Procedures Defined

A. Review Homework Assignment: Performing Acts of Kindness

Assignment Completion and Reward	• Ask students about their progress with completing all five acts of kindness during the week. • Provide a small tangible reward (e.g., candy) for homework completion. • If students did not perform the acts of kindness as planned, problem solve barriers. Stress the importance of continued effort between sessions for changes in happiness to occur.

Reflection	• Ask students to share one or two acts of kindness they carried out.
	• Discuss the significance of acts of kindness in terms of positive feelings about the present; emphasize the benefit to others that came at the cost of the student's time and/or effort.
	  o *How did the people who benefited from your kind act(s) respond?*
	  o *How did you feel following the kind act(s)?*
	• Inform students that their homework for this week will have two parts, one of which they will plan today (use of character strengths in new ways). For the second part, students are encouraged to continue completing activities that increase their happiness by choosing between continuing acts of kindness or returning to their gratitude journal.

B. Survey Assessment of Character Strengths

The VIA Inventory of Strengths for Youth (VIA–Youth) was developed by Park and Peterson (2006) as an extension of their original adult version. The aim of this assessment is to identify individual

(continued)

adolescents' personal ranking of the 24 character strengths with particular emphasis on their top five strengths, known as signature character strengths. The VIA Institute recently developed a shorter assessment of the 24 character strengths in youth ages 10–17. Seligman (2011) discussed how use of one's signature strengths is a key route to sustainable increases in happiness.

Prepare	Prior to this session, register on the website *www.character.org* or *www. authentichappiness.org*. This will permit you access to the online version of the VIA Youth Survey or the VIA–Youth, respectively. You can log on multiple student users on separate computers, simultaneously under your account/logon, thus precluding the student from having to enter personal information or create his or her own account on a website.
Complete the VIA– Youth	• Explain that researchers have developed a survey that helps people identify and rank their character strengths. The top five strengths are called *signature character strengths.* • Explain there is a website on the Internet with surveys designed to help people identify their signature strengths, specifically *www.viacharacter.org* [alternative full-length (198-item) youth VIA survey can be accessed at *www.authentichappiness.org*]. o Once on the website, scroll down and click on the "Take Survey" link. o Select the link for the VIA Survey for Youth. o Follow the online instructions for registering the student and completing the survey. o Read aloud the instructions for completing the questions provided online. • Monitor students as they individually complete the survey; answer questions as necessary and provide encouragement to complete the survey, which may take 15–40 minutes depending on youth reading speed and version of survey selected (brief or original).

C. Discussion: Expected versus Survey-Identified Signature Strengths

Review of Top Character Strengths Yielded from the VIA–Youth	• As a student completes the online survey, print out his or her top five signature character strengths. If a printer is not available, circle the signature strengths on the *VIA Classification of 24 Character Strengths* handout; number them from 1 to 5 as indicated by the website feedback. o *Note:* If a student expresses disagreement with a top five strength as "not true for me," click on the "display all strengths" option and replace the disputed strength with the sixth (or seventh, if needed) strength identified in the assessment. • Give students an opportunity to review the printout (or individualized *VIA Classification of 24 Character Strengths* handout) and their handwritten lists of self-identified strengths (as completed last session). • On an individual and/or small-group level (depending on students' rate of survey completion), discuss the following topics: o *Are your signature strengths from the survey the same or different from the strengths you wrote about yourself before we went online?* o *Reactions to your computer-generated signature strengths?* ▪ Expect surprise, expected, happy, disappointed, or curious.
Identify *Signature* Character Strengths	• Introduce the notion of "signature strengths": *Sometimes the computer-generated strengths don't feel like they are a good fit. That's OK; just don't concentrate on using them. Instead, think about how you use the strengths that do fit you. The ones that fit may feel just right, may be exciting to use, may help you to do well in new activities, may be something you enjoy doing, may be something that gets you pumped up, or something you want to try using in different ways.*

(continued)

- Example of leadership as a signature strength:

    You may be the kind of person who thinks that being a leader is something you can do well, you get excited about the chance to lead groups in class work, in sports, or on trips, or you may already be a leader on your football team but you also want to be student government president and lead a food drive at school for Thanksgiving. Being a leader just feels like it is right for you.

- *Are there any strengths that you feel just don't fit you? Why?*
    o Examples of ways strengths may not fit:
        - Strength doesn't feel "like me."
        - Not comfortable using the strength.
        - Can't think of example situations they could use the strength.
- Assist students to cross off on their printout any strengths that don't seem to fit, as these are not signature strengths.

Current and Future Strengths Use	• *Which of your signature strengths do you use often?* • *Can you think of ways you have used your signature strengths recently?* • Ask students to pick one strength they would like to work on this week and give an example of one way they already use that strength. • Explain the homework assignment to individual or small groups of students.

D. Homework: Use the First Signature Strength in a New Way

Assignment 1	*I want you to use the signature strength you picked in* new ways *each day of the upcoming week.* • Help the student brainstorm ideas of new ways to use the strength; other students can offer ideas, especially if they chose the same strength to target. • Distribute the *New Uses of My First Signature Strength* record form to jot down their plans. Ask students to write down the feelings they had after they used their strength each day, as well as record additional different ways that they used the strength during the week. • Encourage students to try a different way to use the character strength if they encounter obstacles with the plan on their record form. • Store copies of the VIA–Youth results, lists of perceived strengths, and *New Uses of My First Signature Strength* record form in the group binder.
Assignment 2	• Ask students to choose whether they will continue doing acts of kindness or return to their gratitude journal. Note their selection so you can follow-up appropriately next session. • Distribute an *Acts of Kindness Record Form* if relevant. • Review procedures for gratitude journaling if relevant.
Looking Ahead	• Inform students that they will be asked to share their signature strengths and two new uses and related feelings in the next group meeting. • Students should leave the meeting with the *New Uses of My First Signature Strength* record form, as well as the printout of their top five signature strengths, added to their homework folder. • Remind students of the incentives they can receive contingent on homework completion and return of the *New Uses of My First Signature Strength* record form.

Session Protocols for Core Intervention Guide for School Mental Health Providers

USE OF SIGNATURE STRENGTHS IN NEW WAYS AND SAVORING	*Core Session 7:* *Student Group*

Goals	• Explore students' use of their signature strengths in new ways and problem solve obstacles. • Make connections between activities that use signature strengths and positive feelings. • Explore new ways to use signature strengths across life domains. • Learn methods of savoring to expand positive experiences with use of signature strengths.
Overview of Procedures	A. Review Homework: New Uses of the First Signature Strength B. Explore and Plan New Uses of Signature Strengths across Life Domains C. Group Discussion: Savor the Experience D. Homework: Use the Second Signature Strength in New Ways with Savoring
Materials	• Tangible rewards for homework completion (candy, stickers, etc.) • Blackboard, white board, or easel • List of signature character strengths from the previous session • *VIA Classification of 24 Character Strengths* handout • *New Uses of My Second Signature Strength* handout • *Performing Acts of Kindness Record Form* handout

Procedures Defined

A. Review Homework Assignment: New Uses of the First Signature Strength

Assignment Completion and Reward	• Ask students their progress with acts of kindness *or* gratitude journaling. • Ask students about their progress with using a signature strength in new ways each day since the last session. • Provide a small tangible reward (e.g., candy) for homework completion. • If students did not use their character strength as planned, or complete the record form, problem solve barriers. Stress the importance of continued effort between sessions for changes in happiness to occur.
Reflection	• Ask students to share one act of kindness *or* one item on a gratitude entry. • Ask students to share with the group their signature strengths from the online survey, and how well that matched up to the ones they wrote for themselves (refer students to the copies of their VIA–Youth results and their self-generated lists of strengths in the binder if needed). • Ask students to get into pairs and interview their partner about the signature strength they chose to enact for homework. • Each partner should talk about two examples of new ways each used his or her chosen signature strength during last week, and share his or her feelings related to the use of strengths. The partners will then report to the group. • If challenges to using a strength arise, lead a problem-solving discussion with the group regarding how to overcome and avoid identified obstacles.

(continued)

B. Explore and Plan New Uses of Signature Strengths across Life Domains	

People who use their signature strengths in new ways show some of the greatest and most enduring gains in happiness, even compared with the effects of other positive psychology interventions (Seligman et al., 2005). Lasting happiness comes from using signature strengths across life domains. For youth, we focus on school, friendships, and family.

Explore Current Use of Strengths	*In which ways do you currently use your signature strengths?* • Prompt students to pick two strengths (different from the one they worked on for homework) and share examples of how they have shown that strength in school, friendships, and/or with family. • Use a round-robin method so each student has an opportunity to share. • Explain that research findings show that use of character strengths *in new ways* is a good way to increase happiness in the present (emphasis on not just using strengths more, but in *new and different ways* than ever before).

Domains of Life	• Explain that there are three important areas of life for students their age, including school, friendship, and family. To maximize happiness, utilize character strengths in new ways in each area of life.
	  o Provide an example:
	    A student whose signature strength is creativity can use it in school by joining the art club or organizing the layout of the school newspaper, in friendship by thinking of new activities friends can do together, and with family by coming up with new ways to save family memories, such as in a scrapbook.

Plan Future Strengths Use	• Ask students to pick a signature strength that they would like to work on this week (which may not be the same as last week's homework). • Distribute lined paper; ask students to independently make a list of ways to use this signature strength that are unique or different from prior usage. • Monitor the lists to ensure activities listed are manageable and concrete. For instance, if a student's character strength is "fairness," maybe he or she can intervene when he or she sees a younger or smaller sibling getting taken advantage of by an older relative. Such a plan is more feasible than joining the student council between groups. • Write the life domain categories on the board. • Ask for two volunteers to share their lists with the group. • Ask an individual volunteer to state the signature strength and ways in which he or she has thought about using it differently. For each suggested use, ask the group which life domain category the activity would go under—record the activity under the appropriate heading on the board. • Ask the group to brainstorm other ideas for use of this strength; add them to the board under the appropriate life domain. • Clarify any suggestions that may stray from the meaning of the strength and guide students to more targeted suggestions. Keep the *VIA Classification of 24 Character Strengths* handout accessible in the event students need help remembering the meanings of the strengths. • Distribute the *New Uses of My Second Signature Strength* record form. • Ask the volunteer student to write down the ideas that appeal to him or her on the *New Uses of My Second Signature Strength* record form, making sure to note the life domain. Do not plan the days just yet. • Ask the volunteer student to identify potential obstacles to carrying out the strength use plan this week. Problem solve with the group in terms of how those obstacles could be addressed or avoided.

(continued)

- Time permitting, repeat this process with a second volunteer.
- Ask students to form small groups, preferably that include students who selected the same strength to target. Members of the group should help one another complete their *New Uses of My Second Signature Strength* record form by going through their prepared lists of uses of strengths and determining domains as well as brainstorming other ideas and problem solving potential obstacles. Ideally, each small group is facilitated by a co-leader and assisted by the student volunteer(s) who has already prepared his or her record form.
- Once each student in the small group has prepared his or her record form, tell students to write in the days this week they think they can do each of the ways to use their strengths. The days do not have to be in order, but each day of the week should be designated for use of their strength.
- Make a copy of each student's *New Uses of My Second Signature Strength* record form.

C. Group Discussion: Savor the Experience

Bryant and Veroff (2007) defined savoring as attending to, appreciating, and enhancing the positive qualities of one's life. In middle school students, youth who savor (maximize) a positive event are more likely to maintain highly positive emotions about the situation, whereas minimizing a positive event is tied to symptoms of internalizing and externalizing problems (Gentzler et al., 2013).

Introduce Savoring; Relate to Positive Feelings in the Present	Savoring *is the term for when you pay attention to, appreciate, and boost your positive experiences in the present. When you savor, you pay extra close attention to things that you are enjoying now, such as when you pay attention to the taste of a favorite meal, the notes in a favorite song, or a job well done. What are some things that you think would be worth savoring?* • Prompt for preferred foods, vacations, activities, events, friendships, TV shows, and so on. *Savoring makes us happier by stretching out the positive feelings of those activities, foods, events, and so on, to last longer in the present. When you savor, you slow down time by purposefully focusing on the good experience before moving on to something else. Instead of going fast into future stuff, you stay and enjoy the present moment.*

Ways to Savor	*We can make the good feelings we have when using our signature strengths last longer by savoring.*
	 • Introduce two easy ways to savor that take very little time:
	 1. Share the experience with someone else: *You could tell a friend or relative about how you used your strength, and how it felt to use it.*
	     o *You already savored in this way when we went over homework and you interviewed each other . . . you shared your positive experiences.*
	     o *When talking to your partner, did you relive the good feelings that came from using your strength earlier in the week?*
	 2. Absorb yourself: *Take a minute to close your eyes and think about your positive experience, and the specific good feelings you had; you could even congratulate yourself on a job well done.*
	     o *Let's all practice absorbing ourselves now. Think about one of the ways you used your strength for homework. How did it feel? How did others react? Was it something you could congratulate yourself on?*
	     o Instruct everyone to close their eyes for a minute to savor.

(continued)

    o Share how good you feel after reflecting on a use of your strengths. Explain the good feelings connected to your recent actions.

    o Ask for one or two volunteers to share their reflections.

D. Homework: Use the Second Signature Strength in New Ways with Savoring	
Assignment 1	*I want you to use the signature strength you picked in* new ways *each day of the upcoming week, across life domains as you prepared on the* New Uses of My Second Signature Strength *record form.* • Ask students to use their record form to write down the feelings they had after they used their strength each day, record additional different ways that they used the strength during the week, and note how they savored the experiences (e.g., who they talked to or when they thought about it). • Encourage students to try a different way to use the character strength if they encounter obstacles with the plan on their record form. • Store a copy of the *New Uses of My Second Signature Strength* planning form in the group binder.
Assignment 2	• Ask students to choose whether they will perform acts of kindness or complete a gratitude journal. Note their selection so you can follow-up appropriately next session. • Distribute an *Acts of Kindness Record Form* if relevant. • Review procedures for gratitude journaling if relevant.
Looking Ahead	• Inform students that they will be asked to share one to two new uses of the strength, related feelings, and methods of savoring in the next group meeting. • Students should leave the meeting with the *New Uses of My Second Signature Strength* record form added to their homework folder. • Remind students of the incentives they can receive contingent on homework completion and return of the *New Uses of My Second Signature Strength* record form.

Session Protocols for Core Intervention Guide
for School Mental Health Providers

OPTIMISTIC THINKING	Core Session 8: Student Group

Goals	• Make connections among activities that use signature strengths, savoring, and positive feelings. • Define optimistic thinking and how it can impact happiness as related to the future. • Learn the method for developing an optimistic explanatory style.
Overview of Procedures	A. Review Homework: Use Signature Strength in New Ways with Savoring B. Group Discussion: Initial Definition and Importance of Optimism C. Develop an Optimistic Explanatory Style D. Homework: Optimistic Thinking
Materials	• Tangible rewards for homework completion (stickers, candy, pencils, etc.) • Blackboard, white board, or easel • Lined paper • *New Uses of My Third Signature Strength* handout • *Examples of Optimistic Thinking* handout • *My Optimistic Thoughts* handout

Procedures Defined

A. Review Homework Assignment: Use Signature Strength in New Ways with Savoring

Assignment Completion and Reward	• Ask students about their progress with acts of kindness *or* gratitude journaling. • Ask students about their progress with using a signature strength in new ways each day, followed by savoring, since the last session. • Provide a small tangible reward (e.g., candy) for homework completion. • If students did not use their character strength as planned, or savor, or complete the record form, problem solve barriers. Stress the importance of continued effort between sessions for changes in happiness to occur.
Reflection	• Ask students to share one act of kindness *or* one item on a gratitude entry. • Ask students to provide one to two examples of ways they used the signature strength they chose to enact for homework. • Encourage reflection on their feelings related to the use of strengths. • Ask students how they savored the experience and how that may have enhanced positive feelings. • Facilitate group discussion and encouragement over one another's use of strengths and savoring. • If challenges to using a strength arose, lead a problem-solving discussion with the group regarding how to overcome and avoid identified obstacles. • Ask students to choose a different signature strength to target for homework, and independently complete the *Uses of My Third Signature Strength* record form during this week (applying the process learned last week).

(continued)

B. Group Discussion: Initial Definition and Importance of Optimism	
Set the Stage	*What is optimism?* • Facilitate a brief discussion on what students think optimism means. *We've all had people tell us to think more optimistically, to smile, or to be positive. What does thinking optimistically mean to you?* • Record students' responses on the board. Circle and discuss key terms, phrases, and or themes. Provide a common definition, such as: *You feel optimism when you feel that your future holds many positive events because of your talents and effort; bad things that happen will be short-lived.*
Rate Your Optimism	*We are going to rate our own level of optimism.* • Draw a number line from 0 to 10 on a white board. • Distribute small, blank pieces of paper. *Think about how often you have been optimistic in the past few months. On a scale from 0 to 10 with 0 being never optimistic, 5 being sometimes optimistic, and 10 being always optimistic, rate your optimism.* • Ask students to write their ratings on a piece of paper and pass it to the group leader. The group leader will circle each of the numbers indicated by the students on the number line and discuss the overall group range.
Shared Reflection	• In a round-robin fashion, ask each student share his or her number and the reason he or she chose it.

Introduce Links between Optimism and Happiness	*Why may optimism be important?*
	• *Do you think it is valuable to be optimistic?*
	• *Do you think being an optimist can increase happiness? Why or why not?*
	• *How can being optimistic help you in school? In friendships? In family life?*
	• *How is optimism related to your happiness about the future?*
	   o Cover resilience in the discussion. Example script:
	
	    Optimistic thinking leads to resilience: feeling like you can face any bad situation and come out OK.
	
	• *Because of resilience, you are more likely to try when things get hard.*
	• *A person who doesn't think optimistically may instead feel helpless and give up easily, which means missing out on possible success.*
	• *However, a resilient person keeps trying until he or she accomplishes what he or she wants in life.*
	• *Remember, we discussed increasing happiness through purposeful activities. Optimistic thinking is one form of purposeful activity (in this case, a purposeful attitude) and it can help you get involved in other kinds of activities as well.*

C. Develop an Optimistic Explanatory Style	

The focus of this activity is on using Seligman's (1990) description of an optimistic explanatory style to increase optimistic thinking. Rather than completely changing students' explanatory style, the goal of this activity is to teach students how to increase the use of optimistic thinking.

Explain Optimistic Thinking	*Everyone can learn to think more optimistically, even those who already rated themselves highly on optimism.* • Distribute the *Examples of Optimistic Thinking* handout. *Look at your worksheet. Optimistic thinking is broken into two categories: the way you look at good events and the way you look at bad events. Thinking optimistically means:*

(continued)

- *Thinking about* good things *in your life as being* permanent, *such as being caused by your traits and abilities. Look at the "Good Events" column under "Permanent."*
  - *You might say, "I made the goal because I'm talented in sports." A talent is a permanent ability.*
- *Also, you would* see bad events as temporary, *only lasting as long as your mood or effort. Look at the "Bad Events" column under "Temporary."*
  - *That would be like saying, "Even Beckham would have missed that one; I'll probably make the next goal I try for." The missed goal was a one-time thing.*
- *Also, optimists* see good events as widespread—*that is, happening throughout life. Look at the "Good Events" column under "Widespread."*
  - *That would be like thinking, "I do well in my classes because I check my agenda and do my homework every day after school." Good homework habits are something that are part of your routine, and affect your performance in all of your classes.*
- *Optimists* see negative events as specific *to certain areas of life. Look at the "Bad Events" column under "Specific."*
  - *You may think, "I made a poor grade on my math test because I did not understand the ideas that were taught when I was out sick." Math is only one subject, not all of school. The test you did poorly on covered the material you missed, not all of math. When you are present for the lessons, you could do better at a math test.*
- *Optimists* take credit for causing good events *in their lives but* blame other sources for bad events.
  - *Look at the "Good Events" column under "Take Credit." An optimist would think, "I won the contest because of my effort and talent in creative writing." You won the contest because of your hard work and talent, not something other people did.*
  - *Look at the "Bad Events" column under "Blame Other Sources." An optimist would think, "I lost the contest because I needed better materials to prepare myself." You lost the contest because of poor materials, not because you didn't try hard.*

Practice Thinking Optimistically	• Guide students to complete the practice section of the *Examples of Optimistic Thinking* worksheet.
	• Help students to identify events as good or bad and develop optimistic thoughts corresponding to events.

First, read the event and then decide if it is a good or bad situation.

- *If it is a good situation, write an optimistic thought that is* permanent, widespread, *or takes credit. If it is a bad situation, write an optimistic thought that is* temporary, specific, *or blames another source.*
- Point to the *Examples of Optimistic Thinking* worksheet as providing an explanation.

Let's do the first one together.

- *Is this a good or bad situation? It's a good event. Write "good" under the event.*
  - *What's something* permanent *that I can say about it?*
  - *What about* widespread?
  - Taking credit?

Complete the rest on your own and then we'll discuss.

(continued)

- Monitor students' work to make sure that they use this format for all of the answers. Examples of optimistic thoughts include (in order of appearance on the *Examples of Optimistic Thinking* worksheet):
  o This is a good event:
    - Permanent: "I was invited because I am a fun person."
    - Widespread: "I was invited because I am always cheerful."
    - Taking credit: "I was invited because I helped come up with ideas for the theme of the party."
  o This is a bad event:
    - Temporary: "She probably isn't feeling well and will call me as soon as she is better."
    - Specific: "My other friends have called me back, so if there is a problem, it is just between the two of us."
    - Blame other sources: "She has been under a lot of stress with having trouble in school and her parents arguing; she may not feel like talking, and it probably doesn't have anything to do with me."
  o This is a good event:
    - Permanent: "My parents increased my allowance because I have shown that I am a responsible person."
    - Widespread: "My parents have increased my allowance and may make my curfew later because they trust me to be responsible in school, at home, and with my friends."
    - Taking credit: "It was because I made the effort to show them how responsible I can be by taking care of our pet, that my parents increased my allowance."
  o This is a good event:
    - Permanent: "My science group did well because we are smart, hardworking students."
    - Widespread: "I always do well on my class projects because I work well in groups."
    - Taking credit: "I had a large part in why our group did well because I organized our project and acted as the group leader."
  o This is a bad event:
    - Temporary: "I did poorly on my assignment because I only had a little bit of time to work on it. I will start on the next assignment sooner and likely do much better."
    - Specific: "This was a very difficult assignment, not like most of my schoolwork. I have done well on other projects."
    - Blame other sources: "I didn't have enough time for this project because of other responsibilities, which distracted me from doing my best."

Shared Reflection	• After the independent writing time is over, prompt each student to share one to two of their responses with the group.

(continued)

D. Homework: Optimistic Thinking

Assignment 1	*I want you to* purposefully use optimistic thinking one time each day *until the next session. Record the situation and your optimistic thought on the* My Optimistic Thoughts *record form. Let's complete the first line together.* • Distribute the *My Optimistic Thoughts* record form. • Ask two or three students to volunteer a situation from their day (or yesterday). • Ask the first student to describe the situation and then briefly write it under the event or situation category. • Ask the student to decide if it was a good or bad event and fill in that column accordingly. • Ask the student how the situation could be thought of more optimistically; encourage thoughts from other students, particularly if the student struggles to generate optimistic thoughts. *Remember: If the situation is negative, the optimistic thought must be temporary, specific, and/or blaming another source. If it is positive, the thought must be permanent, widespread, and/or taking credit for oneself.*
Assignment 2	• Ask students to use their chosen signature strength in a new way each day and complete the *New Uses of My Third Signature Strength* record form. • Help students brainstorm ways to use their strengths and note ideas on their record form as time allows. • Store a copy of the *New Uses of My Third Signature Strength* planning form in the group binder.
Looking Ahead	• Inform students that they will be asked to share one to two situations that they experienced and then thought about in an optimistic way. • Students should leave the meeting with the *New Uses of My Third Signature Strength* record form and the *My Optimistic Thoughts* record form added to their homework folder. • Remind students of the incentives they can receive contingent on homework completion and return of the *My Optimistic Thoughts* and *New Uses of My Third Signature Strength* record forms.

Session Protocols for Core Intervention Guide
for School Mental Health Providers

HOPE	Student Group

Goals	• Make connections between optimistic thinking and positive feelings. • Define hope (i.e., goal directed) and how it can impact happiness as related to the future. • Learn the method for developing hope by envisioning goals, paths to achieve goals, and motivation for success.
Overview of Procedures	A. Review Homework: Optimistic Thinking B. Initial Appraisal of Hope C. Group Discussion: Definition and Importance of Hope D. Writing Activity: Best Possible Self in the Future E. Homework: Best Possible Self in the Future (Expanded)
Materials	• Tangible rewards for homework completion (stickers, candy, pencils, etc.) • Blackboard, white board, or easel • Lined paper • *Examples of Optimistic Thinking* handout • *New Uses of My Fourth Signature Strength* handout • *My Optimistic Thoughts* handout • *Acts of Kindness Record Form* handout

Procedures Defined

A. Review Homework Assignment: Optimistic Thinking

Assignment Completion and Reward	• Ask students about their progress with using a signature strength in new ways each day, followed by savoring, since the last session. • Ask students about their progress with optimistic thinking each day since the last session. • Provide a small tangible reward (e.g., candy) for homework completion. • If students did not use optimistic thinking as planned or complete the record form, problem solve barriers. Stress the importance of continued effort between sessions for changes in happiness to occur.
Reflection	• Ask students to share one to two examples of ways they used their strength and the feelings that co-occurred or followed. Did savoring stretch out those positive feelings? Were there any problems the group could help with? • Ask the group how they felt using optimistic thinking. o Did it produce any positive feelings about situations? o Was it difficult to do? o Anything they liked or did not like about completing the activity?

(continued)

- Ask volunteers to read some of their situations (approximately two) and their corresponding optimistic thoughts. *Reminder: If the situation is negative, the optimistic thought must be temporary, specific, and/or blaming another source. If it is positive, the thought must be permanent, widespread, and/or taking credit for oneself.*
  - If the student does not follow this format, review the examples on the *Examples of Optimistic Thinking* handout and assist with rewriting the optimistic thought. Group members may provide assistance.
- To show versatility of optimistic thinking, ask the group to think of a different way the situation could be thought of optimistically for two to three student responses.
  - For example, if the event was positive and the student wrote a permanent optimistic thought, challenge students to think of a widespread or taking-credit optimistic thought for the same situation.
- Once each student has had an opportunity to participate, explain the snowball effect of optimistic thinking:

  The great thing about optimistic thinking is that it has a snowball effect. Have you ever heard of a snowball effect? When snowballs roll, they pick up more snow and get bigger. When people start practicing optimistic thinking, it starts to take over how they think. At first, it takes work trying to come up with optimistic thoughts. You have to really think about the situation. But soon it becomes natural and easy. So, keep working on those optimistic thoughts and see if you can get it to snowball.

B. Initial Appraisal of Hope

Set the Stage	*What is hope?* • Facilitate a brief discussion on what students think constitutes hope. • Can provide students with brief definition of hope as "feeling that something desired may happen" or "wishing that certain things will happen" • Record students' responses on the board. • Hope is defined more extensively in the next section.
Rate Your Hope	*We are going to rate our own level of hope.* • Draw a number line from 0 to 10 on the board. • Distribute small, blank pieces of paper. *Think about how often you have felt hope in the past few months. On a scale from 0 to 10 with 0 being* never hopeful, *5 being* sometimes hopeful, *and 10 being* always hopeful, *rate your level of hope.* • Ask students to write their ratings on a piece of paper and fold it over.
Shared Reflection	• In a round-robin fashion, ask each to student share his or her number and the reason he or she chose it.

C. Group Discussion: Definition and Importance of Hope

Snyder and colleagues (2005) define hopeful thinking as comprising both the ability to envision viable methods for goal attainment and belief in one's ability to utilize those methods in reaching specific goals. The following discussion is based on their work.

Present Definition in Line with Hope Theory	*Now that we have shared our ideas about "what is hope," I'm going to tell you how psychologists have defined hope:* *Having hope means believing that you can become motivated and find ways to meet your goals. This is like telling yourself, "I'll find a way to get this done or make this happen!" When an obstacle gets in your way, having hope means believing you can find another way to meet your needs and coming up with ideas on what those other*

(continued)

ways might be. When you are hopeful, you believe that you can reach your goals because you have the ability and can get the resources—you are motivated. You might say to yourself, "Nothing can stop me!" For example, if you want to play basketball but you don't make the school team, then you may organize a recreational team in your neighborhood so that you can play and practice somewhere besides school. Or, if you want to make a new friend and the first person you ask to go to the movies says "no," then you identify another classmate and try a different approach.

Introduce Links between Hope and Happiness	Present discussion questions to the group and ensure the topics below the questions are a part of the conversation:
	
	 Thinking about hope like this, how can it be important or not important in your life? In school? In friendships? With family?
	
	 • School:
	    o Motivation to do well, work harder, be more successful.
	    o Find different ways to meet goals such as get better grades, meet deadlines, or meet entrance criteria for academic programs.
	 • Athletics:
	    o Greater performance because you get "psyched" that you can win, compete, or make it to the end.
	    o Confidence in your abilities.
	    o Willingness to practice harder because you think it will help you win.
	 • Social relationships:
	    o Make new friends.
	    o Work to maintain positive relationships with family and friends.
	 • Emotions:
	    o Good feelings about yourself (self-esteem) and beliefs that you can do well (self-efficacy) because you are motivated and believe you can find ways to meet your goals.
	    o Develop strategies to deal with stress and are motivated to use them because you believe one way will work.
	    o More likely to problem solve when difficult situations occur.
	
	 How do you think hope could impact people's happiness about their future?
	
	 • Allow a few minutes for student volunteers to offer ideas.
	 • Summarize student responses:
	
	 Hope can help us focus on positive goals for our future. It limits feelings of helplessness through believing that there are ways to meet goals.
	
	 • Tie in with optimism:
	
	 Hope works like optimistic thinking about the future, in that people see the things they do now as leading to future benefits across life domains (widespread across school, friends, and family parts of life) and that they are lasting (or permanent parts of the future). On the other hand, misfortunes or problems are seen as temporary and limited to a particular situation, thereby minimizing impact on the future. When thinking that way, people are more likely to believe there are many different ways to meet goals and feel more motivated to work toward those positive future goals.

(continued)

D. Writing Activity: Best Possible Self in the Future

Envisioning and writing about life goals through an exercise termed one's "Best-Possible Self" (a version of the future self that accomplished desired goals) leads to greater happiness (King, 2001; Sheldon & Lyubomirsky, 2006b). This activity focuses on goals, paths to achieve goals, and motivation that provides a concrete way of practicing hopeful thinking.

Provide Rationale	Remind students that they have the ability to change their levels of hope by using hopeful thinking about their futures.
Write about Best Possible Self in the Future	• Introduce activity: *I would like you to think about your life in the future. Take a few minutes to imagine that everything has gone as well as it possibly could. You have worked hard and succeeded at accomplishing all of your life goals.* [Pause for approximately 2 minutes.] *Now write about what you imagined* (adapted from King, 2001). • Provide each student with lined paper. • Allow about 5 minutes for students to write their thoughts and then ask them to share what they have written so far with the group. • Encourage students to provide more detail in describing how they will meet their goals. • Make copies of what they have written thus far; retain a copy in the group binder and return the original to students for storage in their group folder.

E. Homework: Best Possible Self in the Future (Expanded)

Assignment 1	*I want you to continue writing about your best possible selves in the future. Review your story each night and add new thoughts and ideas. You can also make changes to what you have already written.* Focus on identifying ways you can achieve the goals you imagine for your future.
Assignment 2	• Ask students to select an additional positive psychology activity that they have found to be the most personally meaningful. • Offer these choices: acts of kindness, gratitude journals, use another signature strength in a new way each day, or optimistic thinking. Note their selection so you can follow-up appropriately during the next session. • Distribute the corresponding record form as relevant.
Looking Ahead	• Inform students that they will be asked to share at least one goal and one to two ideas for how to reach that goal in the next group meeting. • Students should leave the meeting with the "Best-Possible Self in the Future" story and whatever record form is needed to complete the second assignment added to their homework folder. • Remind students of the incentives they can receive contingent on homework completion and return of their enhanced "Best-Possible Self in the Future" story.

Session Protocols for Core Intervention Guide for School Mental Health Providers

PROGRAM TERMINATION	*Core Session 10:* *Student Group*

Goals	• Make connections between goal-directed thoughts and positive feelings. • Review the theoretical framework for increasing personal happiness. • Review the activities and exercises learned in the group. • Encourage a personal reflection. • Gather students' feedback on exercises perceived to be most helpful and activities they plan to continue.
Overview of Procedures	A. Review Homework: "Best-Possible Self in the Future" and Self-Selected Activity B. Group Discussion: Review of Happiness Framework C. Personal Reflection: Progress during Group D. Wrap-Up and Solicit Student Feedback
Materials	• Tangible rewards for homework completion (stickers, candy, pencils, etc.) • Blackboard, white board, or easel • Lined paper • *What Determines Happiness?* figure • *Happiness Flowchart* figure • *Program Summary Sheet* handout • *Certificate of Completion* • *Program Feedback Request* handout

Procedures Defined

A. Review Homework Assignment: "Best-Possible Self in the Future" and Self-Selected Activity

Assignment Completion and Reward	• Ask students about their progress with the self-selected activity (use strength in new ways, optimistic thinking, acts of kindness, gratitude journaling). • Briefly check students' progress with reviewing and adding to their "Best-Possible Self in the Future" story (this is discussed in greater detail during the reflection). • Provide a small tangible reward (e.g., candy) for homework completion. • If students did not revisit their "Best-Possible Self in the Future" story, problem solve barriers and explain that they will have another opportunity to do so now, at the start of the session. Stress the importance of continued activity practice outside group meetings for changes in happiness to occur.
Reflection, Part 1: Hope	• Ask students to take a few minutes to reread their updated "Best-Possible Self in the Future" writing activity and reflect on their feelings, strengths, plans, accomplishments, and so forth. • Ask students to share their stories with the group, with one to two reflections. ○ Point out the multiple domains of life in which they envisioned their best-possible future selves (e.g., school, athletics, physical health, emotions, relationships). ○ *What changes/additions to your ideas about your best possible self in the future occurred since last session?* ○ *Which goals in life seem most important to you? What ways can you go about achieving those goals?*

(continued)

- Ask whether students felt any different after thinking about their future in a positive manner.
  - *Are you more motivated to work on future goals?*
  - Initiate reflections on group members' stories with identifications or reaffirmations of motivations and goal orientation within the story.
- Encourage group members to reflect on the positives features of one another's stories.
  - Something they admired or liked in the story.
  - Goals they share with the presenter.
  - Other ideas for ways of achieving goals.
- Once each student has had a turn, ask students how this activity has impacted their hope for the future, if at all.

Reflection, Part 2: Independence with Positive Activities	• Ask students to share one to two examples of the activity they chose to do for the second part of homework (gratitude journal, acts of kindness, character strengths, or optimistic thinking). • Why did they choose that activity? • What changes in mood occurred with or after that activity? *You were successful in purposefully selecting and completing a positive activity all on your own, through practicing the strategies you learned in this group. Today is the end of the Well-Being Promotion Program. Your success between our meetings shows how you are ready to continuing practicing the positive activities in your daily life.*

B. Group Discussion: Review of the Happiness Framework

The goal of this program wrap-up is to review some of the primary concepts taught:
- Happiness can be best increased through *the purposeful activities* that we do each day (show the *What Determines Happiness?* figure).
- Lasting happiness comes from positive thoughts and feelings about one's past experiences, present behaviors, and positive views of the future (show the *Happiness Flow Chart* figure).
- Specific activities learned in this group create the positive thoughts and feelings that lead to lasting happiness.
- Continued practice of these activities (purposeful behaviors!), in particular the ones that the student felt "fit" him or her best, is essential to maintain gains in happiness.

Group Review and Reflection	*In the past 10 meetings, we have completed multiple exercises that were designed to improve happiness by changing the activities (thoughts and behaviors) that we do on purpose* [show the *What Determines Happiness?* figure]. • List the exercises on the board for students to access during this discussion (list: "You at Your Best," "Gratitude Journaling," "Gratitude Visits," "Acts of Kindness," "Using Signature Strengths in New Ways," "Savoring," "Optimistic Thinking," and "Best-Possible Self in the Future"). *Which exercises are meant to promote positive feelings about one's past?* • "Gratitude Journaling." • "Gratitude Visits." • "You at Your Best" (could also fit with present, to identify strengths). *How did gratitude improve your satisfaction with your past?* *Which exercises are intended to promote positive emotions in the present?* • "Acts of Kindness."*

(continued)

- "Using Signature Character Strengths in New Ways."
- "Savoring" (positive experiences when using character strengths).

  How did these activities make you feel happier in the moment, feel better about your current life?

  Which exercises are meant to improve your view of the future?

- "Optimistic Thinking."
- Hope ("Best-Possible Self in the Future").

  How did these exercises improve your feelings about the future?

Application to Future Situations; Summarize Activities	• Distribute the *Well-Being Promotion Program Summary Sheet.* To promote application of learned material to future situations, ask students to identify situations/times in which it would be a good idea to use the activities to increase positive thoughts about the past, present, and future in their own future lives (i.e., upon completion of the group).
	○ For instance, in addition to practicing grateful thinking at all times, they may want to enact a gratitude visit or complete a gratitude journal at times they are feeling regret or disappointment with their life circumstances. They may want to do acts of kindness, use strengths in new ways, or savor when they catch themselves feeling "blah" about their day. When they catch themselves feeling hopeless about their future, they should prompt themselves to practice hopeful and/or optimistic thinking.
	○ After students identify perceived emotions that cue them to increase positive thoughts about a specific time period (past, present, and future), ask students to read aloud the definition of activities that correspond to this period (use a round-robin format).
	• *Note:* Students should record their character strengths in their summary sheet during the discussion of planning to improve daily experiences.
	• *Which of these activities did you feel gave you the biggest happiness boost?*
	• *Which do you plan to continue in the future?*
	• *Why that particular activity?*
	• To capitalize on intrinsic motivation, students should plan to keep up those activities that felt natural and enjoyable and are consistent with their values. They should feel free to set aside any activities they completed mostly to gain access to rewards or out of guilt/obligation.

C. Personal Reflection: Progress during Group

It is important to have students think through and reflect on their personal growth during the intervention. Provide them with the following instructions.

Personal Reflection	*Take a few minutes to think of the ways you have changed over the past 10 weeks.* Allow a couple of minutes for students to reflect.
	In general, how have your feelings about your life changed?
	• Follow-up prompts for topics if not included in students' responses:
	○ *Any changes in happiness?*
	○ *What about your feelings about yourself?*
	○ *People in your life?*
	○ *Your past?*
	○ *Your current life?*
	○ *Your future?*

(continued)

D. Wrap-Up and Solicit Student Feedback

- Provide students with the *Certificate of Completion* and express appreciation for their continued efforts over the weeks.
- Distribute the *Program Feedback Request*; ask students to write down their thoughts about their satisfaction with the program/group before leaving.
- Collect postintervention outcome data using the same indicators of subjective well-being administered preintervention (baseline). Data collapsed across participants (i.e., mean scores at each time point) should be compared to assess progress.

What Determines Happiness?*

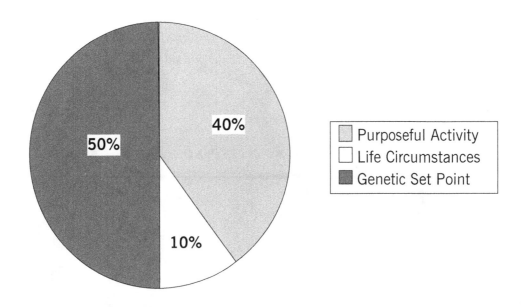

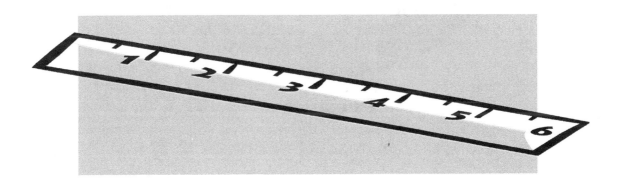

*Based on research reported in Lyubomirsky, Sheldon, and Schkade (2005).

Happiness Flowchart

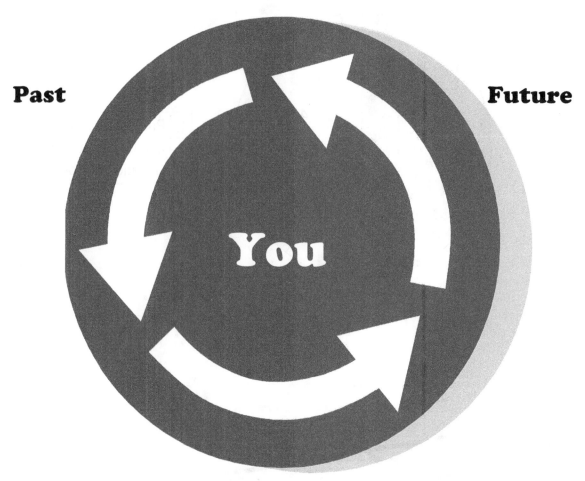

Overview of Program Activities

What Determines Happiness?

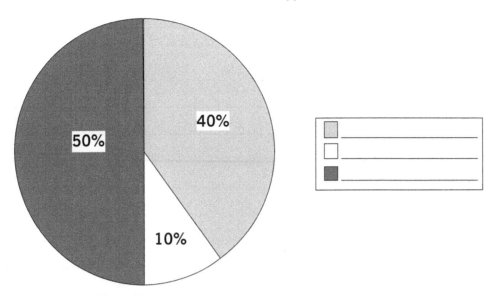

What Is the Purpose of This Well-Being Promotion Group?

1. During our weekly group meetings, which of the three areas that determine happiness are we going to focus on in order to improve our happiness? _____

_____

_____

2. How many times each week are we going to meet? _____

_____

_____

3. How many weeks will we meet? _____

_____

_____

4. What do I need to bring with me to the meetings? _____

_____

_____

Confidentiality

What Is Confidentiality?

_____

_____

_____

_____

_____

_____

_____

_____

_____

_____

How Will I Keep What Students Say in This Group Confidential?

_____

_____

_____

_____

_____

_____

_____

_____

_____

_____

_____

Gratitude Visit Planning Form

People who have been especially kind or helpful to me:

1. _____

2. _____

3. _____

4. _____

5. _____

Person I will make a gratitude visit to: _____

Date: _____   Time: _____

**Reminder: Tell the person that you want to make plans to spend time with him or her. Don't tell him or her about your gratitude letter before the visit. To have the gratitude visit work really well, remember to read your letter out loud to the person. Read slowly with expression and make eye contact.

Performing Acts of Kindness Record Form

Day of the week: _____   Date: _____

<table>
<tr><td rowspan="5">Acts of Kindness</td><td></td></tr>
<tr><td></td></tr>
<tr><td></td></tr>
<tr><td></td></tr>
<tr><td></td></tr>
</table>

VIA Classification of 24 Character Strengths*

Virtue	Strength	Description (features of the character strength)
Wisdom and Knowledge	Creativity	Thinks of new ways to do things; has unique ideas or actions
	Curiosity	Interested in exploring and discovering things; asks a lot of questions
	Love of learning	Likes to become an expert in things; enjoys reading, school, and other chances to learn new information and skills
	Judgment/open-mindedness	Thinks things through from all angles; looks for evidence; does not jump to conclusions
	Perspective	Sees both sides of a story; offers good advice to other people
Courage	Honesty/authenticity	Tells the truth; a "real" person who is down to earth and genuine
	Bravery	Speaks up for what is right; faces challenges head-on
	Persistence/perseverance	Completes tasks; focused and hard-working
	Zest	Energetic; committed; full of excitement for life
Humanity	Kindness	Generous; does favors and good deeds for other people
	Love	Cares and shares with other people; values close relationships
	Social intelligence	Senses thoughts and feelings of self and other people; fits in with different groups while making others feel at ease
Justice	Fairness	Treats all people the same; gives everyone a chance without judging others harshly
	Leadership	Organizes group activities; encourages other people to make sure things get done and that everyone feels included
	Teamwork	Works well with other people; loyal to the group; does own share of work so the team succeeds
Temperance	Forgiveness	Gives people a second chance after they do something wrong; believes in mercy not revenge
	Humility/modesty	Lets achievements speak for themselves; does not seek attention, brag, or feel they are better than everyone else
	Prudence	Makes choices carefully; avoids doing things that he or she might later wish to take back
	Self-regulation	In control of his or her emotions, desires, and behaviors
Transcendence	Appreciation of beauty and excellence	Notices and is in awe of beautiful and special things in the world, such as in nature, art, science, and skilled performances
	Gratitude	Gives thanks for good things that happen; does not take things for granted
	Hope	Believes that good things will happen in the future; works hard to achieve those goals
	Humor	Likes to laugh, tease, and make other people smile
	Spirituality	Believes in a higher purpose and meaning of the universe; may be religious

*The classification system in this handout is reported in Park and Peterson (2006).

New Uses of My First Signature Strength

Signature Strength: _____

Day of the Week	New Use	Feelings

New Uses of My Second Signature Strength

Signature Strength: _____

Day of the Week	Life Domain	New Use	Feelings
			Savor:
			Savor:
			Savor:
			Savor:
			Savor:
			Savor:
			Savor:

**Remember to savor: Make your good feelings last by telling someone about using your strength or taking a minute to close your eyes and think about the experience.

New Uses of My Third Signature Strength

Signature Strength: _____

Day of the Week	Life Domain	New Use	Feelings
			Savor:
			Savor:
			Savor:
			Savor:
			Savor:
			Savor:
			Savor:

**Remember to savor: Make your good feelings last by telling someone about using your strength or taking a minute to close your eyes and think about the experience.

New Uses of My Fourth Signature Strength

Signature Strength:

Day of the Week	Life Domain	New Use	Feelings
			Savor:
			Savor:
			Savor:
			Savor:
			Savor:
			Savor:
			Savor:

**Remember to savor: Make your good feelings last by telling someone about using your strength or taking a minute to close your eyes and think about the experience.

New Uses of My Fifth Signature Strength

Signature Strength:

Day of the Week	Life Domain	New Use	Feelings
			Savor:
			Savor:
			Savor:
			Savor:
			Savor:
			Savor:
			Savor:

**Remember to savor: Make your good feelings last by telling someone about using your strength or taking a minute to close your eyes and think about the experience.

New Uses of My Signature Strength (Child)

Strength:

New Ways I Can Use This Strength:
1.
2.
3.

Day of the Week	New Use	Feelings

Examples of Optimistic Thinking

Examples

Good Events	Bad Events	Event
Permanent	**Temporary**	
I made the goal because I'm talented in sports.	Even Beckham would have missed that one—I'll probably make the next goal I try for.	I was invited to the biggest party of the year.
Widespread	**Specific**	
I do well in my classes because I check my agenda and do my homework after school.	I made a poor grade on my math test because I did not understand the ideas that were taught when I was out sick.	My good friend hasn't called me back in days.
		My parents increased my allowance.
Take Credit	**Blame Other Sources**	
I won the contest because of my effort and talent in creative writing.	I lost the contest because I needed better materials to prepare myself.	My teacher said my science group did the best in the class.
		I had to finish a giant assignment in 3 days and I got a D on it.

Practice

Event	Optimistic Thought

My Optimistic Thoughts

Date	Event or Situation	Is the Event Good or Bad?	Optimistic Thought*

*Remember: Optimistic thoughts for good events are widespread, permanent, and take credit. Optimistic thoughts for bad events are temporary, specific, and blame other sources.

Program Summary Sheet

Name: _____ Date: _____

When I want to feel more positive about my past:
- Gratitude journal
  - Five things I'm grateful for, write down one time each week.
- Gratitude visit
  - Write a letter of thanks to someone who has been kind to me; read the letter to the person.

When I want to feel more positive about my daily life:
- Do acts of kindness
  - Five kind acts for other people in 1 day.
- Use my signature character strengths, which are:

  - _____   _____

  - _____   _____

  - _____

- Savor my successes
  - Tell someone about it or absorb myself (take a few minutes to focus on it).

When I want to feel more positive about my future:
- Optimistic thinking
  - View good situations as permanent, widespread, and take credit for them.
  - View bad situations as temporary, specific, and not totally my fault.
- Hopeful thinking
  - Focus on goals and ways to achieve those goals.

Program Feedback Request

Your Thoughts on the Well-Being Promotion Program

1. What do you feel are some of the most important things you learned in the program?

   _____

   _____

   _____

2. What did you like *best* about the program?

   _____

   _____

   _____

3. What did you like *least* about the program?

   _____

   _____

   _____

4. Which activities that you learned in the meetings are you likely to continue to do on your own?

   ____ "You at your best" writing   ____ Gratitude journal

   ____ Gratitude visit   ____ Acts of kindness

   ____ Savoring   ____ Using my signature strengths in new ways

   ____ Optimistic thinking   ____ "Best-possible self in the future" writing

   ____ None

5. What suggestions do you have to improve the program?

   _____

   _____

   _____

   _____

6. Any additional comments?

   _____

   _____

   _____

Certificate of Completion

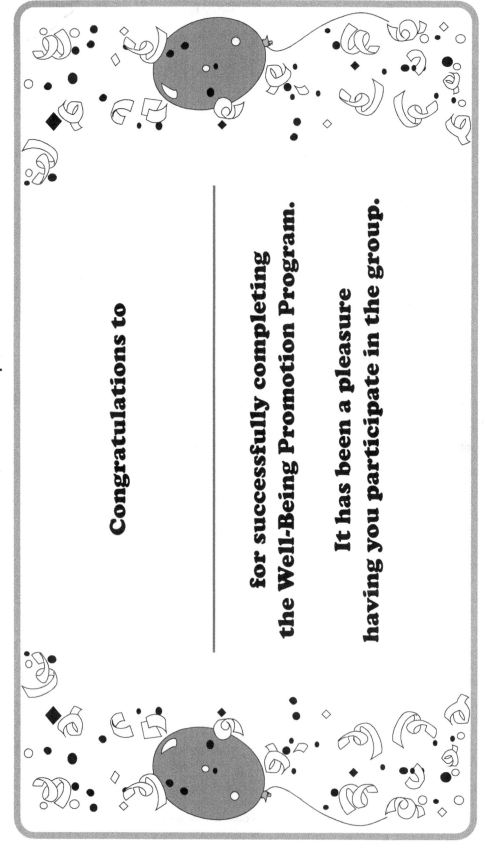

Congratulations to

_____

**for successfully completing
the Well-Being Promotion Program.**

**It has been a pleasure
having you participate in the group.**

Follow-Up Sessions to Promote Maintenance of Gains from the Core Program

PROGRAM REVIEW; SPOTLIGHT ON GRATITUDE	*Follow-Up Session 1: Student Group*

Goals	• Review framework for increasing personal happiness. • Review activities and exercises learned in the intervention. • Discuss progress and activities students have continued since termination. • Practice method for using gratitude to create a focus on positive interpretations of past events.
Overview of Procedures	A. Personal Reflection: Positive Psychology Strategies Used Since Program Termination B. Group Discussion: Review of the Happiness Framework C. Group Discussion: Review of Student Progress and Continued Activities D. Overview of Activities for Further Practice E. Revisit Gratitude Journals
Materials	• Tangible rewards for homework completion (stickers, candy, pencils, etc.) • Blackboard, white board, or easel • Lined paper • *What Determines Happiness?* figure • *Happiness Flowchart* figure • *Program Summary Sheet* handout • Students' gratitude notebooks/journals

Procedures Defined

A. Personal Reflection: Positive Psychology Strategies Used Since Program Termination

Independent Activity	• Welcome students back to group, provide them with notebook paper. • Ask students to write about the positive activities or exercises they engaged in or used the most frequently *in general* since the last meeting. • Ask students to write about the positive strategies they used *in response to difficult situations or during times of distress* since the last meeting. • Inform students that they will have the opportunity to share with the group later their continued use of purposeful activities to maintain happiness. • Ask students about the extent to which they have discussed the Well-Being Promotion Program activities/strategies with their parents since the last meeting.

B. Group Discussion: Review of the Happiness Framework

Group Review and Reflection	• Prior to the session starting, consider listing the exercises on the board for students to access during this discussion (list: "You at Your Best," "Gratitude Journaling," "Gratitude Visits," "Acts of Kindness," "Using Signature Strengths in New Ways," "Savoring," "Optimistic Thinking," "Best-Possible Self in the Future"). *Throughout the 10 weeks of our group meetings, we completed multiple exercises that were designed to improve happiness by changing the activities (thoughts and*

(continued)

behaviors) that we do on purpose. [Reference the What Determines Happiness? figure.]

The exercises we did during the group meetings helped you learn how to purposely create positive ways to use your strengths in the present, how to create positive thoughts about your past, and how to think in ways that create positive views of the future. [Reference the Happiness Flowchart figure.]

It has been a while since we talked about these things, so let's review the main ideas. Which of the exercises are meant to cause positive feelings about your past?

- Gratitude journaling.
- Gratitude visits.
- "You at Your Best" (could also fit with present, to identify strengths).

Since our last meeting, how has gratitude impacted your satisfaction with your past?

Which of the exercises are meant to promote positive emotions in the present?

- "Acts of Kindness."
- "Using Signature Character Strengths in New Ways."
- "Savoring" (positive experiences when using character strengths).

Since our last meeting, in what ways have these activities impacted your feelings and satisfaction with how things are going now, in your current life?

Which exercises did you do that are meant to improve your view of the future?

- "Optimistic Thinking."
- Hope ("Best-Possible Self in the Future").

Since our last meeting, in what ways have these activities impacted your feelings about your future?

C. Group Discussion: Review of Student Progress and Continued Activities

Savoring Successes

Positive Activities as Coping Strategies

Let's talk some more about the activities that you have used since we ended our weekly group meetings, specifically the situations you recalled and wrote about at the beginning of today's meeting.

- Consider reminding students that sharing and reliving success, such as through the use of strengths in everyday life, or benefiting another person through acts of kindness, is an example of savoring in action.

What activities have you used the most often, in general, since we last met?

What are some situations, perhaps times of stress or negative mood, when you used the activities we learned to intentionally increase positive thoughts about the past, present, or future?

- For instance, in addition to practicing grateful thinking pretty much daily, students may have enacted a gratitude visit or completed a gratitude journal at times they felt regret or disappointment with their life circumstances. They may have performed acts of kindness, used their strengths in a new way, or savored when they caught themselves feeling "blah" about their day.
- Encourage each student to share at least one example with the group. If a student cannot identify a time he or she has used a happiness-increasing activity in the face of distress, ask the student to share a minor or major stressor that has occurred since the last meeting, and have him or her receive assistance from group members to generate ideas of activities likely to increase mood in such negative situations.

(continued)

Personal Reflection of Growth	*Take a few minutes to think of the ways you changed over the course of our 10 weekly meetings, and how you have changed or stayed the same since we stopped meeting each week.*
	• Pose these questions to the group:
	  o *How have your feelings about your life changed?*
	  o *Any changes in happiness?*
	  o *What about your feelings about yourself?*
	  o *People in your life?*
	  o *Your past?*
	  o *Your future?*

D. Overview of Activities for Further Practice

Need for Continued Practice	• Continued practice of positive activities (purposeful behaviors!), in particular the ones that the student felt "fit" him or her best, is essential to maintain gains in happiness. *One way to keep improving our lives and feelings is to continue to practice the strategies you learned during our weekly meetings, in particular those that have felt "natural" to you (those activities you have continued to use the most on your own), as well as those exercises and strategies that, upon reflection, you realize have been the most helpful in terms of having a positive impact on your mood. For our remaining time together today, we'll practice grateful thinking. When we meet again for follow-up and review in a couple of weeks, we'll focus on another—using signature strengths in new ways and optimistic thinking.*

E. Revisit Gratitude Journals

Practice Gratitude Journaling	*Remember a while back we learned that keeping a gratitude journal is a way for you to express thanks for the things in life for which you are grateful. Gratitude is linked to feelings of happiness through refocusing our thoughts on the positive parts of our past, which increases positive attitudes about our histories and lives. I would like you to take a few minutes to think about your day and write down five things in your life that you are grateful for, including both small and large things, events, people, talents, or anything else you can think of. Some examples may include generosity of my friends, my teacher giving me extra help, family dinner, your favorite band/singer, and so on.* • Give students about 5 minutes to list five things for which they are grateful. • Prompt the student to be specific with identifying positive situations. • Prompt each student to share one to two of their responses with the group after the independent writing time is over.
Plan for Generalization	*How do you intend to continue gratitude journaling in your daily life?* • Encourage students to continue journaling on a regular basis, for example, each night before bed, Sunday nights when preparing for the week, or during a shared writing activity with a parent.

Follow-Up Sessions to Promote Maintenance of Gains
from the Core Program

PROGRAM REVIEW; SPOTLIGHT ON USE OF CHARACTER STRENGTHS AND OPTIMISTIC THINKING	*Follow-Up Session 2: Student Group*

Goals	• Review progress with gratitude journals. • Review activities and exercises learned in the group. • Review and rehearse method for planning new uses of signature strengths. • Review method for thinking optimistically.
Overview of Procedures	A. Progress with Gratitude Journals B. Group Discussion: Review of the Happiness Framework C. Explore and Plan Uses of the Fifth Signature Strength in New Ways D. Review and Practice: Optimistic Explanatory Style E. Wrap Up and Gratitude for Student Participation
Materials	• Tangible rewards for homework completion (stickers, candy, pencils, etc.). • Blackboard, white board, or easel • *What Determines Happiness?* figure • *Happiness Flowchart* figure • *Classification of 24 Character Strengths* handout • *New Uses of My Fifth Signature Strength* handout • *My Optimistic Thoughts* handout

Procedures Defined

A. Progress with Gratitude Journals

Assignment Completion	*Last time we were together, we discussed gratitude and developed plans for writing down our thoughts in gratitude journals. Please share your progress with continuing to write in your gratitude journals.* • Pose these questions to the group: 　○ *How often did you journal? At what time and where?* 　○ *What types of things did you acknowledge you were grateful for?* 　○ *How did focusing on those events and situations impact your mood?* 　○ *What obstacles did you face when attempting to journal?* 　○ *To what extent were your parents involved in your gratitude journaling?*

B. Group Discussion: Review of the Happiness Framework

Group Review and Reflection	*Throughout our group meetings, we have completed multiple exercises that were designed to improve happiness by changing the activities (thoughts and behaviors) that we do on purpose.* [Show the *What Determines Happiness?* figure.] *The exercises we did during the group meetings helped you learn how to purposely create positive ways to use your strengths in the present, how to create positive thoughts about your past, and how to think in ways that create positive views of the future.* [Show the *Happiness Flowchart* figure.] *Let's review the main ideas. Which of the exercises are meant to cause positive feelings about your past?*

(continued)

- "Gratitude Journaling."
- "Gratitude Visits."
- "You at Your Best" (could also fit with present, to identify strengths).

  Since we last met, how has gratitude impacted your satisfaction with your past?

  Which of the exercises are meant to promote positive emotions in the present?

- "Acts of Kindness."
- "Using Signature Character Strengths in New Ways."
- "Savoring" (positive experiences when using character strengths).

  Since we last met, in what ways have these activities impacted your feelings and satisfaction with how things are going now, in your current life?

  Which exercises did you do that are meant to improve your view of the future?

- "Optimistic Thinking."
- Hope ("Best-Possible Self in the Future").

  Since we last met, in what ways have these activities impacted your feelings about your future?

C. Explore and Plan Uses of the Fifth Signature Strength in New Ways

Using Signature Strengths across Life Domains

- Review the rationale for using signature strengths in new ways.

  Remember a while back we learned that using our character strengths in new and different ways than we have before is a good way to increase happiness in the present. We also learned that in order to use character strengths in new ways to effectively increase happiness, they should be used in multiple areas of life, including school, friendships, and family.

- Ask each student to refer to his or her list of signature strengths.
  - Prompt each student to indicate which strengths he or she has targeted for increased use in prior sessions.
  - Students should then identify a fifth strength to focus on this week; student can "redo" a strength targeted prior if he or she desires.
- Provide students with the *New Uses of My Fifth Signature Strength* handout. Ask them to work in small groups to make a list of ways they may use this strength that are different from, or unique, to prior usage.
- Write the life domain categories on the white board and prompt students to think of ways they can use their signature strength in each domain.
- As students work, group leaders should make sure that the activities being listed are manageable and concrete. Group leaders should brainstorm ideas alongside students and solicit ideas from other students.
- Clarify any suggestions that may stray from the content of the signature strength and guide students to more targeted ideas. Copies of the *VIA Classification of 24 Character Strengths* handout should be on hand to help students remember the meanings of the strengths.

(continued)

Plan for Implementation and Generalization	• Ask students to use their chosen *signature strength* in new ways each day of the upcoming week *across life domains as was prepared on their* New Uses of My Fifth Signature Strength *record form.* Ask them to use the form daily to write down their feelings after using the strength, to promote self-reflection and savoring. Encourage students to find a different way to use the strength if they encounter obstacles with the first plan.
	Typically, you've shared your homework completion with me and the other members of the group. After you complete your plan for using this strength in new ways, who can you share your experiences and feelings with?
	• Prompt students to consider family members, friends, educators, and possibly other group members.
	• Remind students that sharing successes with others helps us savor our positive experiences.
	After your plan for next week is completed, how do you intend to continue using your signature strengths in your daily life?
	• Encourage students to continue to use all or any of their signature strengths in new ways.

D. Review and Practice: Optimistic Explanatory Style

Practice Thinking Optimistically	*Remember a while back we learned about optimistic thinking, which involves thinking about good things in your life as being* permanent, *such as being caused by your traits and abilities, and thinking about bad events as* temporary, *only lasting as long as your mood or effort. Also, optimistic thinking involves seeing good events as* widespread, *or seeing good things as happening throughout life, and seeing bad events as* specific *to certain areas of life. Finally, optimistic thinking involves* taking credit *for causing good events in our lives, but* blaming other factors *for bad events.*
	• Illustrate with own example of a positive situation (e.g., observation of current group of students' progress with happiness promotion skills); ask students to help generate the optimistic attributions.
	Optimistic thinking leads to resilience, the feeling that you can face any situation and come out OK. Thus, optimistic thinking is a purposeful attitude that can increase our happiness. Let's think of good or bad situations from the last few weeks, where you did or could have practiced optimistic thinking.
	• Distribute the *My Optimistic Thoughts* handout to students. Have one or two students volunteer a situation from the last 2–4 weeks. Ask the speaker to decide if it was a good or bad event, and ask him or her how the situation could be thought of more optimistically. Ask the group to assist the speaker generate thoughts about the situation that are optimistic.
Plan for Generalization	*How do you intend to keep practicing optimistic thinking in your daily life?*
	• Encourage students to continue using optimistic thinking regularly in their lives, for both positive and negative situations and events.

E. Wrap-Up and Gratitude for Student Participation

Program Termination	• Ask students about their final thoughts on the interventions beyond character strengths and optimistic thinking that they plan to continue.
	• Remind them of the importance of including significant others at home (parents) and school (teachers, classmates) in their happiness efforts.
	• Express gratitude for the students' continued efforts to take control over their actions and thoughts that are related to feeling happy.

Supplemental Individual Student Sessions: Multidimensional Interview of Students' Determinants of Subjective Well-Being

INTRODUCTION TO INTERVENTION	*Supplemental Session 1: Individual Student*

Goals	• Establish rapport with student. • Introduce student to intervention purpose and meeting logistics. • Gather baseline data on life satisfaction. • Start student thinking about factors that influence personal happiness. • Address questions and clarify misconceptions (as needed).
Overview of Procedures	A. Introduction to Counselor and Intervention B. Activity: Multidimensional Assessment of Life Satisfaction C. Introductory Exploration of Student's Personal Determinants of Happiness
Materials	• Blank copy of the screening measure completed prior (e.g., BMSLSS) • Blank copy of the SLSS and MSLSS for completion in session • (*For younger students*) Games and activities to play to establish rapport

Procedures Defined

A. Introduction to Counselor and Intervention

Clarify Professional Role	• Name the child prefers to go by . . . spelling? • Your name (including spelling). • Title (*counselor*); if applicable, explain trainee status. • (For younger students): *Do you know what a counselor is?* Example: *A counselor is someone who people talk to. They can talk about things that are going well, and things that are going not so well, in their life. As your counselor, I'm here to help you feel as happy as possible and to be successful. I'm here to listen and help you learn ways to feel your best. So, I'll get to see you each week for the next few months. We'll talk about you and ways to help you become and stay very happy.*
Purpose of Intervention	• Ask student if he or she knows why he or she gets to meet with you. If student does not know, provide a clear and accurate explanation. Example: *A few weeks ago, your teacher asked you to fill out a brief questionnaire that asked you to indicate your happiness with different areas of life—home, friends, school—and overall life. Thank you for completing that! Your answers told us that although things are going OK for you, you have some room for growth in your happiness.* *School counselors will meet with students who have parent permission to work on happiness with a counselor. I'm so glad you brought back your permission slip. I'm excited to help you learn ways of thinking and acting and getting along with others so you can become happier!*

(continued)

Provide an Overview of the Session Content	• Explain the meeting logistics. Example: *We will meet each week during first or second period, likely in this room.* • Provide student with an advanced organizer for the content and goal of the Well-Being Promotion Program, and the initial meetings. *In our first few meetings, I'd like to know more about you, including how happy you are currently. We will talk about what influences your well-being. Well-being is your overall happiness. It is how happy you are with your whole life. It is also how often you feel good and bad feelings.* • If collaboration with teachers or parents is intended, explain that to the student. Example: *I would also like to chat with some of your teachers about their goals for your happiness. Is that OK with you? Then, I will take all of the information and we can set goals for what areas of life we want to make better and which areas we want to keep the same. Also, I will touch base with your parents to let them know what we will be working on in our weekly meetings.* • If intervention is intended for implementation in small groups, explain that to the student. *Then, together with other students in your class/grade/school, we'll learn things that help most children feel happy.*

Establish Rapport	• To start the verbal communication process, engage the student in a discussion of easy-to-talk-about topics; reinforce sharing of information and highlight similarities.
	Before we move to talking about your current feelings, it would be helpful to know more about you in general.
	  o *Interests?*
	    ■ *Music; TV shows; movies; athletic teams*
	  o *Things you do for fun after school (sports, clubs?) and on the weekend?*
	  o *Favorite and least favorite school subjects and activities?*
	  o *Family life? (siblings, pets?)*
	• Point out similarities between student and self, in interests and background
	Do you have any questions for me so far?
	• *Note:* Younger students, such as those in elementary and maybe middle school, may speak more freely when or after engaged in a fun activity.
	If you'd like, we can play a game today while we're talking. Or, play a game and then talk. I have _____ game and _____ game . . . would you like to play one?
	• When comfortable, interject the general questions above during the game.

(continued)

B. Activity: Multidimensional Assessment of Life Satisfaction

Comprehensive Assessment of Multidimensional Life Satisfaction

- Administer the SLSS and MSLSS (provide completion instructions).

To get started, it would be helpful to know how you are feeling about your life currently. Please take a few minutes and complete this survey about how you have felt the past few weeks. Read the instructions, then indicate the extent to which you disagree or agree with each statement.

- Allow student to complete the SLSS and MSLSS independently; stay nearby in case there are any questions about words in the items, or questions about the response metric.
- After student indicates he or she is finished, check to make sure he or she selected one response only to each of the 47 items . . . prompt the student to complete any skipped items, and to select the best answer if he or she circled two options for one item.

Thank you for completing that survey. When we meet next, I'd like to talk more about your happiness levels in each area of life, like happiness at home, school, and with your friends.

C. Introductory Exploration of Student's Personal Determinants of Happiness

Set the Stage

- Explain that the meeting will end soon, and you are interested in learning the primary areas of life that impact the student's personal happiness.

Explore Student's Perception of Primary Contributors to Life Satisfaction

In our last few minutes today, I'm curious about the main things you're thinking of when judging your overall happiness—that is, your satisfaction with your life in general. Like on question 1, you circled a "_____" on the scale of 1–6.

- Reference one of the global satisfaction items from the SLSS, such as:

	Strongly disagree	Moderately disagree	Mildly disagree	Mildly agree	Moderately agree	Strongly agree
My life is going well.	1	2	3	4	5	6
My life is just right.	1	2	3	4	5	6
I have a good life.	1	2	3	4	5	6

What were you thinking about when you decided how happy you were with your whole life?

o *What types of things make you happy?*
o *What else makes you happier?*

Optional questions for teenagers (some younger children have struggled with the abstract nature of these questions).

o *Overall, what do you think would have to change in order to move your happiness rating/level up 1 whole point (e.g., from a 5 to a 6)?*
o *What else do you think would make you happier? Are there things that your parents, teachers, classmates, or friends could do?*

[Summarize] is that correct? Would you like to add something else that would help me better understand what influences your satisfaction with your life?

(continued)

| **Provide Preview of Next Meeting** | • End meeting with an affirming statement and preview of the next session. |

Provide Preview of Next Meeting

• End meeting with an affirming statement and preview of the next session.

I've enjoyed talking with you today, and getting to know you a bit! I am looking forward to seeing you again next week.

• Remind student of the planned contact with parents and teachers, as applicable.

I'll also try to introduce myself to a teacher, and contact your parent. Some parents like to receive a quick e-mail that tells the activities done in a meeting.

   ○ *Who do you live with at home?*

   ○ *Parent e-mail address:* _____

   ○ *If e-mail unknown, phone number:* _____

So I'll be back next week, and every week for about 10 weeks, on _____ (day) during _____ (class period). One of the student office assistants will bring you a pass so you may be excused from class. We'll typically meet in _____ (place).

Next week, we'll talk more about your happiness in different areas of life.

Supplemental Individual Student Sessions: Multidimensional Interview of Students' Determinants of Subjective Well-Being

COMPREHENSIVE ASSESSMENT OF DETERMINANTS OF LIFE SATISFACTION	*Supplemental Session 2: Individual Student*

Goals	• Get to know student in the context of his or her current status on the common determinants of happiness. • Continue student reflection on factors that influence personal happiness.
Procedures	A. Semistructured Interview—Determinants of Personal Happiness
Materials	• Prior to the session, score SLSS and MSLSS; flag for clarification any items to which the student responded in an unusual or interesting way.

Procedures Defined

A. Semistructured Interview—Determinants of Personal Happiness

Preparation	• Before this meeting, score the SLSS and MSLSS. In the relevant section of this general interview protocol (e.g., family, friendships, personality), add questions to follow-up on survey items that the student responded to in a notable manner (e.g., inconsistent with other responses, particular satisfaction or dissatisfaction).
General	*This week, I'd like to know more about things in your family and your activities that may affect your happiness.* • Review themes from last meeting; prompt for additional student reflections. *Last week you mentioned that for you, your happiness depends on _____ [recap top determinants], and sometimes _____ [recap minor themes].* o *Any thoughts on what other types of things might make you happy or unhappy?*
Personality and Self	*How would your friends describe you? Like in terms or your personality—your typical mood or behavior)?* • *For instance, would your friends describe you as friendly, quiet, curious, funny, hardworking, caring, stressed out?* • *What about these traits (your personality) makes you happy or unhappy with your life?*
Coping Strategies	• Gather information about preexisting use of strategies for cultivating happiness, including strategies to calm (maintain emotional well-being) in the face of stressors. *I'd like to know more about what you try to do to get or stay happy.* *What are some of the ways that you handle problems or deal with challenges/ stressors?*

(continued)

Family	Who lives in your home? How happy are these people in your family?

• On a scale of 1–5, how would you rate the well-being (overall happiness; satisfaction with life) of each person living in your home?

	Not at all happy	Slightly	Medium	Often happy	Delighted
Mom/Stepmom or partner	1	2	3	4	5
Dad/Stepdad or partner	1	2	3	4	5
Sibling 1 (*name:* _____)	1	2	3	4	5
Sibling 2 (*name:* _____)	1	2	3	4	5
Sibling 3 (*name:* _____)	1	2	3	4	5
Other person in home (*name:* _____)	1	2	3	4	5

Relationships

• Gather information about interpersonal relationships, first in an open-ended manner, and then in a specific fashion about particular people if needed.

I'd like to know more about how you are getting along with people in your life. Which of your relationships (with people at home, school, or elsewhere) are going well?

o *In what ways do they make you feel happy?*

Which of your relationships are not going so well (or that you are having a hard time with)?

o *In what ways do they make you feel unhappy?*
o (If relationships at home are not brought up): *In general, how well do you get along with your parents? Siblings?*
o (If relationships at school are not brought up): *Which people at school make you happy or unhappy? Teachers? Classmates? In what ways?*

Life Circumstances

• Gather information about life circumstances.

Last, think about the events in your life (good or bad) that may affect your happiness.

o *What are some of the things that are going on in your life (good events or situations, even those that may be out of your control) that have made you happy?*
o *Which things that are going on in your life (events or situations, even those possibly out of your control) have made you not happy?*
o *Any other things going on that affect your happiness with your life?*

Recap

[Summarize themes from student responses during this interview.] *Is that correct? Is there anything else in your life that makes you happy or unhappy? For instance, perhaps how your religion, or your pets, or sports or after-school activities, influences your happiness?*

Provide Preview of Next Meeting

• End the meeting with an affirming statement and preview of the next meeting.

I've enjoyed talking with you again today! Next week, we'll start learning strategies that help students feel happier. [If relevant: *As a reminder, a few other students in your class/grade/school will be included in our meetings, so that we can all learn together and support one another.*]

Supplemental Teacher and Classroom Sessions
Facilitating Student–Teacher and Student–Student Relationships

PSYCHOEDUCATION FOR TEACHERS	*Supplemental Session: Teacher*
Goals	• Establish rapport with teacher. • Introduce teacher to the field of positive psychology and key constructs. • Discuss baseline level of subjective well-being among target students. • Convey importance of positive student–teacher relationships. • Share strategies for teachers to communicate support. • Introduce teacher to content of student intervention. • Address questions and clarify misconceptions (as needed).
Overview of Procedures	A. Brief Presentation: Positive Psychology and Key Constructs in Intervention B. Baseline Subjective Well-Being of Target Students for Program C. Clarify Purpose of Intervention D. Provide an Overview of the Student-Focused Intervention E. Plan for Behavior Management during Classwide or Small-Group Sessions F. Homework: Teacher Preparation for Participation G. Provide Time for Expression of Questions and Concerns
Materials	• *Overview of Program Activities* handout for teacher • *Building Strong Student–Teacher Relationships* handout for teacher • Copy of intervention manual • (*If baseline measure administered and scored*): Graphed average student subjective well-being levels

Procedures Defined

A. Brief Presentation: Positive Psychology and Key Constructs in Intervention

Welcome the teacher, provide a copy of the teacher handouts, and thank him or her for making time to participate in the program. Introduce self and other co-facilitators, such as other mental health providers or trainees at your school, before beginning the presentation.

> *In order to provide you with a better understanding of the kinds of concepts and activities that your students will be learning and engaging in throughout participation in the Well-Being Promotion Program, we will first share with you information related to the field the program is based upon: positive psychology. We will also share some strategies for what you can do outside of our weekly meetings with the students, in order to improve your own happiness and strengthen your relationships with your students.*

Deliver the PowerPoint presentation that you prepared in advance. Presentation goals:
- Communicate the importance of students' happiness.
- Introduce positive psychology and define key targets.
- Explain what positive psychology interventions are, and outline which are targeted to students in the subsequent sessions of the program.
- Convey the importance of classroom relationships to students' happiness; share the research-based ties between teacher social support and student subjective well-being.

(continued)

- Discuss how teachers currently communicate support and care to students.
- Suggest strategies for conveying support as suggested by prior research (specifically, Suldo et al., 2009).
- Encourage teachers to complete the weekly exercises along with their students.

As a summary of the presentation content, for teacher reference after the informational meeting, distribute the handouts *Overview of Program Activities* and *Building Strong Student–Teacher Relationships.*

Note: If presentation equipment is unavailable, consider allowing the teacher to reference the handouts through the discussion (rather than focus on a presentation screen). Use the handouts as an outline and guide for the discussion; the goals for the discussion remain the same as above.

Throughout and once completed, provide opportunities to pose questions.

B. Baseline Subjective Well-Being of Target Students for Program

Before this first meeting, administer and score baseline measure(s) of subjective well-being to students targeted for inclusion. Commonly used measures of global life satisfaction and satisfaction in primary domains of life include:

- Students Life Satisfaction Scale (SLSS; seven-items; global).
- Multidimensional Students' Life Satisfaction Scale (MSLSS; 40 items across five domains).
- Brief Multidimensional Students' Life Satisfaction Scale (BMSLSS; six items—five domain specific and one global).

All are available free from the author (Scott Huebner) at *www.psych.sc.edu/faculty/Scott_Huebner.*

- If the program is intended as a Tier 2 intervention for students with room for growth in life satisfaction, then data from the schoolwide screening (e.g., via the BMSLSS) conducted to identify the targeted students should be graphed.
- If the program is intended to be administered classwide (e.g., as a Tier 1 wellness-promotion program for all students), consider administering more comprehensive measures such as the SLSS and MSLSS to all students in the class.
- The PANAS-C (Laurent et al., 1999) can also be used to index positive and negative affect.

Share with the teacher graphed averages that contain his or her students' current (i.e., preintervention, baseline) levels of life satisfaction, and highlight domains that are relatively high and low. Note these measures will be readministered at the program conclusion. Average scores pre- and postintervention will be compared in order to evaluate students' level of response.

C. Clarify Purpose of Intervention

Ensure that the teacher understands that the Well-Being Promotion Program was designed to maximize students' happiness and overall well-being. Explain:

Optimal well-being involves being happy (satisfied with life) in addition to not having mental health problems. The Well-Being Promotion Program that we are implementing with your students was designed to maximize students' happiness, not to intervene with mental health problems. Research tells us that we all have genetically set ranges of happiness, and the key to increasing happiness within our range is through purposeful activities. The purpose of the Well-Being Promotion Program is to increase your students' happiness by talking about key concepts we covered in the presentation and engaging in activities focused on them, such as gratitude and character strengths.

(continued)

238

D. Provide an Overview of the Student-Focused Intervention

Describe the main components of the Well-Being Promotion Program. Explain:

The happiness-increasing interventions we will teach your students will be taught in a classwide format, with one group leader (me) and co-facilitators (you). [If applicable, also identify the mental health provider or trainee at your school who may also assist in a co-facilitator role.] *We will meet once weekly during one period of the school day, for about 10 weeks. The first meeting is just between us (the current meeting). After that, the weekly meetings with the students will include leader-guided group discussions and activities. Students will also be assigned homework at the conclusion of each meeting in order to facilitate further practice with concepts and skills learned. Regarding the focus of the meetings, the first two student meetings are mainly focused on establishing team building, a positive group environment, and introducing the students to the program. The fourth and fifth meetings focus on gratitude and include activities such as students writing about things for which they're grateful and expressing thanks to people who have been kind to them in the past. The sixth meeting focuses on acts of kindness and includes activities such as increasing the frequency of performing kind acts. The seventh, eighth, ninth, and 10th meetings focus mainly on identifying one's character strengths and include activities such as identifying perceived strengths, objectively identifying them through completing a survey, and using strengths in new ways. The 11th and final meeting includes a review of the program, including activities and skills learned in the program.*

E. Plan for Behavior Management during Classwide or Small-Group Sessions

Given the young developmental stage that is the intervention target, and the fact that groups can be as large as entire classrooms (pending sufficient availability of group co-leaders), it is advisable to develop an explicit behavior management system for use during the student sessions (meetings 2–11). This can entail extension of a current classwide system perceived by teachers as effective, or development of a new strategy for use only during the program meetings.

- To develop a behavioral management system for use prior to Session 2, inquire:
  - *What are the current classroom/school rules?*
  - *What behavior management system is currently in place in the classroom or school?*
  - *How often is feedback provided to students regarding compliance with classroom rules?*
  - *What incentives/tangibles do students seem to find motivating? Which of the options are acceptable to the classroom teacher(s)?*

F. Homework: Teacher Preparation for Participation

To prepare for participation as a co-facilitator of the Well-Being Promotion Program throughout the intervention period, encourage the teacher to become further familiar with the positive psychology constructs covered during the PowerPoint presentation.

- Distribute the full text article from Suldo and colleagues (2009) in *School Psychology Review.*
  - Encourage teacher to plan strategies (new ones introduced weekly) for communicating teacher support.
- Encourage teachers to visit *www.authentichappiness.org.*
  - *Personal levels of subjective well-being, gratitude, hope?*
  - *Own signature strengths?*
- Provide teacher with complete intervention manual.
  - Discuss plan for reading, and communicating about, session plans in advance of group leaders/facilitators meetings with students.

(continued)

G. Provide Time for Expression of Questions and Concerns

Ensure several minutes to recap the information shared today, answer any of the teacher's remaining questions, problem solve concerns, and establish the most effective methods for communication between student meetings.

Supplemental Teacher and Classroom Sessions
Facilitating Student–Teacher and Student–Student Relationships

GETTING TO KNOW CLASSMATES THROUGH TEAM BUILDING	*Supplemental Session: Class*

Goals	• Establish a supportive group environment with clear behavioral expectations. • Identify classmates' common life experiences. • Learn to work together and contribute to a group project. • Understand the importance of working in a team and supporting one another. • Underscore ties between social relationships and personal happiness.
Overview of Procedures	A. Introduction to Leaders and Rules B. Get-to-Know-You Exercise: Commonalities between Classmates C. Team-Building Exercise: Creative Coloring D. Group Discussion: Challenges and Benefits to Working Together E. Introduction to the Well-Being Promotion Program
Materials	• Different-colored markers, crayons, or colored pencils for each student • A large sheet of paper

Procedures Defined

A. Introduction to Leaders and Rules

Introduction to Leaders	• Explain to students who you are, and an overview of why you are there. *Hello!* [Each facilitator provides name and explains professional role at the school.] *We have the same goal: increasing all children's happiness. We'll be with you each* [specify regular meeting time, such as Friday afternoon] *for the next several weeks to talk about happiness. We'll help you do activities that have been shown to help all kinds of young people feel better about their lives. We'll talk more about those types of activities next week. Today, we're hoping to just get to know one another better.*
Establish Behavioral Expectations	• Below is an example behavior management system aligned with the larger school positive behavioral intervention and support system. *But first, we want to give you some tips on how to behave during our meetings so that you'll get the most benefit from the activities, and earn rewards for good behavior. The CHAMPS for this lesson are:* ○ *C—Conversation level is a "2"—we'll be doing group work.* ○ *H—To ask for help, please raise your hand.* ○ *A—Activity . . . listen to the adult speaking (leader or your teacher) or the classmate we've asked to share, or do the activity we assign.* ○ *M—Movement . . . please sit at your desk until we ask you to move.* ○ *P—Participation looks like eyes on the speaker or assignment.* ○ *S—And that's how you'll be successful.* *Every 5 minutes, we will put stars next to the names of the students who are following those CHAMPS. At the end of our meeting, all students who have earned at least five stars will get a reward: stickers or candy! Any questions?*

(continued)

B. Get-to-Know-You Exercise: Commonalities between Classmates

This first exercise is an ice-breaker designed to help group participants get to know some of the things they have in common with their peers. The potential commonalities start with innocuous situations, and progress to more sensitive situations. Point out how no student is ever alone; there is almost always at least one other person who shares his or her unique situation.

Commonalities between Classmates

We would like to do an activity to help us get to know one another. I know you guys know one another, but you're new to us. And, you may discover some situations you have in common with one another that you weren't aware of.

- Ask students to stand in a large circle or in a line. Then, they should take a step forward if their answer is "yes" to a situation.
- *Take a step forward if you . . .*
  - *Have a pet.*
  - *You have at least one brother or sister.*
  - *Like to play sports.*
  - *Like video games.*
  - *Like to sing or dance.*
  - *Have a nickname.*
  - *Have ever gotten into an argument with a friend.*
  - *Have ever been picked on or teased.*
  - *Have ever been unfriendly to another kid.*
  - *Have ever felt really happy.*
  - *Have ever felt really unhappy.*
- Along the way, ask students if they knew they had that in common with their classmate; they can tell you more about their classmate's situation if they're aware of details.
- Initiate reflections from group members with regard to asking them if they realized they had so much in common with one another, and surprising identifications among classmates.

C. Team-Building Exercise: Creative Coloring

The next activity was design to increase cooperative play between small groups of children.

Creative Coloring (Jones, 1998)

Sometimes in life we must accept help from others or rely on our friends and family for help if we are to get it done well. Think about suppertime or a big holiday dinner. If one person tries to make dinner and clean up, there is a lot of work to be done and it's a hard task. But when a whole team of people pitch in and help, making dinner and cleaning can be done in no time. Each person is a part of the puzzle and can offer different talents to use in the mealtime process.

In this activity, each student will be a part of a team that can make a big project easy. Each student will contribute his or her own skills to create the big picture.

- In each small group, give each student a different-colored marker, crayon, or colored pencil.
- Tell students that the color they have will be the only color they can use for the project.

Your group must create a picture, using all the colors. Each student may only use his or her color. You are not allowed to share or trade. Work together to create a nice picture, with each student using only the crayon in your hand.

(continued)

- **Modifications:**
    - For smaller groups, each student may have more than one color.
    - Rather than creating own picture, have the group color in a page from a coloring book.
    - For added teamwork, ask the group to decide how to determine which color each person will use.

D. Group Discussion: Challenges and Benefits to Working Together

Pose the following thought questions:

- *Was this a difficult project for the group? Why or why not?*
- *How did you work as a team to complete the project?*
- *How does everyone in the team feel about the picture that was created?*
- *Is it easier to do things on your own or with others?*
- *Why is it important to be able to work with and support others as members of a team?*

E. Introduction to Well-Being Promotion Program

We are going to be spending some time with your class over the next few months. In our time together, we'll talk about ways to feel happier by acting differently, including by supporting one another and noticing nice things about the people in our class, including our teachers and classmates. Each meeting, we look forward to hearing about the ways that working together and treating one another kindly has made you feel. Your teacher is also going to point out (and tell us about) times where you have treated one another particularly nicely, or worked together successfully. Scientists know that happier people are especially close to many people; happy people's close friends include people in their school, like classmates and teachers, and people at home, like parents and brothers and sisters. So it's important to us that you care for one another, and let others know about that care.

Overview of Program Activities

Frequently Asked Questions

What is positive psychology?

- The study of factors and traits that make people thrive. Positive psychology emphasizes the presence of positive indicators of mental health, such as personal happiness.

Why are we trying to make your students happier?

- Happier kids earn better grades, perform better on standardized tests, have more positive attitudes toward school and learning, have better social relationships, are physically healthier, and have fewer symptoms of mental health problems like depression and anxiety.

Why are we working with your students? Or some students in particular?

- If we are working with your entire class, we would like all of your students to participate in this universal wellness initiative because we expect they will experience an increase in happiness due to taking part in the Well-Being Promotion Program.
- If we are working with a subset of your class, we have invited students to participate based on their responses on the short survey of life satisfaction that all students recently completed. The selected students' responses indicated that they are less than completely satisfied with life. They are eligible to take part in the Well-Being Promotion Program that is intended to increase students' happiness, including from "pleased" to "delighted" with life. We would like them to participate because we expect they will experience an increase in happiness due to taking part in the Well-Being Promotion Program.

What does the Well-Being Promotion Program include?

- The program consists of meetings between school mental health providers and students. A schedule of what your students will be focusing on with their counselor:
  - Meeting 1: Building Strong Student–Teacher Relationships
  - Meeting 2: Getting to Know Students in the Class (Student Team Building)
  - Meeting 3: You at Your Best (Happiness Introduction)
  - Meeting 4: Gratitude Journaling
  - Meeting 5: Gratitude Visits
  - Meeting 6: Acts of Kindness
  - Meeting 7: Introduction to Character Strengths
  - Meeting 8: Assessment of Character Strengths
  - Meeting 9: Using First Signature Strength in New Ways
  - Meeting 10: Using Second Signature Strength in New Ways
  - Meeting 11: Program Review

Your class's program leader (or student's counselor) is: _____

Contact details: _____

Your class or student will typically meet with the leader/counselor on: _____

Building Strong Student–Teacher Relationships

Students' perceptions of social support from teachers reflect how much students feel respected, cared for, and valued by their teachers. Happier students report greater social support. *Emotional support* and *instrumental support* are the aspects of teacher support most highly related to students' happiness. **Emotional support** = students' perceptions of how often teachers care about them, treat them fairly, and make it OK to ask questions. **Instrumental support** = how much students perceive teachers make sure students have what they need for school, take time to help them learn to do something well, and spend time with them when they need help.

Sometimes, students and adults have different ideas about what types of adult actions are supportive. For example, children may focus on tangible goods as "proof" of care, whereas adults go out of their way to keep children safe (actions that may go unnoticed to children). When researchers* interview children about what support from teachers "looks like," many children report the same ideas, suggesting some strategies teachers may want to consider in an effort to promote positive student–teacher relationships:

- *Communicate care for well-being* through:
  - Asking personal questions (e.g., asking a withdrawn student if everything is OK).
  - Being pleasant and/or respectful.
  - Allowing free time during the day.
  - Giving candy.

- *Utilize best teaching practices* through:
  - Showing concern for both the individual student's and the entire class's understanding of academic material, then providing additional learning experiences as needed.
  - Using diverse teaching strategies, especially those consistent with a child's preferred method of learning.

- *Show explicit interest in students' academic achievement* through:
  - Recognizing student accomplishments.
  - Helping students to improve grades.
  - Providing rewards for good academic performance.
  - Explaining errors made on assignments.
  - Ensuring academic workload can be completed in a reasonable amount of time.

- *Show equity of support* through:
  - Appearing objective in your approach to (1) selecting students to participate in class, and (2) providing rewards to students.
  - Explicitly stating intent to treat all students the same.
  - Disciplining students by taking time to correctly identify the wrongdoer, rather than punishing the entire class.

(continued)

---

*The findings reported in this handout are based on research conducted by school psychologists at the University of South Florida, as reported in Suldo, S. M., Friedrich, A. A., White, T., Farmer, J., Minch, D., & Michalowski, J. (2009). Teacher support and adolescents' subjective well-being: A mixed-methods investigation. *School Psychology Review, 38,* 67–85.

- *Make students feel comfortable asking questions* through:
  - Creating a physical and emotional classroom environment in which questions appear to be encouraged—for example, through the use of posters, "question boxes" where students can privately place questions for later answer, and so on.
  - Creating a supportive emotional environment by responding positively to questions and appreciating students' interest in learning answers.
  - Creating a logistical arrangement by providing permission, time, and diverse mechanisms for students to pose questions.

Research suggests that boys differ from girls in their views of which teacher behaviors communicate care.

For GIRLS, teacher actions noted most as showing care:	For BOYS, teacher acts noted most as showing care:
• Taking actions to help students improve their moods. • Expressing an interest in students' well-being. • Sharing their personal experiences with students. • Having contact with students outside of class. • Taking an interest in students' academic progress. • Use of varied teaching strategies.	• Giving students rewards (e.g., candy, free time, treats). • Helping students improve their grades. • Explicitly stating permission to ask questions. • Responding to questions in a positive manner.
What NOT to do for girls? GIRLS appear especially sensitive to feeling low support when they perceive:	**What NOT to do for boys? BOYS appear particularly sensitive to:**
• A negative emotional environment. • Negative responses to students' questions. • Strict grading policies. • Setting firm rules and expectations. • Insufficient assistance for learning.	• Teachers assigning an overwhelming workload.

Supplemental Parent Information Session

PSYCHOEDUCATION FOR PARENTS	*Supplemental Session: Parent*
Goals	• Establish rapport with parents. • Introduce parents to the field of positive psychology and key constructs. • Introduce parents to the content of student intervention. • Address questions and clarify misconceptions (as needed).
Overview of Procedures	A. Brief Presentation: Positive Psychology and Key Targets in Intervention B. Clarify Purpose of the Group C. Provide Overview of Student-Focused Intervention
Materials	• Computer, projector, and screen for presentation • Parent handout: *Overview of Program Activities and Positive Psychology*

Procedures Defined

A. Brief Presentation: Positive Psychology and Key Targets in Intervention

Welcome the parents and note who is in attendance. Once all have arrived, give parents a copy of the parent handout and thank them for attending the informational session. Introduce self and other group leaders to parents before beginning the presentation.

To give you a better understanding of the kinds of concepts and activities that your children will be learning and engaging in throughout participation in the Well-Being Promotion Program, we will first share with you information related to the field the program is based upon: positive psychology.

Deliver the PowerPoint presentation that you prepared in advance. Presentation goals:

- Communicate the importance of parents' and children's happiness.
- Introduce positive psychology and define key targets.
- Explain what positive psychology interventions are, then demonstrate by leading the parents to complete one (e.g., gratitude journaling, acts of kindness planning, savoring).
- Encourage parents to complete the weekly exercises at home along with their child.
- Outline the positive psychology targets their child will focus on each week in the group.

As a summary of the presentation content, for parent reference after the informational meeting, distribute the *Overview of Positive Psychology and Program Activities* handout.

If presentation equipment is unavailable, consider allowing parents to reference the handout through the discussion (rather than focus on a presentation screen). Use the handout as an outline and guide for the discussion; the goals for the discussion remain the same as above.

Throughout presentation and once completed, provide opportunities for parents to pose questions.

B. Clarify Purpose of the Group

Ensure that parents understand that their child has been asked to participate in the group in order to maximize happiness and overall well-being, not because he or she has been identified as mentally ill, for instance, with elevated levels of depression or other problems. Sample script:

(continued)

Optimal well-being involves being happy (satisfied with life) in addition to not having mental health problems. We have asked your child to participate in the group program in order to maximize his or her happiness, not because of mental health problems. Research tells us that we all have genetically set ranges of happiness, and the key to increasing happiness within our range is through purposeful activities. The purpose of the weekly group is to increase your child's happiness to the top of his or her possible range by talking about key concepts we covered in the presentation, and doing exercises focused on those targets, such as gratitude, character strengths, optimism, and hope.

C. Provide Overview of Student-Focused Intervention

Describe the main components of the Well-Being Promotion Program. Sample script:

The happiness-increasing interventions we will teach your children will be taught in a small-group format, with roughly six to seven students per group, as well as one group leader and a co-facilitator. All leaders are trained in the program and are mental health practitioners or trainees. For example, I am a school psychologist [school social worker, counselor] here at the school. Your child and other students in the group will meet once weekly during one period of the school day, for 10 weeks. Additionally, once the program ends, your children will attend once-monthly check-in meetings to review skills learned in the program. These check-ins will also occur during one period of the school day, for 2–3 months. The weekly meetings will include leader-guided group discussions and activities. Students will also be assigned homework at the end of each meeting, intended to provide more practice with concepts and skills learned.

In order to keep you apprised of what your children are learning, each week you will receive a handout via e-mail or a hard copy that will be sent home with your child. The handout of the week will provide an overview of the skills learned and types of activities performed that week in the student meetings, as well as tell you the homework tasks assigned. It will also provide suggestions for things you can do and talk about at home to help your children further acquire the skills taught in the group meetings.

Regarding the focus of the meetings, the main goal of the first is to establish a positive group environment and introduce the students to the program. The second and third meetings focus on gratitude and include activities such as students writing about things they're grateful for and expressing thanks to people who have been kind to them in the past. The fourth meeting focuses on acts of kindness and includes activities such as increasing the frequency of performing kind acts. The fifth, sixth, and seventh meetings focus mainly on identifying and using one's character strengths. These meetings include activities such as identifying perceived strengths, objectively identifying them through completing a survey, and using strengths in new ways. Also, the seventh meeting teaches students how to savor positive experiences. The eighth meeting focuses on optimism and includes an activity that teaches students to think optimistically. The ninth meeting focuses on hope and includes an activity in which students write about their best possible selves in the future, including their personal goals and paths to attaining these goals. The tenth and final meeting includes a review of the program, including activities and skills learned in the program. The check-in meetings also review the skills and concepts learned in addition to reviewing students' progress and experiences since the conclusion of the program, and provide an opportunity to rehearse specific activities they learned through participating in the program.

Encourage parents to ask questions about the intervention. Provide more details about the scheduling logistics or intervention content as necessary to address questions.

Overview of Program Activities and Positive Psychology

Consider and Discuss

- *What do you hope your child will gain from the Well-Being Promotion Program?*

Why Parents' Happiness Is Crucial to Children's Happiness

- Research has demonstrated that youth's happiness ratings are correlated, or have a positive relationship with, parents' happiness ratings.
  - As parents' life satisfaction increases, so does their child's.
  - Reciprocal relationship: your child's level of life satisfaction may influence yours too.
- Research has found numerous benefits of happiness, including better physical health, academic and occupational success, and rewarding social relationships.

Consider and Discuss

- *What is your understanding of "positive psychology"? What have you heard before?*

Key Features of Positive Psychology

- The study of factors and traits that make people thrive.
- Positive psychology gained in popularity in the last 15 years, and grew out of discontent with a focus on mental health problems.
- Emphasizes both the absence of mental health problems and the presence of well-being.

Key Terms in Positive Psychology

- **Subjective well-being:** A scientific term for happiness, and common indicator of wellness. Often the primary outcome of interventions designed to improve happiness. High subjective well-being reflects high life satisfaction (judging your life to be going well on the whole), and experiencing more positive emotions than negative emotions.
- **Gratitude:** A tendency to appreciate positive aspects of life, feel grateful for positive things in life, and convey thankfulness and appreciate others. Crucial to making and maintaining positive relationships with others.
- **Kindness:** A character strength involving motivation to act kindly toward others, to follow through on plans to be kind, and to recognize kindness in others. Acts of kindness, or behaving in ways that benefit others or make them happy at personal expense, have been shown to cause increases in happy moods and life satisfaction.
- **Character strengths:** Set of 24 individual positive traits within six broader classes of virtues. Each person has a unique profile of strengths and signature strengths, which are traits most frequently used and appreciated in one's life. Research has shown that using signature strengths in everyday life can improve overall subjective well-being.
- **Savoring:** Focusing on and enjoying past, present, and/or future positive events. Savoring involves anticipation, reminiscing, and prolonging the enjoyable moment. It can be increased through behavioral, social, and cognitive strategies. Linked to higher subjective well-being.

(continued)

- **Optimism:** A tendency to expect positive outcomes and emphasize the positive aspects of situations. Also refers to viewing positive situations as widespread and due to personal factors, while crediting negative events to temporary and external factors. Related to the prevention and reduction of mental health problems, as well as better school adjustment and resilience.
- **Hope:** A positive motivational state involving goal-directed thoughts and strategies, and paths to achieving goals. Linked to positive mental health and well-being.

What Are "Positive Psychology Interventions"?

- Brief, easy, often self-administered exercises designed to mimic the actions and thoughts of naturally very happy people.
- These exercises have emerged within the last decade, and are growing in popularity in line with increasing evidence that they work to increase subjective well-being as intended.
- Positive psychology interventions for children and teens have targeted gratitude, character strengths, kindness, optimism, and hope.
- Overall, research on these interventions has found positive results, including increases in life satisfaction and improved mood.

Activity: "Sweet Savoring"

- *Instructions:* For the next 2–3 minutes, think about an enjoyable experience you have had, either recently or in the past.
- *Do:* Take a minute to close your eyes; think about your experience during that situation and the good feelings you had then.
  - Use your senses—consider sight, smell, hearing, touch, and taste.
  - Remember and relive the experience . . .
- *Share:* Pair up and spend a few minutes talking with your partner about your experience.
- *Reflect:* What feelings did you have with completing this activity? Feelings when reliving the experience in your thoughts? Feeling when sharing (reminiscing) with another adult?

Additional Thoughts

- When your child shares with you the strategies he or she is learning through the program, and you practice them too (either independently or with your child), you may cause even greater improvements in well-being for both of you.
- Visit *www.viacharacter.org* or *www.authentichappiness.org* to learn more about ways to maximize your well-being.

What Does the Well-Being Promotion Program Include?

- The program consists of meetings between school mental health providers and students.
- A schedule of what your child will be focusing on in each meeting:
  - Meeting 1: Introduction to Program ("You at Your Best" activity)
  - Meeting 2: Gratitude Journaling
  - Meeting 3: Gratitude Visits
  - Meeting 4: Acts of Kindness
  - Meeting 5: Introduction to Character Strengths
  - Meeting 6: Identifying Signature Strengths
  - Meeting 7: Using Signature Strengths in New Ways
  - Meeting 8: Optimistic Thinking
  - Meeting 9: Hope and Goal-Directed Thinking
  - Meeting 10: Program Review
  - Follow-Up Meetings (Program Review, Focus on specific exercises)

References

Abramson, L. Y., Seligman, M. E., & Teasdale, J. D. (1978). Learned helplessness in humans: Critique and reformulation. *Journal of Abnormal Psychology*, 87(1), 49–74.

Achenbach, T. M., McConaughy, S. H., Ivanova, M. Y., & Rescorla, L. A. (2011). *Manual for the ASEBA Brief Problem Monitor*. Burlington: University of Vermont, Research Center for Children, Youth, and Families.

Achenbach, T. M., & Rescorla, L. A. (2001). *Manual for the ASEBA school-age forms and profiles*. Burlington: University of Vermont, Research Center for Children, Youth, and Families.

Adelman, H., & Taylor, L. (2009). Ending the marginalization of mental health in schools: A comprehensive approach. In R. W. Christner & R. B. Mennuti (Eds.), *School-based mental health* (pp. 25–54). New York: Routledge.

Albrecht, N. J., Albrecht, P. M., & Cohen, M. (2012). Mindfully teaching in the classroom: A literature review. *Australian Journal of Teacher Education*, 37(12), 1–14.

Algozzine, K., & Algozzine, B. (2007). Classroom instructional ecology and school-wide positive behavior support. *Journal of Applied School Psychology*, 24(1), 29–47.

Andrews, F. M., & Withey, S. B. (1976). *Social indicators of well-being: Americans' perceptions of life quality*. New York: Plenum Press.

Antaramian, S. P., Huebner, E. S., Hills, K. J., & Valois, R. F. (2010). A dual-factor model of mental health: Toward a more comprehensive understanding of youth functioning. *American Journal of Orthopsychiatry*, 80(4), 462–472.

Asgharipoor, N., Farid, A. A., Arshadi, H., & Sahebi, A. (2010). A comparative study on the effectiveness of positive psychotherapy and group cognitive-behavioral therapy for the patients suffering from major depressive disorder. *Iranian Journal of Psychiatry and Behavioral Sciences*, 6(2), 33–41.

Ash, C., & Huebner, E. S. (1998). Life satisfaction reports of gifted middle-school students. *School Psychology Quarterly*, 13(4), 310–321.

Athey, M., Kelly, S. D., & Dew-Reeve, S. E. (2012). Brief Multidimensional Students' Life Satisfaction Scale—PTPB Version: Psychometric properties and relations to mental health. *Administration and Policy in Mental Health and Mental Health Services Reviewer*, 39(1–2), 30–40.

Austin, D. (2005). *The effects of a strengths development intervention program upon the self-perceptions of students' academic abilities*. Asusa, CA: Azusa Pacific University.

Baker, J. A. (1999). Teacher–student interaction in urban at-risk classrooms: Differential behavior, relationship quality, and student satisfaction with school. *Elementary School Journal*, 100(1), 57–70.

Bandura, A. (1997). Sources of self-efficacy. In *Self-efficacy: The exercise of control* (pp. 79–115). New York: Freeman.

Bartels, M., & Boomsma, D. I. (2009). Born to be happy?: The etiology of subjective well-being. *Behavior Genetics*, 39(6), 605–615.

Bartels, M., Cacioppo, J. T., van Beijsterveldt, T. C. E. M., & Boomsma, D. I. (2013). Exploring the association between well-being and psychopathology in adolescents. *Behavior Genetics*, 43(3), 177–190.

Bavelas, J., De Jong, P., Franklin, C., Froerer, A., Gingerich, W., Kim, J., et al. (2013). *Solution focused therapy treatment manual for working with individuals* (2nd ed.). Santa Fe, NM: Solution-Focused Brief Therapy Association. Retrieved from *www.sfbta.org/PDFs/researchDownloads/fileDownloader.asp?fname=SFBT_Revised_Treatment_Manual_2013.pdf.*

Ben-Arieh, A. (2008). The child indicators movement: Past, present, and future. *Child Indicators Research, 1*(1), 3–16.

Benn, R., Akiva, T., Arel, S., & Roeser, R. W. (2012). Mindfulness training effects for parents and educators of children with special needs. *Developmental Psychology, 48*(5), 1476–1487.

Biegel, G. M., Brown, K. W., Shapiro, S. L., & Schubert, C. M. (2009). Mindfulness-based stress reduction for the treatment of adolescent psychiatric outpatients: A randomized clinical trial. *Journal of Consulting and Clinical Psychology, 77*(5), 855–866.

Boehm, J. K., & Lyubomirsky, S. (2008). Does happiness promote career success? *Journal of Career Assessment, 16*(1), 101–116.

Boehm, J. K., Lyubomirsky, S., & Sheldon, K. M. (2011). A longitudinal experimental study comparing the effectiveness of happiness-enhancing strategies in Anglo Americans and Asian Americans. *Cognition and Emotion, 25*(7), 1263–1272.

Bögels, S. M., Hellemans, J., van Deursen, S., Römer, M., & van der Meulen, R. (2014). Mindful parenting in mental health care: Effects on parental and child psychopathology, parental stress, parenting, coparenting, and marital functioning. *Mindfulness, 5*(5), 536–551.

Bond, C., Woods, K., Humphrey, N., Symes, W., & Green, L. (2013). Practitioner review: The effectiveness of solution focused brief therapy with children and families: A systematic and critical evaluation of the literature from 1990–2010. *Journal of Child Psychology and Psychiatry, 54*(7), 707–723.

Bono, G., Froh, J. J., & Forrett, R. (2014). Gratitude in school: Benefits to students and schools. In M. J. Furlong, R. Gilman, & E. S. Huebner (Eds.), *Handbook of positive psychology in the schools* (pp. 67–81). New York: Routledge.

Bookwala, J., & Schulz, R. (1996). Spousal similarity in subjective well-being: The cardiovascular health study. *Psychology and Aging, 11*(4), 582–590.

Bradshaw, C. P., Koth, C. W., Thornton, L. A., & Leaf, P. J. (2012). Altering school climate through schoolwide positive behavioral interventions and supports: Findings from a group-randomized effectiveness trial. *Prevention Science, 10*(2), 100–115.

Bradshaw, C. P., Mitchell, M. M., & Leaf, P. J. (2010). Examining the effects of schoolwide positive behavioral interventions and supports on student outcomes: Results from a randomized controlled effectiveness trial in elementary schools. *Journal of Positive Behavior Interventions, 12*(3), 133–148.

Brantley, A., Huebner, E. S., & Nagle, R. J. (2002). Multidimensional life satisfaction reports of adolescents with mild mental disabilities. *Mental Retardation, 40*(4), 321–329.

Brickman, P., Coates, D., & Janoff-Bulman, R. (1978). Lottery winners and accident victims: Is happiness relative? *Journal of Personality and Social Psychology, 36*(8), 917–927.

Brownell, T., Schrank, B., Jakaite, Z., Larkin, C., & Slade, M. (2015). Mental health service user experience of positive psychotherapy. *Journal of Clinical Psychology, 71*(1), 85–92.

Brunwasser, S. M., Gillham, J. E., & Kim, E. S. (2009). A meta-analytic review of the Penn Resiliency Program's effect on depressive symptoms. *Journal of Consulting and Clinical Psychology, 77*(6), 1042–1054.

Bryant, F. B., & Veroff, J. (2007). *Savoring: A new model of positive experience.* Mahwah, NJ: Erlbaum.

Caplan, G. (1964). *Principles of preventive psychiatry.* New York: Basic Books.

Caprara, G. V., Barbaranelli, C., Steca, P., & Malone, P. S. (2006). Teachers' self-efficacy beliefs as determinants of job satisfaction and students' academic achievement: A study at the school level. *Journal of School Psychology, 44*(6), 473–490.

Carr, E. G., Dunlap, G., Horner, R. H., Koegel, R. L., Turnbull, A. P., Sailor, W., et al. (2002). Positive behavior support evolution of an applied science. *Journal of Positive Behavior Interventions, 4*(1), 4–16.

Casas, F., & Rees, G. (2015). Measures of children's subjective well-being: Analysis of the potential for cross-national comparisons. *Child Indicator Research, 8*(1), 49–69.

Casas, F., Sarriera, J. C., Alfaro, J., Gonzalez, M., Bedin, L., Abs, D., et al. (2015). Reconsidering life domains that contribute to subjective well-being among adolescents with data from three countries. *Journal of Happiness Studies, 16*(2), 491–513.

Challen, A., Noden, P., West, A., & Machin, S. (2011). *UK Resilience Programme evaluation: Final report* (Research reports, DFE-RR097). London: Department for Education.

Challen, A. R., Machin, S. J., & Gillham, J. E. (2014). The UK Resilience Programme: A school-based universal nonrandomized pragmatic controlled trial. *Journal of Consulting and Clinical Psychology, 82*(1), 75–89.

Chan, D. W. (2010). Gratitude, gratitude intervention and subjective well-being among Chinese school teachers in Hong Kong. *Educational Psychology, 30*(2), 139–153.

Chan, D. W. (2011). Burnout and life satisfaction: Does gratitude intervention make a difference among Chinese school teachers in Hong Kong? *Educational Psychology, 31*(7), 809–823.

Chan, D. W. (2013). Subjective well-being of Hong

Kong Chinese teachers: The contribution of gratitude, forgiveness, and the orientations to happiness. *Teaching and Teacher Education, 32,* 22–30.

Chappel, A., Suldo, S. M., & Ogg, J. (2014). Associations between adolescents' family stressors and life satisfaction. *Journal of Child and Family Studies, 23*(1), 76–84.

Clunies-Ross, P., Little, E., & Kienhuis, M. (2008). Self-reported and actual use of proactive and reactive classroom management strategies and their relationship with teacher stress and student behaviour. *Educational Psychology, 28*(6), 693–710.

Coatsworth, J. D., Duncan, L. G., Nix, R. L., Greenberg, M. T., Gayles, J. G., Bamberger, K. T., et al. (2015). Integrating mindfulness with parent training: Effects of the mindfulness-enhanced strengthening families program. *Developmental Psychology, 51*(1), 26–35.

Cohn, M. A., & Fredrickson, B. L. (2010). In search of durable positive psychology interventions: Predictors and consequences of long-term positive behavior change. *Journal of Positive Psychology, 5*(5), 355–366.

Cook, C. R., Frye, M., Slemrod, T., Lyon, A. R., Renshaw, T. L., & Zhang, Y. (2015). An integrated approach to universal prevention: Independent and combined effects of PBIS and SEL on youth's mental health. *School Psychology Quarterly, 30*(2), 166–183.

Crede, J., Wirthwein, L., McElvany, N., & Steinmayr, R. (2015). Adolescents' academic achievement and life satisfaction: The role of parents' education. *Frontiers in Psychology, 6*(52), 1–8.

Crenshaw, M. (1998). *Adjudicated violent youth, adjudicated non-violent youth vs. non-adjudicated, non-violent youth on selected psychological measures.* Unpublished master's thesis, University of South Carolina, Columbia, SC.

Critchley, H., & Gibbs, S. (2012). The effects of positive psychology on the efficacy beliefs of school staff. *Educational and Child Psychology, 29*(4), 64–76.

Csikszentmihalyi, M. (2014). *Applications of flow in human development and education: The collected works of Mihaly Csikszentmihalyi.* Dordrecht, The Netherlands: Springer.

Csikszentmihalyi, M., & Hunter, J. (2003). Happiness in everyday life: The uses of experience sampling. *Journal of Happiness Studies, 4*(2), 185–199.

Csillik, A. (2015). Positive motivational interviewing: Activating clients' strengths and intrinsic motivation to change. *Journal of Contemporary Psychotherapy, 45*(2), 119–128.

Cummins, R. A., & Lau, A. L. D. (2005). *Personal Wellbeing Index—School Children (PWI-CS)—Manual.* Melbourne, Australia: Australian Centre on Quality of Life, School of Psychology, Deakin University. Available at *www.deakin.edu.au/research/acqol/instruments/wellbeing-index.*

Curry, J. F. (2014). Future directions in research on psychotherapy for adolescent depression. *Journal of Clinical Child and Adolescent Psychology, 43*(3), 510–526.

Damon, W., Menon, J., & Bronk, K. C. (2003). The development of purpose during adolescence. *Applied Developmental Science, 7*(3), 119–128.

Davis, M. H. (1983). Measuring individual differences in empathy: Evidence for a multidimensional approach. *Journal of Personality and Social Psychology, 44*(1), 113–126.

Derogatis, L. R., & Spencer, M. S. (1982). *The Brief Symptom Inventory (BSI): Administration, scoring, and procedures manual–1.* Baltimore: Johns Hopkins University School of Medicine, Clinical Psychometrics Research Unit.

Dew, T., & Huebner, E. S. (1994). Adolescents' perceived quality of life: An exploratory investigation. *Journal of School Psychology, 33*(2), 185–199.

Diener, E., & Chan, M. (2011). Happy people live longer: Subjective well-being contributes to health and longevity. *Applied Psychology: Health and Well-Being, 3*(1), 1–43.

Diener, E., Emmons, R. A., Larsen, R. S., & Griffin, S. (1985). The Satisfaction with Life Scale. *Journal of Personality Assessment, 49*(1), 71–75.

Diener, E., Scollon, C. N., & Lucas, R. E. (2009). The evolving concept of subjective well-being: The multifaceted nature of happiness. In E. Diener (Ed.), *Assessing well-being: The collected works of Ed Diener* (pp. 67–100). New York: Springer.

Diener, E., & Seligman, M. E. P. (2002). Very happy people. *Psychological Science, 13*(1), 81–84.

Dinisman, T., Fernandes, L., & Main, G. (2015). Findings from the first wave of the ISCWeB project: International perspectives on child subjective well-being. *Child Indicators Research, 8*(1), 1–4.

Doll, B., Brehm, K., & Zucker, S. (2014). *Resilient classrooms: Creating healthy environments for learning* (2nd ed.). New York: Guilford Press.

Doll, B., Cummings, J. A., & Chapla, B. A. (2014). Best practices in population-based school mental health services. In P. L. Harrison & A. Thomas (Eds.), *Best practices in school psychology: Systems level perspectives* (pp. 149–163). Bethesda, MD: National Association of School Psychologists.

Domitrovich, C. E., Bradshaw, C. P., Poduska, J. M., Hoagwood, K., Buckley, J. A., Olin, S., et al. (2008). Maximizing the implementation quality of evidence-based preventive interventions in schools: A conceptual framework. *Advances in School Mental Health Promotion, 1*(3), 6–28.

Donaldson, S. I., Dollwet, M., & Rao, M. A. (2015). Happiness, excellence, and optimal human functioning revisited: Examining the peer-reviewed literature linked to positive psychology. *Journal of Positive Psychology, 10*(3), 185–195.

Dowdy, E., Furlong, M. J., Raines, T. C., Bovery, B., Kauffman, B., Kamphaus, R. W., et al. (2015). Enhancing school-based mental health services with a preventive and promotive approach to universal screening for complete mental health. *Journal of Educational and Psychological Consultation, 25*(2–3), 178–197.

Duan, W., Ho, S. M. Y., Bai, Y., Tang, X., Zhang, Y., Li, T., et al. (2012). Factor structure of the Chinese Virtues Questionnaire. *Research on Social Work Practice, 22*(6), 680–688.

Duan, W., Ho, S. M. Y., Tang, X., Li, T., & Zhang, Y. (2014). Character strength-based intervention to promote satisfaction with life in the Chinese university context. *Journal of Happiness Studies, 15*(6), 1347–1361.

Duckworth, A. L., Quinn, P. D., & Seligman, M. E. (2009). Positive predictors of teacher effectiveness. *Journal of Positive Psychology, 4*(6), 540–547.

Dunlap, G., Kincaid, D., & Jackson, D. (2013). Positive behavior support: Foundations, systems, and quality of life. In M. L. Wehmeyer (Ed.), *The Oxford handbook of positive psychology and disability* (pp. 303–316). New York: Oxford University Press.

Durlak, J. A., & DuPre, E. P. (2008). Implementation matters: A review of research on the influence of implementation on program outcomes and the factors affecting implementation. *American Journal of Community Psychology, 41*(3–4), 327–350.

Durlak, J. A., Weissberg, R. P., Dymnicki, A. B., Taylor, R. D., & Schellinger, K. B. (2011). The impact of enhancing students' social and emotional learning: A meta-analysis of school-based universal interventions. *Child Development, 82*(1), 405–432.

Eber, L., Weist, M., & Barrett, S. (2013). An introduction to the interconnected systems framework. In S. Barrett, L. Eber, & M. Weist (Eds.), *Advancing education effectiveness: Interconnecting school mental health and school-wide positive behavior support* (pp. 3–17). Retrieved from *www.pbis.org/common/cms/files/Current%20Topics/Final-Monograph.pdf*.

Eklund, K., Dowdy, E., Jones, C., & Furlong, M. (2011). Applicability of the dual-factor model of mental health for college students. *Journal of College Student Psychotherapy, 25*(1), 79–92.

Emmons, R. A., & McCullough, M. E. (2003). Counting blessings versus burdens: An experimental investigation of gratitude and subjective well-being in daily life. *Journal of Personality and Social Psychology, 84*(2), 377–389.

Emmons, R. A., & Stern, R. (2013). Gratitude as a psychotherapeutic intervention. *Journal of Clinical Psychology, 69*(8), 846–855.

Ferraioli, S. J., & Harris, S. L. (2013). Comparative effects of mindfulness and skills-based parent training programs for parents of children with autism: Feasibility and preliminary outcome data. *Mindfulness, 4*(2), 89–101.

Fisher, D. L., & Fraser, B. J. (1981). Validity and use of the My Class Inventory. *Science Education, 65*(2), 145–156.

Fleming, J. L., Mackrain, M., & LeBuffe, P. A. (2013). Caring for the caregiver: Promoting the resilience of teachers. In S. Goldstein & R. B. Brooks (Eds.), *Handbook of resilience in children* (pp. 387–397). New York: Springer.

Forgatch, M. S., & Patterson, G. R. (2005). *Parents and adolescents living together. Part 2: Family problem solving* (2nd ed). Champaign, IL: Research Press.

Fox, J. (2008). *Your child's strengths: Discover them, develop them, use them.* New York: Viking Adult.

Fox Eades, J. M. (2008). *Celebrating strengths: Building strengths-based schools.* Coventry, UK: CAPP Press.

Franklin, J., & Doran, J. (2009). Does all coaching enhance objective performance independently evaluated by blind assessors?: The importance of the coaching model and content. *International Coaching Psychology Review, 4*(2), 128–144.

Fredrickson, B. L. (2001). The role of positive emotions in positive psychology: The broaden-and-build theory of positive emotions. *American Psychologist, 56*(3), 218–226.

Fredrickson, B. L. (2009). *Positivity: Groundbreaking research to release your inner optimist and thrive.* Oxford, UK: Oneworld.

Fredrickson, B. L. (2013). Updated thinking on positivity ratios. *American Psychologist, 68*(9), 814–822.

Friedrich, A., Thalji, A., Suldo, S. M., Chappel, A., & Fefer, S. (2010, March). *Increasing thirteen year-olds' happiness through a manualized group intervention.* Paper presented at the National Association of School Psychologists Annual Conference, Chicago, IL.

Frisch, M. B. (1998). Quality of life therapy and assessment in health care. *Clinical Psychology: Science and Practice, 5*(1), 19–39.

Frisch, M. B. (2013). Evidence-based well-being/positive psychology assessment and intervention with quality of life therapy and coaching and the Quality of Life Inventory (QOLI). *Social Indicators Research, 114*(2), 193–227.

Froh, J. J., Bono, G., Fan, J. Emmons, R. A., Henderson, K., Harris, C, et al. (2014). Nice thinking!: An educational intervention that teaches children to think gratefully. *School Psychology Review, 43*(2), 132–152.

Froh, J. J., Fan, J., Emmons, R. A., Bono, G., Huebner, E. S., & Watkins, P. (2011). Measuring gratitude in youth: Assessing the psychometric properties of adult gratitude scales in children and adolescents. *Psychological Assessment, 23*(2), 311–324.

Froh, J. J., Kashdan, T. B., Ozimkowski, K. M., & Miller, N. (2009). Who benefits the most from a gratitude intervention in children and adolescents?: Examining positive affect as a moderator. *Journal of Positive Psychology, 4*(5), 408–422.

Froh, J. J., Sefick, W. J., & Emmons, R. A. (2008). Counting blessings in early adolescents: An experimental study of gratitude and subjective well-being. *Journal of School Psychology, 46*(2), 213–233.

Fung, B. K. K., Ho, S. M. Y., Fung, A. S. M., Leung, E. Y. P., Chow, S. P., Ip, W. Y., et al. (2011). The development of a strength-focused mutual support group for caretakers of children with cerebral palsy. *East Asian Archives of Psychiatry, 21*(2), 64–72.

Furlong, M. J. (2015). *Social Emotional Health Survey System.* Santa Barbara: Center for School-Based Youth Development, University of California, Santa Barbara. Available at *www.michaelfurlong.info/research/covitality.html.*

Furlong, M. J., Dowdy, E., Carnazzo, K., Bovery, B., & Kim, E. (2014). Covitality: Fostering the building blocks of complete mental health. *NASP Communiqué, 42*(8), 24, 27–28. Available at *www.readperiodicals.com/201406/3346560221.html.*

Furlong, M. J., You, S., Renshaw, T. L., O'Malley, M. D., & Rebelez, J. (2013). Preliminary development of the Positive Experiences at School Scale for Elementary School Children. *Child Indicators Research, 6*(4), 753–775.

Furlong, M. J., You, S., Renshaw, T. L., Smith, D. C., & O'Malley, M. D. (2014). Preliminary development and validation of the Social and Emotional Health Survey for Secondary School Students. *Social Indicators Research, 117*(3), 1011–1032.

Furrer, C., & Skinner, E. (2003). Sense of relatedness as a factor in children's academic engagement and performance. *Journal of Educational Psychology, 95*(1), 148–162.

Garland, E. L., Fredrickson, B., Kring, A. M., Johnson, D. P., Meyer, P. S., & Penn, D. L. (2010). Upward spirals of positive emotions counter downward spirals of negativity: Insights from the broaden-and-build theory and affective neuroscience on the treatment of emotion dysfunctions and deficits in psychopathology. *Clinical Psychology Review, 30*(7), 849–864.

Geldhof, G. J., Bowers, E. P., Boyd, M. J., Mueller, M. K., Napolitano, C. M., Schmid, K. L., et al. (2014). Creation of short and very short measures of the five Cs of positive youth development. *Journal of Research on Adolescence, 24*(1), 163–176.

Gentzler, A. L., Morey, J. N., Palmer, C. A., & Yi, C. Y. (2013). Young adolescents' responses to positive events: Associations with positive affect and adjustment. *Journal of Early Adolescence, 33*(5), 663–683.

Gentzler, A. L., Ramsey, M. A., Yi, C. Y., Palmer, C. A., & Morey, J. N. (2014). Young adolescents' emotional and regulatory responses to positive life events: Investigating temperament, attachment, and event characteristics. *Journal of Positive Psychology, 9*(2), 108–121.

Gibbs, S., & Miller, A. (2014). Teachers' resilience and well-being: A role for educational psychology. *Teachers and Teaching, 20*(5), 609–621.

Gillham, J. (2011, July). *Positive psychology in schools: 3 year follow-up.* Paper presented at the World Congress on Positive Psychology, Philadelphia, PA.

Gillham, J. E., Abenavoli, R. M., Brunwasser, S. M., Linkins, M., Reivich, K. J., & Seligman, M. E. P. (2013). Resilience education. In S. David, I. Boniwell, & A. Conley Ayers (Eds.), *The Oxford handbook of happiness* (pp. 609–630). Oxford, UK: Oxford University Press.

Gillham, J. E., Hamilton, J., Freres, D. R., Patton, K., & Gallop, R. (2006). Preventing depression among early adolescents in the primary care setting: A randomized controlled study of the Penn Resiliency Program. *Journal of Abnormal Child Psychology, 34*(2), 203–219.

Gillham, J. E., Jaycox, L. H., Reivich, K. J., Seligman, M. E. P., & Silver, T. (1990). *The Penn Resiliency Program.* Unpublished manual, University of Pennsylvania, Philadelphia, PA.

Gillham, J. E., Reivich, K. J., Brunwasser, S. M., Freres, D. R., Chajon, N. D., Kash-MacDonald, M., et al. (2012). Evaluation of a group cognitive-behavioral depression prevention program for young adolescents: A randomized effectiveness trial. *Journal of Clinical Child and Adolescent Psychology, 41*(5), 621–639.

Gillham, J. E., Reivich, K. J., Freres, D. R., Chaplin, T. M., Shatté, A. J., Samuels, B., et al. (2007). School-based prevention of depressive symptoms: A randomized controlled study of the effectiveness and specificity of the Penn Resiliency Program. *Journal of Consulting and Clinical Psychology, 75*(1), 9–19.

Gilman, R., Easterbrooks, S. R., & Frey, M. (2004). A preliminary study of multidimensional youth life satisfaction among deaf/hard of hearing youth across environmental settings. *Social Indicators Research, 66*(1–2), 143–164.

Gilman, R., & Huebner, E. S. (1997). Children's reports of their life satisfaction. *School Psychology International, 18*(3), 229–243.

Gilman, R., Huebner, E. S., Tian, L., Park, N., O'Byrne, J., Schiff, M., et al. (2008). Cross-national adolescent multidimensional life satisfaction reports: Analyses of mean scores and response style differences. *Journal of Youth and Adolescence, 37*(2), 142–154.

Govindji, R., & Linley, P. A. (2007). Strengths use, self-concordance and well-being: Implications for strengths coaching and coaching psychologists. *International Coaching Psychology Review, 2*(2), 143–153.

Grant, A. M. (2014). The efficacy of executive coaching in times of organisational change. *Journal of Change Management, 14*(2), 258–280.

Gray, L., & Taie, S. (2015). *Public school teacher attrition and mobility in the first five years: Results from the first through fifth waves of the 2007–08 Beginning Teacher Longitudinal Study* (NCES 2015-337). Washington, DC: National Center for Education

Statistics. Retrieved June 6, 2015, from *http://nces. ed.gov/pubsearch*.

Green, L. S., Oades, L. G., & Grant, A. M. (2006). Cognitive behavioral, solution-focused life coaching: Enhancing goal striving, well-being, and hope. *Journal of Positive Psychology, 1*(3), 142–149.

Green, S., Grant, A., & Rynsaardt, J. (2007). Evidence-based life coaching for senior high school students: Building hardiness and hope. *International Coaching Psychology Review, 2*(1), 24–32.

Greenberg, M. T., Weissberg, R. P., O'Brien, M. U., Fredericks, L., Resnick, H., & Elias, M. J. (2003). Enhancing school-based prevention and youth development through coordinated social, emotional, and academic learning. *American Psychologist, 58*(6–7), 466–474.

Greenspoon, P. J., & Saklofske, D. H. (2001). Toward an integration of subjective well-being and psychopathology. *Social Indicators Research, 54*(1), 81–108.

Gresham, F. M., & Elliott, S. N. (1990). *The Social Skills Rating System*. Minneapolis, MN: Pearson Assessments.

Gresham, F. M., & Elliott, S. N. (2008). *Social Skills Improvement System—Rating Scales*. Minneapolis, MN: Pearson Assessments.

Griffin, M., & Huebner, E. S. (2000). Multidimensional life satisfaction reports of students with serious emotional disturbance. *Journal of Psychoeducational Assessment, 18*(2), 111–124.

Hamre, B. K., Pianta, R. C., Downer, J. T., & Mashburn, A. J. (2008). Teachers' perceptions of conflict with young students: Looking beyond problem behaviors. *Social Development, 17*(1), 115–136.

Harter, S. (1982). The Perceived Competence Scale for Children. *Child Development, 53*(1), 87–97.

Harter, S. (1985). *Manual for the Self-Perception Profile for Children*. Denver, CO: University of Denver.

Hawn Foundation. (2008). *Mindfulness education*. Miami Beach, FL: Author.

Headey, B., Muffels, R., & Wagner, G. G. (2014). Parents transmit happiness along with associated values and behaviors to their children: A lifelong happiness dividend? *Social Indicators Research, 116*(3), 909–933.

Helliwell, J. F., Layward, R., & Sachs, J. (Eds.). (2015). *World happiness report 2015*. New York: Sustainable Development Solutions Network.

Herman, K. C., Reinke, W. M., Frey, A. J., & Shepard, S. A. (2014). *Motivational interviewing in schools: Strategies for engaging parents, teachers, and students*. New York: Springer.

Hexdall, C. M., & Huebner, E. S. (2007). Subjective well-being in pediatric oncology patients. *Applied Research in Quality of Life, 2*(3), 189–208.

Hills, K. J., & Robinson, A. (2010). Enhancing teacher well-being: Put on your oxygen masks! *Communique, 39*(4), 1–17.

Ho, S. M. Y., & Cheung, M. W. L. (2007). Using the combined etic–emic approach to develop a measurement of interpersonal subjective well-being in Chinese populations. In A. D. Ong & M. H. M. van Dulmen (Eds.), *Oxford handbook of methods in positive psychology* (pp. 139–152). New York: Oxford University Press.

Ho, S. M. Y., Duan, W., & Tang, S. C. M. (2014). The psychology of virtue and happiness in Western and Asian thought. In N. E. Snow & F. V. Trivigno (Eds.), *The philosophy and psychology of character and happiness* (pp. 215–238). New York: Routledge.

Hoppmann, C. A., Gerstorf, D., Willis, S. L., & Schaie, K. W. (2011). Spousal interrelations in happiness in the Seattle Longitudinal Study: Considerable similarities in levels and change over time. *Developmental Psychology, 47*(1), 1–8.

Horner, R. H., Sugai, G., & Anderson, C. M. (2010). Examining the evidence base for school-wide positive behavior support. *Focus on Exceptional Children, 42*(8), 1–14.

Horner, R. H., Sugai, G., Smolkowski, K., Eber, L., Nakasato, J., Todd, A., et al. (2009). A randomized, wait-list controlled effectiveness trial assessing school-wide positive behavior support in elementary schools. *Journal of Positive Behavior Interventions, 11*(3), 133–144.

Hoy, B., Thalji, A., Frey, M., Kuzia, K., & Suldo, S. M. (2012, February). *Bullying and students' happiness: Social support as a protective factor*. Poster presented at the annual conference of the National Association of School Psychologists, Philadelphia, PA.

Hoy, B. D., Suldo, S. M., & Raffaele Mendez, L. (2013). Links between parents' and children's levels of gratitude, life satisfaction, and hope. *Journal of Happiness Studies, 14*(4), 1343–1361.

Huebner, E. S. (1991a). Further validation of the Student's Life Satisfaction Scale: Independence of satisfaction and affect ratings. *Journal of Psychoeducational Assessment, 9*(4), 363–368.

Huebner, E. S. (1991b). Initial development of the Student's Life Satisfaction Scale. *School Psychology International, 12*(3), 231–240.

Huebner, E. S. (1994). Preliminary development and validation of a multidimensional life satisfaction scale for children. *Psychological Assessment, 6*(2), 149–158.

Huebner, E. S., & Alderman, G. L. (1993). Convergent and discriminant validation of a children's life satisfaction scale: Its relationship to self- and teacher-reported psychological problems and school functioning. *Social Indicators Research, 30*(1), 71–82.

Huebner, E. S., Brantley, A., Nagle, R. J., & Valois, R. F. (2002). Correspondence between parent and adolescent ratings of life satisfaction for adolescents with and without mental disabilities. *Journal of Psychoeducational Assessment, 20*(1), 20–29.

Huebner, E. S., Drane, J. W., & Valois, R. F. (2000). Levels and demographic correlates of adolescent life satisfaction reports. *School Psychology International, 21*(3), 281–292.

Huebner, E. S., & Hills, K. J. (2013). Assessment of life satisfaction with children and adolescents. In D. Saklofske, C. R. Reyolds, & V. Schwean (Eds.), *Oxford handbook of psychological assessment of children and adolescents* (pp. 773–787). Oxford, UK: Oxford University Press.

Huebner, E. S., Hills, K. J., & Jiang, X. (2013). Assessment and promotion of life satisfaction in youth. In C. Proctor & P. A. Linley (Eds.), *Research, applications and interventions for children and adolescents: A positive psychology perspective* (pp. 23–42). New York: Springer.

Huebner, E. S., Hills, K. J., Siddall, J., & Gilman, R. (2014). Life satisfaction and schooling. In M. Furlong, R. Gilman, & E. S., Huebner (Eds.), *Handbook of positive psychology in the schools* (2nd ed., pp. 192–207). New York: Routledge.

Huebner, E. S., Nagle, R. J., & Suldo, S. (2003). Quality of life assessment in child and adolescent health care: The use of the Multidimensional Students' Life Satisfaction Scale. In M. J. Sirgy, D. Rahtz, & A. C. Samli (Eds.), *Advances in quality of life theory and research* (pp. 179–190). Dordrecht, The Netherlands: Kluwer Academic Press.

Huebner, E. S., Seligson, J., Valois, R. F., & Suldo, S. M. (2006). A review of the Brief Multidimensional Students' Life Satisfaction Scale. *Social Indicators Research, 79*(3), 477–484.

Huebner, E. S., Valois, R. F., Paxton, R., & Drane, J. W. (2005). Middle school students' perceptions of quality of life. *Journal of Happiness Studies, 6*(1), 15–24.

Huebner, E. S., Zullig, K., & Saha, R. (2012). Factor structure and reliability of an abbreviated version of the Multidimensional Students' Life Satisfaction Scale. *Child Indicators Research, 5*(4), 651–657.

Hurley, D. B., & Kwon, P. (2012). Results of a study to increase savoring the moment: Differential impact on positive and negative outcomes. *Journal of Happiness Studies, 13*(4), 579–588.

Institute of Education Sciences & National Science Foundation. (2013, August). *Common guidelines for education research and development* (A report from the Joint Committee of the IES, U.S. Department of Education, and the National Science Foundation). Retrieved May 11, 2015, from *http://ies.ed.gov/pdf/CommonGuidelines.pdf.*

Ito, A., Smith, D. C., You, S., Shimoda, Y., & Furlong, M. J. (2015). Validation of the Social Emotional Health Survey—Secondary for Japanese Students. *Contemporary School Psychology, 19*(4), 243–252.

Jennings, P. A., Frank, J. L., Snowberg, K. E., Coccia, M. A., & Greenberg, M. T. (2013). Improving classroom learning environments by Cultivating Awareness and Resilience in Education (CARE): Results of a randomized controlled trial. *School Psychology Quarterly, 28*(4), 374–390.

Jennings, P. A., & Greenberg, M. T. (2009). The prosocial classroom: Teacher social and emotional competence in relation to student and classroom outcomes. *Review of Educational Research, 79*(1), 491–525.

Jiang, X., Huebner, E. S., & Siddall, J. (2013). A short-term longitudinal study of differential sources of school-related social support and adolescents' school satisfaction. *Social Indicators Research, 114*(3), 1073–1086.

Johnstone, J., Rooney, R. M., Hassan, S., & Kane, R. T. (2014). Prevention of depression and anxiety symptoms in adolescents: 42 and 54 months follow-up of the Aussie Optimism Program—Positive Thinking Skills. *Frontiers in Psychology, 5*(364), 1–10.

Jones, A. (1998). Creative coloring. In *104 activities that build* (pp. 26–27). Richland, WA: Rec Room.

Jones, C. N., You, S., & Furlong, M. J. (2013). A preliminary examination of covitality as integrated wellbeing in college students. *Social Indicators Research, 111*(2), 511–526.

Jose, P. E., Lim, B. T., & Bryant, F. B. (2012). Does savoring increase happiness?: A daily diary study. *Journal of Positive Psychology, 7*(3), 176–187.

Joseph, S., & Murphy, D. (2013). Person-centered approach, positive psychology, and relational helping: Building bridges. *Journal of Humanistic Psychology, 53*(1), 26–51.

Joseph, S., & Wood, A. (2010). Assessment of positive functioning in clinical psychology: Theoretical and practical issues. *Clinical Psychology Review, 30*(7), 830–838.

Joshanloo, M., & Weijers, D. (2014). Aversion to happiness across cultures: A review of where and why people are averse to happiness. *Journal of Happiness Studies, 15*(3), 717–735.

Kabat-Zinn, J. (1990). *Full catastrophe living: Using the wisdom of your body and mind to face stress, pain and illness.* New York: Dell.

Kabat-Zinn, J. (2003). Mindfulness-based interventions in context: Past, present, and future. *Clinical Psychology: Science and Practice, 10*(2), 144–156.

Kahneman, D., & Deaton, A. (2010). High income improves evaluation of life but not emotional well-being. *Proceedings of the National Academy of Sciences, 107*(38), 16489–16493.

Kalak, N., Lemola, S., Brand, S., Holsboer-Trachsler, E., & Grob, A. (2014). Sleep duration and subjective psychological well-being in adolescence: A longitudinal study in Switzerland and Norway. *Neuropsychiatric Disease and Treatment, 10*(3), 1199–1207.

Kamphaus, R. W., & Reynolds, C. R. (2007). *BASC-2 Behavioral and Emotional Screening System manual.* Bloomington, MN: Pearson.

Kam, C., & Greenberg, M. T. (1998). *Technical measurement report on the Teacher Social Competence Rating Scale.* Unpublished technical report, Prevention Research Center for the Promotion of Human Development, Pennsylvania State University.

Kan, C., Karasawa, M., & Kitayama, S. (2009). Minimalist in style: Self, identity, and well-being in Japan. *Self and Identity, 8*(2–3), 300–317.

Kehoe, J., & Fischer, N. (2002). *Mind power for children: The guide for parents and teachers.* Vancouver, BC, Canada: Zoetic.

Kelly, R. M., Hills, K. J., Huebner, E. S., & McQuillin, S. D. (2012). The longitudinal stability and dynamics of group membership in the dual-factor model of mental health: Psychosocial predictors of mental health. *Canadian Journal of School Psychology, 27*(4), 337–355.

Kern, M. L., Waters, L. E., Adler, A., & White, M. A. (2015). A multidimensional approach to measuring well-being in students: Application of the PERMA framework. *Journal of Positive Psychology, 10*(3), 262–271.

Keyes, C. L. M. (2006). Mental health in adolescence: Is America's youth flourishing? *American Journal of Orthopsychiatry, 76*(3), 395–402.

Keyes, C. L. M. (2009). The nature and importance of positive mental health in America's adolescents. In R. Gilman, E. S. Huebner, & M. J. Furlong (Eds.), *Handbook of positive psychology in the schools* (pp. 9–23). New York: Routledge.

Kim, E., Dowdy, E., & Furlong, M. J. (2014). An exploration of using a dual-factor model in school-based mental health screening. *Canadian Journal of School Psychology, 29*(2), 127–140.

Kim, J. S., & Franklin, C. (2009). Solution-focused brief therapy in schools: A review of the outcome literature. *Children and Youth Services Review, 31*(4), 464–470.

King, L. A. (2001). The health benefits of writing about life goals. *Personality and Social Psychology Bulletin, 27*(7), 798–807.

Klassen, R. M., & Chiu, M. M. (2010). Effects on teachers' self-efficacy and job satisfaction: Teacher gender, years of experience, and job stress. *Journal of Educational Psychology, 102*(3), 741–756.

Koestner, R. F., & Veronneau, M. H. (2001). *The Children's Intrinsic Needs Satisfaction Scale.* Unpublished questionnaire, McGill University, Montreal, Quebec, Canada.

Kosher, H., Ben-Arieh, A., Jiang, X., & Huebner, E. S. (2014). Advances in children's rights and the science of subjective well-being: Implications for school psychologists. *School Psychology Quarterly, 29*(1), 7–20.

Kovacs, M. (1992). *Children's Depression Inventory (CDI) manual.* New York: Multi-Health Systems.

Kurtz, J. L. (2008). Looking to the future to appreciate the present: The benefits of perceived temporal scarcity. *Psychological Science, 19*(12), 1238–1241.

Kusché, C. A., Greenberg, M. T., & Beilke, R. (1988). *Seattle Personality Questionnaire for Young School-Aged Children.* Unpublished measure, University of Washington, Department of Psychology.

Lam, C. C., Lau, N. S., Lo, H. H., & Woo, D. M. S. (2015). Developing mindfulness programs for adolescents: Lessons learned from an attempt in Hong Kong. *Social Work in Mental Health, 13*(4), 365–389.

Lambert, R. G., McCarthy, C., O'Donnell, M., & Wang, C. (2009). Measuring elementary teacher stress and coping in the classroom: Validity evidence for the classroom appraisal of resources and demands. *Psychology in the Schools, 46*(10), 973–988.

Lau, N.-S., & Hue, M.-T. (2011). Preliminary outcomes of a mindfulness-based programme for Hong Kong adolescents in schools: Well-being, stress and depressive symptoms. *International Journal of Children's Spirituality, 16*(4), 315–330.

Laurent, J., Cantanzaro, S. J., Joiner, T. E., Rudolph, K. D., Potter, K. I., Lambert, S., et al. (1999). A measure of positive and negative affect for children: Scale development and preliminary validation. *Psychological Assessment, 11*(3), 326–338.

Lawlor, M. S., Schonert-Reichl, K. A., Gadermann, A. M., & Zumbo, B. D. (2014). A validation study of the Mindful Attention Awareness Scale adapted for children. *Mindfulness, 5*(6), 730–741.

Lawson, A., Moore, R., Portman-Marsh, N., & Lynn, J. (2013). Random Acts of Kindness (RAK) school-based pilot implementation: Year two evaluation report executive summary. Retrieved from *http://rak-materials.s3.amazonaws.com/reports/RAK_Final_EOY_Pilot_Program_Report.docx.*

Layous, K., Chancellor, J., & Lyubomirsky, S. (2014). Positive activities as protective factors against mental health conditions. *Journal of Abnormal Psychology, 123*(1), 3–12.

Layous, K., Lee, H., Choi, I., & Lyubomirsky, S. (2013). Culture matters when designing a successful happiness-increasing activity: A comparison of the United States and South Korea. *Journal of Cross-Cultural Psychology, 44*(8), 1294–1303.

Layous, K., & Lyubomirsky, S. (2014). The how, why, what, when, and who of happiness: Mechanisms underlying the success of positive interventions. In J. Gruber & J. T. Moskowitz (Eds.), *Positive emotion: Integrating the light sides and dark side* (pp. 473–495). New York: Oxford University Press.

Layous, K., Nelson, S. K., & Lyubomirsky, S. (2013). What is the optimal way to deliver a positive activity intervention?: The case of writing about one's best possible selves. *Journal of Happiness Studies, 14*(2), 635–654.

Layous, K., Nelson, S. K., Oberle, E., Schonert-Reichl, K. A., & Lyubomirsky, S. (2012). Kindness counts: Prompting prosocial behavior in preadolescents boosts peer acceptance and well-being. *PLoS ONE, 7*(12), e51380.

Lee, B. J., & Yoo, M. S. (2015). Family, school, and community correlates of children's subjective well-being: An international comparative study. *Child Indicators Research, 8*(1), 151–175.

Lee, S., You, S., & Furlong, M. J. (2016). Validation of

the Social Emotional Health Survey—Secondary for Korean students. *Child Indicators Research, 9*(1), 73–92.

Lenzi, M., Dougherty, D., Furlong, M. J., Sharkey, J., & Dowdy, E. (2015). The configuration protective model: Factors associated with adolescent behavioral and emotional problems. *Journal of Applied Developmental Psychology, 38*, 49–59.

Leong, F. T. L., Leung, K., & Cheung, F. M. (2010). Integrating cross-cultural psychology research methods into ethnic minority psychology. *Cultural Diversity and Ethnic Minority Psychology, 16*(4), 590–597.

Lewinsohn, P. M., Redner, J. E., & Seeley, J. R. (1991). The relationship between life satisfaction and psychosocial variables: New perspectives. In F. Strack, M. Argyle, & N. Schwarz (Eds.), *Subjective well-being: An interdisciplinary perspective* (pp. 141–169). Elmsford, NY: Pergamon Press.

Linkins, M., Niemiec, R. M., Gillham, J., & Mayerson, D. (2015). Through the lens of strength: A framework for educating the heart. *Journal of Positive Psychology, 10*(1), 64–68.

Linley, P. A., Garcea, N., Hill, J., Minhas, G., Trenier, E., & Willars, J. (2010). Strengthspotting in coaching: Conceptualisation and development of the Strengthspotting Scale. *International Coaching Psychology Review, 5*(2), 165–176.

Lippman, L. H., Moore, K. A., Guzman, L., Ryberg, R., McIntosh, H., Ramos, M. F., et al. (2014). *Flourishing children*. New York: Springer.

Long, A. C., Renshaw, T. L., Hamilton, M., Bolognino, B. S., & Lark, C. (2015, February). *Teacher psychological resources as they relate to classroom management practices*. Poster presented at the annual convention of the National Association of School Psychologists, Orlando, FL.

Lovibond, S. H., & Lovibond, P. F. (1995). *Manual for the Depression Anxiety Stress Scales* (2nd ed.) Sydney: Psychology Foundation.

Lu, L. (2006). "Cultural fit": Individual and societal discrepancies in values, beliefs, and subjective well-being. *Journal of Social Psychology, 146*(2), 203–221.

Luiselli, J. K., Putnam, R. F., Handler, M. W., & Feinberg, A. B. (2005). Whole-school positive behaviour support: Effects on student discipline problems and academic performance. *Educational Psychology, 25*(2–3), 183–198.

Lykken, D. T. (1999). *Happiness: What studies on twins show us about nature, nurture, and the happiness set point*. New York: Golden Books.

Lyons, M. D., & Huebner, E. S. (2015). Academic characteristics of early adolescents with higher levels of life satisfaction. *Applied Research in Quality of Life*. Published online.

Lyons, M. D., Huebner, E. S., & Hills, K. J., (2013). The dual-factor model of mental health: A short-term longitudinal study of school-related outcomes. *Social Indicators Research, 114*(2), 549–565.

Lyons, M. D., Otis, K. L., Huebner, E. S., & Hills, K. J. (2014). Life satisfaction and maladaptive behaviors in early adolescents. *School Psychology Quarterly, 29*(4), 553–566.

Lyubomirsky, S. (2008). *The how of happiness: A scientific approach to getting the life you want*. New York: Penguin.

Lyubomirsky, S., & Layous, K. (2013). How do simple positive activities increase well-being? *Current Directions in Psychological Science, 22*(1), 57–62.

Lyubomirsky, S., & Lepper, H. S. (1999). A measure of subjective happiness: Preliminary reliability and construct validation. *Social Indicators Research, 46*(2), 137–155.

Lyubomirsky, S., Sheldon, K. M., & Schkade, D. (2005). Pursuing happiness: The architecture of sustainable change. *Review of General Psychology, 9*(2), 111–131.

Lyubomirsky, S., Tkach, C., & Sheldon, K. M. (2004). [Pursuing sustained happiness through random acts of kindness and counting one's blessings: Tests of two six-week interventions]. Unpublished raw data.

Madden, W., Green, S., & Grant, A. M. (2011). A pilot study evaluating strengths-based coaching for primary school students: Enhancing engagement and hope. *International Coaching Psychology Review, 6*(1), 71–83.

Manassis, K., Lee, T. C., Bennett, K., Zhao, X. Y., Mendlowitz, S., Duda, S., et al. (2014). Types of parental involvement in CBT with anxious youth: A preliminary meta-analysis. *Journal of Consulting and Clinical Psychology, 82*(6), 1163–1172.

Manicavasagar, V., Horswood, D., Burckhardt, R., Lum, A., Hadzi-Pavlovic, D., & Parker, G. (2014). Feasibility and effectiveness of a web-based positive psychology program for youth mental health: Randomized controlled trial. *Journal of Medical Internet Research, 16*(6), 23–39.

Marion, D., Laursen, B., Zettergren, P., & Bergman, L. R. (2013). Predicting life satisfaction during middle adulthood from peer relationships during mid-adolescence. *Journal of Youth and Adolescence, 42*(8), 1299–1307.

Marques, S. C., Lopez, S. J., & Pais-Ribeiro, J. L. (2011). "Building hope for the future": A program to foster strengths in middle-school students. *Journal of Happiness Studies, 12*(1), 139–152.

Marques, S. C., Pais-Ribeiro, J. L., & Lopez, S. J. (2007). Validation of a Portuguese version of the Students' Life Satisfaction Scale. *Applied Research in Quality of Life, 2*(2), 83–94.

Marsh, H. W., Barnes, J., Cairns, L., & Tidman, M. (1984). Self-Description Questionnaire: Age and sex effects in the structure and level of self-concept for preadolescent children. *Journal of Educational Psychology, 76*(5), 940–956.

Martens, B. K., Witt, J. C., Elliott, S. N., & Darveaux, D. X. (1985). Teacher judgments concerning the acceptability of school-based interventions. *Professional Psychology: Research and Practice, 16*(2), 191–198.

Maslach, C., & Goldberg, J. (1999). Prevention of burnout: New perspectives. *Applied and Preventive Psychology, 7*(1), 63–74.

Masten, A. S. (2014). Invited commentary: Resilience and positive youth development frameworks in developmental science. *Journal of Youth and Adolescence, 43*(6), 1018–1024.

Masten, A. S., Cutuli, J. J., Herbers, J. E., & Reed, M. J. (2009). Resilience in development. In C. R. Snyder & S. J. Lopez (Eds.), *The Oxford handbook of positive psychology* (2nd ed., pp. 117–131). New York: Oxford University Press.

Masten, A. S., Roisman, G. I., Long, J. D., Burt, K. B., Obradović, J. R., Boelcke-Stennes, K., et al. (2005). Developmental cascades: Linking academic achievement and externalizing and internalizing symptoms over 20 years. *Developmental Psychology, 41*(5), 733–746.

McCabe, K., Bray, M. A., Kehle, T. J., Theodore, L. A., & Gelbar, N. W. (2011). Promoting happiness and life satisfaction in school children. *Canadian Journal of School Psychology, 26*(3), 177–192.

McCabe-Fitch, K. A. (2009). *Examination of the impact of an intervention in positive psychology on the happiness and life satisfaction of children.* Unpublished doctoral dissertation, University of Connecticut, Storrs.

McCullough, G., & Huebner, E. S. (2003). Life satisfaction reports of adolescents with learning disabilities and normally achieving adolescents. *Journal of Psychoeducational Assessment, 21*(4), 311–324.

McCullough, M. E., Emmons, R. A., & Tsang, J. A. (2002). The grateful disposition: A conceptual and empirical topography. *Journal of Personality and Social Psychology, 82*(1), 112–127.

McCullough, M. M. (2015). *Improving elementary teachers' well-being through a strength-based intervention: A multiple baseline single-case design.* Unpublished master's thesis, University of South Florida, Tampa, FL.

McDermott, D., & Hastings, S. (2000). Children: Raising future hopes. In C. R. Snyder (Ed.), *Handbook of hope: Theory, measures, and applications* (pp. 185–199). San Diego, CA: Academic Press.

McGrath, H., & Noble, T. (2011). *Bounce Back! A well-being and resilience program* (2nd ed.). Melbourne, Australia: Pearson Education.

McIntosh, K., Bennett, J. L., & Price, K. (2011). Evaluation of social and academic efforts of school-wide positive behaviour support in a Canadian school district. *Exceptionality Education International, 21*(1), 46–60.

McIntosh, K., Filter, K. J., Bennett, J. L., Ryan, C., & Sugai, G. (2010). Principles of sustainable prevention: Designing scale-up of school-wide positive behavior support to promote durable systems. *Psychology in the Schools, 47*(1), 5–21.

McLaughlin, K. A., Gadermann, A. M., Hwang, I., Sampson, N. A., Al-Hamzawi, A., Andrade, L. H., et al. (2012). Parent psychopathology and offspring mental disorders: Results from the WHO World Mental Health Surveys. *British Journal of Psychiatry, 200*, 290–299.

McMahan, M. M. (2013). *A longitudinal examination of high school students' group membership in a dual-factor model of mental health: Stability of mental health status and predictors of change* (doctoral dissertation). Retrieved from PsycInfo (Accession Number: 2013-99200-311).

McNulty, J. K., & Fincham, F. D. (2012). Beyond positive psychology?: Toward a contextual view of psychological processes and well-being. *American Psychologist, 67*(2), 101–110.

Merkas, M., & Brajsa-Zganec, A. (2011). Children with different levels of hope: Are there differences in their self-esteem, life satisfaction, social support, and family cohesion? *Child Indicators Research, 4*(3), 499–514.

Merrell, K. W., Carrizales, D., Feuerborn, L., Gueldner, B. A., & Tran, O. K. (2007). *Strong kids: A social and emotional learning curriculum for students in grades 3–5.* Baltimore: Brookes.

Miller, D. N., Nickerson, A. B., Chafouleas, S. M., & Osborne, K. M. (2008). Authentically happy school psychologists: Applications of positive psychology for enhancing professional satisfaction and fulfillment. *Psychology in the Schools, 45*(8), 679–692.

Miller, W. R., & Rollnick, S. (2013). *Motivational interviewing: Helping people change* (3rd ed.). New York: Guilford Press.

Mitchell, J., Vella-Brodrick, D., & Klein, B. (2010). Positive psychology and the Internet: A mental health opportunity. *E-Journal of Applied Psychology, 6*(2), 30–41.

Mitchell, M. M., & Bradshaw, C. P. (2013). Examining classroom influences on student perceptions of school climate: The role of classroom management and exclusionary discipline strategies. *Journal of School Psychology, 51*(5), 599–610.

Miyamoto, Y., & Ryff, C. D. (2011). Cultural difference in the dialectical and non-dialectical emotional styles and their implications for health. *Cognition and Emotion, 25*(1), 22–39.

Montgomery, C., & Rupp, A. A. (2005). A meta-analysis for exploring the diverse causes and effects of stress in teachers. *Canadian Journal of Education, 28*(3), 458–486.

Moor, I., Lampert, T., Rathmann, K., Kuntz, B., Kolip, P., Spallek, J., et al. (2014). Explaining educational inequalities in adolescent life satisfaction: Do health behaviour and gender matter? *International Journal of Public Health, 59*(2), 309–317.

Moore, S. A., Wildales-Benetiz, O., Carnazzo, K. W.,

Kim, E. K., Moffa, K., & Dowdy, E. (2015). Conducting universal complete mental health screening via student self-report. *Contemporary School Psychology, 19*(4), 253–267.

Mychailyszyn, M. P., Brodman, D. M., Read, K. L., & Kendall, P. C. (2012). Cognitive-behavioral school-based interventions for anxious and depressed youth: A meta-analysis of outcomes. *Clinical Psychology: Science and Practice, 19*(2), 129–153.

National Association of School Psychologists. (2010). *National Association of School Psychologists Principles for Professional Ethics*. Bethesda, MD: Author. Available at *www.nasponline.org*.

Navarro, D., Montserrat, C., Malo, S., Gonzalez, M., Casas, F., & Crous, G. (2015). Subjective well-being: What do adolescents say? *Child and Family Social Work*. Published online.

Nelson, J. R., Martella, R. M., & Marchand-Martella, N. (2002). Maximizing student learning: The effects of a comprehensive school-based program for preventing problem behaviors. *Journal of Emotional and Behavioral Disorders, 10*(3), 136–148.

Nelson, R. B., Schnorr, D., Powell, S., & Huebner, S. (2013). Building resilience in schools. In R. B. Mennuti, C. R. Christner, & A. Freeman (Eds.), *Cognitive-behavioral interventions in educational settings* (2nd ed., pp. 643–681). New York: Routledge.

Nowack, K. M. (1990). Initial development of an inventory to assess stress and health risk. *American Journal of Health Promotion, 4*(3), 173–180.

Oberle, E., Schonert-Reichl, K. A., & Zumbo, B. D. (2011). Life satisfaction in early adolescence: Personal, neighborhood, school, family, and peer influences. *Journal of Youth and Adolescence, 40*(7), 889–901.

Odou, N., & Vella-Brodrick, D. A. (2013). The efficacy of positive psychology interventions to increase well-being and the role of mental imagery ability. *Social Indicators Research, 110*(1), 111–129.

O'Grady, P. (2013). *Positive psychology in the elementary school classroom*. New York: Norton.

Olenik, C., Zdrojewski, N., & Bhattacharya, S. (2013). *Scan and review of youth development measurement tools*. Washington, DC: United States Agency for International Development. Available at *www.usaid. gov/sites/default/files/documents/2155/USAID%20 Life%20Skills%20Measurement%20Review%20 FINAL%20EXTERNAL%20REPORT.pdf*.

Orkibi, H., Ronen, T., & Assoulin, N. (2014). The subjective well-being of Israeli adolescents attending specialized school classes. *Journal of Educational Psychology, 106*(2), 515–526.

Otake, K., Shimai, S., Tanaka-Matsumi, J., Otsui, K., & Fredrickson, B. L. (2006). Happy people become happier through kindness: A counting kindnesses intervention. *Journal of Happiness Studies, 7*(3), 361–375.

Owens, R. L., & Patterson, M. M. (2013). Positive psychology interventions for children: A comparison of gratitude and best possible selves approaches. *Journal of Genetic Psychology, 174*(4), 403–428.

Oyserman, D., Bybee, D., & Terry, K. (2006). Possible selves and academic outcomes: How and when possible selves impel action. *Journal of Personality and Social Psychology, 91*(1), 188–204.

Park, N., & Huebner, E. S. (2005). A cross-cultural study of the levels and correlates of life satisfaction of adolescents. *Journal of Cross-Cultural Psychology, 36*(4), 444–456.

Park, N., & Peterson, C. (2006). Moral competence and character strengths among adolescents: The development and validation of the Values in Action Inventory of Strengths for Youth. *Journal of Adolescence, 29*(6), 891–909.

Park, N., Peterson, C., & Seligman, M. E. P. (2004). Strengths of character and well-being. *Journal of Social and Clinical Psychology, 23*(5), 603–619.

Parks, A. C., & Biswas-Diener, R. (2013). Positive interventions: Past, present, and future. In T. B. Kashdan & J. Ciarrochi (Eds.), *Mindfulness, acceptance, and positive psychology: The seven foundations of well-being* (pp. 140–165). Oakland, CA: Context Press/ New Harbinger.

Patterson, G. R., & Forgatch, M. S. (2005). *Parents and adolescents living together: Part 1. The basics* (2nd ed). Champaign, IL: Research Press.

Perez-Blasco, J., Viguer, P., & Rodrigo, M. F. (2013). Effects of a mindfulness-based intervention on psychological distress, well-being, and maternal self-efficacy in breast-feeding mothers: Results of a pilot study. *Archives of Women's Mental Health, 16*(3), 227–236.

Peterson, C., & Seligman, M. E. P. (2004). *Character strengths and virtues: A classification and handbook*. Washington, DC: American Psychological Association.

Powdthavee, N., & Vignoles, A. (2008). Mental health of parents and life satisfaction of children: A within-family analysis of intergenerational transmission of well-being. *Social Indicators Research, 88*(3), 397–422.

Proctor, C., Linley, P. A., & Maltby, J. (2009a). Youth life satisfaction measures: A review. *Journal of Positive Psychology, 4*(2), 128–144.

Proctor, C., Linley, P. A., & Maltby, J. (2009b). Youth life satisfaction: A review of the literature. *Journal of Positive Psychology, 10*(5), 583–630.

Proctor, C., Linley, P. A., & Maltby, J. (2010). Very happy youths: Benefits of very high life satisfaction among adolescents. *Social Indicators Research, 98*(3), 519–532.

Proctor, C., Tsukayama, E., Wood, A. M., Maltby, J., Fox Eades, J., & Linley, P. A. (2011). Strengths Gym: The impact of a character strengths-based intervention on the life satisfaction and well-being of adolescents. *Journal of Positive Psychology, 6*(5), 377–388.

Quinlan, D., Vella-Brodrick, D., Caldwell, J., & Swain, N. (2016). *It just makes my hopes rise: The student and teacher experience of strengths in the classroom.* Manuscript in preparation.

Quinlan, D., Vella-Brodrick, D., Gray, A., & Swain, N. (2016). *Teachers' strengths spotting matter: Student outcomes in a classroom strengths intervention.* Manuscript in preparation.

Quinlan, D. M., Swain, N., Cameron, C., & Vella-Brodrick, D. A. (2015). How "other people matter" in a classroom-based strengths intervention: Exploring interpersonal strategies and classroom outcomes. *Journal of Positive Psychology, 10*, 77–89.

Rashid, T. (2005) *Positive Psychotherapy Inventory.* Unpublished manuscript, University of Pennsylvania.

Rashid, T. (2015). Positive psychotherapy: A strength-based approach. *Journal of Positive Psychology, 10*(1), 25–40.

Rashid, T., & Anjum, A. (2008). Positive psychotherapy for young adults and children. In J. R. Z. Abela & B. L. Hankin (Eds.), *Handbook of depression in children and adolescents* (pp. 250–287). New York: Guilford Press.

Rashid, T., Anjum, A., Lennox, C., Quinlan, D., Niemiec, R. M., Mayerson, D., et al. (2013). Assessment of character strengths in children and adolescents. In C. Proctor & P. A. Linley (Eds.), *Research, applications, and interventions for children and adolescents: A positive psychology perspective* (pp. 81–115). New York: Springer.

Raskin, N. J., Rogers, C. R., & Witty, M. C. (2014). Client-centered therapy. In R. J. Corsini & D. Wedding (Eds.), *Current psychotherapies* (10th ed., pp. 95–150). Belmont, CA: Thomson Brooks/Cole.

Rees, G., & Dinisman, T. (2015). Comparing children's experiences and evaluations of their lives in 11 different countries. *Child Indicators Research, 8*(1), 5–31.

Reinke, W. M., Herman, K. C., & Stormont, M. (2013). Classroom-level positive behavior supports in schools implementing SW-PBIS: Identifying areas for enhancement. *Journal of Positive Behavior Interventions, 15*(1), 39–50.

Reinke, W. M., Stormont, M., Herman, K. C., Puri, R., & Goel, N. (2011). Supporting children's mental health in schools: Teacher perceptions of needs, roles, and barriers. *School Psychology Quarterly, 26*(1), 1–13.

Renshaw, T. L., & Cohen, A. S. (2014). Life satisfaction as a distinguishing indicator of college student functioning: Further validation of the two-continua model of mental health. *Social Indicators Research, 117*(1), 319–334.

Renshaw, T. L., Furlong, M. J., Dowdy, E., Rebelez, J., Smith, D. C., O'Malley, M. D., et al. (2014). Covital-

ity: A synergistic conception of adolescents' mental health. In M. J. Furlong, R. Gilman, & E. S. Huebner (Eds.), *Handbook of positive psychology in schools* (2nd ed., pp. 12–32). New York: Routledge/Taylor & Francis.

Renshaw, T. L., Long, A. C. J., & Cook, C. R. (2015). Assessing teachers' positive psychological functioning at work: Development and validation of the teacher Subjective Wellbeing Questionnaire. *School Psychology Quarterly, 30*(2), 289–306.

Reynolds, C. R., & Kamphaus, R. (2004). *Behavior Assessment System for Children* (2nd ed.). Circle Pines, MN: American Guidance Services.

Reynolds, S., Wilson, C., Austin, J., & Hooper, L. (2012). Effects of psychotherapy for anxiety in children and adolescents: A meta-analytic review. *Clinical Psychology Review, 32*(4), 251–262.

Robertson-Kraft, C., & Duckworth, A. L. (2014). True grit: Trait-level perseverance and passion for long-term goals predicts effectiveness and retention among novice teachers. *Teachers College Record, 116*(3), 1–27.

Roeser, R. W., Schonert-Reichl, K. A., Jha, A., Cullen, M., Wallace, L., Wilensky, R., et al. (2013). Mindfulness training and reductions in teacher stress and burnout: Results from two randomized, waitlist-control field trials. *Journal of Educational Psychology, 105*(3), 787–804.

Rooney, R., Hassan, S., Kane, R., Roberts, C. M., & Nesa, M. (2013). Reducing depression in 9–10 year old children in low SES schools: A longitudinal universal randomized controlled trial. *Behaviour Research and Therapy, 51*(12), 845–854.

Rosenberg, M. (1965). Society and the adolescent self-image. Princeton, NJ: Princeton University Press.

Roth, R., & Suldo, S. M., & Ferron, J. (2016). *Improving middle school students' subjective well-being: Efficacy of a multicomponent positive psychology intervention targeting small groups of youth.* Manuscript submitted for publication.

Ruini, C., Ottolini, F., Tomba, E., Belaise, C., Albieri, E., Visani, D., et al. (2009). School intervention for promoting psychological well-being in adolescence. *Journal of Behavior Therapy and Experimental Psychiatry, 40*(4) 522–532.

Rust, T., Diessner, R., & Reade, L. (2009). Strengths only or strengths and relative weaknesses?: A preliminary study. *Journal of Psychology: Interdisciplinary and Applied, 143*(5), 465–476.

Rye, M. S., Fleri, A. M., Moore, C. D., Worthington, E. L., Wade, N. G., Sandage, S. J., et al. (2012). Evaluation of an intervention designed to help divorced parents forgive their ex-spouse. *Journal of Divorce and Remarriage, 53*(3), 231–245.

Ryff, C. D., & Keyes, C. L. M. (1995). The structure of psychological well-being revisited. *Journal of Personality and Social Psychology, 69*(4), 719–727.

Ryff, C. D., Love, G. D., Miyamoto, Y., Markus, H. R.,

Curhan, K. B., Kitayama, S., et al. (2014). Culture and the promotion of well-being in east and west: Understanding varieties of attunement to the surrounding context. In G. A. Fava & C. Ruini (Eds.), *Increasing psychological well-being in clinical and educational settings* (pp. 1–21). Dordrecht, The Netherlands: Springer.

Saha, R., Huebner, E. S., Hills, K. J., Malone, P. S., & Valois, R. F. (2014). Social coping and life satisfaction in adolescents. *Social Indicators Research, 115*(1), 241–252.

Saha, R., Huebner, E. S., Suldo, S. M., & Valois, R. F. (2010). A longitudinal study of adolescent life satisfaction and parenting. *Child Indicators Research, 3*, 149–165.

Sarriera, J. C., Casas, F., Bedin, L., Abs, D., Strelhow, M. R., Gross-Manos, D., et al. (2015). Material resources and children's subjective well-being in eight countries. *Child Indicators Research, 8*(2), 199–209.

Scales, P. C., Benson, P. L., Moore, K. A., Lippman, L., Brown, B., & Zaff, J. F. (2008). Promoting equal developmental opportunity and outcomes among America's children and youth: Results from the National Promises Study. *Journal of Primary Prevention, 29*(1), 121–144.

Scheier, M. F., & Carver, C. S. (1985). Optimism, coping, and health: Assessment and implications of generalized outcome expectancies. *Health Psychology, 4*(2), 219–247.

Scheier, M. F., Carver, C. S., & Bridges, M. W. (1994). Distinguishing optimism from neuroticism (and trait anxiety, self-mastery, and self-esteem): A reevaluation of the Life Orientation Test. *Journal of Personality and Social Psychology, 67*(6), 1063–1078.

Schonert-Reichl, K. A., & Lawlor, M. S. (2010). The effects of a mindfulness-based education program on pre- and early adolescents' well-being and social and emotional competence. *Mindfulness, 1*(3), 137–151.

Schonert-Reichl, K. A., Oberle, E., Lawlor, M. S., Abbott, D., Thomson, K., Oberlander, T. F., et al. (2015). Enhancing cognitive and social–emotional development through a simple-to-administer mindfulness-based school program for elementary school children: A randomized controlled trial. *Developmental Psychology, 51*(1), 52–66.

Schueller, S. M. (2010). Preferences for positive psychology exercises. *Journal of Positive Psychology, 5*(3), 192–203.

Schwarz, B., Mayer, B., Trommsdorff, G., Ben-Arieh, A., Friedlmeier, M., Lubiewska, K., et al. (2012). Does the importance of parent and peer relationships for adolescents' life satisfaction vary across cultures? *Journal of Early Adolescence, 32*(1), 55–80.

Schwarzer, R., & Jerusalem, M. (1995). Generalized Self-Efficacy scale. In J. Weinman, S. Wright, & M. Johnston, *Measures in health psychology: A user's portfolio* (pp. 35–37). Windsor, UK: NFER-NELSON.

Seligman, M. E. P. (1990). *Learned optimism: How to change your mind and your life.* New York: Random House.

Seligman, M. E. P. (2002). *Authentic happiness: Using the new positive psychology to realize your potential for lasting fulfillment.* New York: Free Press.

Seligman, M. E. P. (2011). *Flourish: A visionary new understanding of happiness and well-being.* New York: Free Press.

Seligman, M. E. P., & Csikszentmihalyi, M. (2000). Positive psychology: An introduction. *American Psychologist, 55*(1), 5–14.

Seligman, M. E. P., Ernst, R. M., Gillham, J., Reivich, K., & Linkins, M. (2009). Positive education: Positive psychology and classroom interventions. *Oxford Review of Education, 35*(3), 293–311.

Seligman, M. E. P., Kaslow, N. J., Alloy, L. B., Peterson, C., Tanenbaum, R. L., & Abramson, L. Y. (1984). Attributional style and depressive symptoms among children. *Journal of Abnormal Psychology, 93*(2), 235–238.

Seligman, M. E. P., Steen, T. A., Park, N., & Peterson, C. (2005). Positive psychology progress: Empirical validation of interventions. *American Psychologist, 60*(5), 410–421.

Seligman, M. P., Reivich, K., Jaycox, L., & Gillham, J. (1995). *The optimistic child.* Boston: Houghton Mifflin.

Seligson, J. L., Huebner, E. S., & Valois, R. F. (2003). Preliminary validation of the Brief Multidimensional Students' Life Satisfaction Scale (BMSLSS). *Social Indicators Research, 61*(5), 121–145.

Seligson, J. L., Huebner, E. S., & Valois, R. F. (2005). An investigation of a brief life satisfaction scale with elementary school children. *Social Indicators Research, 73*(3), 355–374.

Senf, K., & Liau, A. K. (2013). The effects of positive interventions on happiness and depressive symptoms with an examination of personality as a moderator. *Journal of Happiness Studies, 14*(2), 591–612.

Shapira, L. B., & Mongrain, M. (2010). The benefits of self-compassion and optimism exercises for individuals vulnerable to depression. *Journal of Positive Psychology, 5*(5), 377–389.

Shek, D. T. L., & Liu, T. T. (2014). Life satisfaction in junior secondary school students in Hong Kong: A 3-year longitudinal study. *Social Indicators Research, 117*(3), 777–794.

Sheldon, K. M., Boehm, J. K., & Lyubomirsky, S. (2013). Variety is the spice of happiness: The hedonic adaptation prevention (HAP) model. In S. A. David, I. Boniwell, & A. C. Ayers (Eds.), *Oxford handbook of happiness* (pp. 901–914). Oxford, UK: Oxford University Press.

Sheldon, K. M., & Lyubomirsky, S. (2006a). Achieving sustainable gains in happiness: Change your actions, not your circumstances. *Journal of Happiness Studies, 7*(1), 55–86.

Sheldon, K. M., & Lyubomirsky, S. (2006b). How to increase and sustain positive emotion: The effects of expressing gratitude and visualizing best possible selves. *Journal of Positive Psychology, 1*(2), 73–82.

Sheldon, K. M., & Lyubomirsky, S. (2012). The challenge of staying happier: Testing the hedonic adaptation prevention model. *Personality and Social Psychology Bulletin, 38*(5), 670–680.

Shonin, E., Van Gordon, W., Compare, A., Zangeneh, M., & Griffiths, M. D. (2015). Buddhist-derived loving-kindness and compassion meditation for the treatment of psychopathology: A systematic review. *Mindfulness, 6*(5), 1161–1180.

Shoshani, A., & Steinmetz, S. (2014). Positive psychology at school: A school-based intervention to promote adolescents' mental health and well-being. *Journal of Happiness Studies, 15*(6), 1289–1311.

Sin, N. L., & Lyubomirsky, S. (2009). Enhancing well-being and alleviating depressive symptoms with positive psychology interventions: A practice-friendly meta-analysis. *Journal of Clinical Psychology: In Session, 65*(5), 467–487.

Siu, O. L., Cooper, C. L., & Phillips, D. R. (2014). Intervention studies on enhancing work well-being, reducing burnout, and improving recovery experiences among Hong Kong health care workers and teachers. *International Journal of Stress Management, 21*(1), 69–84.

Skinner, E. A., Kindermann, T. A., & Furrer, C. J. (2009). A motivational perspective on engagement and disaffection: Conceptualization and assessment of children's behavioral and emotional participation in academic activities in the classroom. *Educational and Psychological Measurement, 69*(3), 493–525.

Snyder, C. R. (2005). Measuring hope in children. In K. A. Moore & L. H. Lippman (Eds.), *What do children need to flourish?: Conceptualizing and measuring indicators of positive development* (pp. 61–73). New York: Springer.

Snyder, C. R., Harris, C., Anderson, J. R., Holleran, S. A., Irving, L. M., Sigmon, S. T., et al. (1991). The will and the ways: Development and validation of an individual-differences measure of hope. *Journal of Personality and Social Psychology, 60*(4), 570–585.

Snyder, C. R., Hoza, B., Pelham, W. E., Rapoff, M., Ware, L., Danovsky, M., et al. (1997). The development and validation of the children's hope scale. *Journal of Pediatric Psychology, 22*(3), 399–421.

Snyder, C. R., Rand, K. L., & Sigmon, D. R. (2005). Hope theory: A member of the positive psychology family. In C. R. Snyder & S. J. Lopez (Eds.), *Handbook of positive psychology* (pp. 257–276). New York: Oxford University Press.

Song, M. (2003). *Two studies on the Resilience Inventory (RI): Toward the goal of creating a culturally sensitive measure of adolescence resilience.* Unpublished doctoral dissertation, Harvard University.

Spence, S. H. (1998). A measure of anxiety symptoms among children. *Behavior Research and Therapy, 36*(5), 545–566.

Spilt, J. L., Koomen, H. M., & Thijs, J. T. (2011). Teacher wellbeing: The importance of teacher–student relationships. *Educational Psychology Review, 23*(4), 457–477.

Sprick, R. (2009). *CHAMPS: A proactive and positive approach to classroom management* (2nd ed.). Eugene, OR: Pacific Northwest.

Stansberry Beard, K. S., Hoy, W. K., & Woolfolk Hoy, A. (2010). Academic optimism of individual teachers: Confirming a new construct. *Teaching and Teacher Education, 26*(5), 1136–1144.

Steel, P., Schmidt, J., & Shultz, J. (2008). Refining the relationship between personality and subjective well-being. *Psychological Bulletin, 134*(1), 138–161.

Steinberg, L. (2004). *The ten basic principles of good parenting.* New York: Simon & Schuster.

Stewart-Brown, S., Tennant, A., Tennant, R., Platt, S., Parkinson, J., & Weich, S. (2009). Internal construct validity of the Warwick–Edinburgh Mental Well-Being Scale (WEMWBS): A Rasch analysis using data from the Scottish Health Education Population Survey. *Health and Quality of Life Outcomes, 7*, 15.

Stiglbauer, B., Gnambs, T., Gamsjäger, M., & Batinic, B. (2013). The upward spiral of adolescents' positive school experiences and happiness: Investigating reciprocal effects over time. *Journal of School Psychology, 51*(2), 231–242.

Strait, G. G., Smith, B. H., McQuillin, S., Terry, J., Swan, S., & Malone, P. S. (2012). A randomized trial of motivational interviewing to improve middle school students' academic performance. *Journal of Community Psychology, 40*(8), 1032–1039.

Sugai, G., Horner, R. H., Algozzine, R., Barrett, S., Lewis, T., Anderson, C., et al. (2010). *School-wide positive behavior support: Implementers' blueprint and self-assessment.* Eugene: University of Oregon. Retrieved August 15, 2015, from *www.pbis.org.*

Sugai, G., & Horner, R. R. (2006). A promising approach for expanding and sustaining school-wide positive behavior support. *School Psychology Review, 35*(2), 245.

Suldo, S. M., Bateman, L., & Gelley, C. D. (2014). Understanding and promoting school satisfaction in children and adolescents. In M. J. Furlong, R. Gilman, & E. S. Huebner (Eds.), *Handbook of positive psychology in schools* (2nd ed., pp. 365–380). New York: Routledge.

Suldo, S. M., Dedrick, R. F., Shaunessy-Dedrick, E., Fefer, S. A., & Ferron, J. (2015). Development and initial validation of the Coping with Academic Demands Scale (CADS): How students in accelerated high school curricula cope with school-related stressors. *Journal of Psychoeducational Assessment, 33*(4), 357–374.

Suldo, S. M., Dedrick, R. F., Shaunessy-Dedrick, E., Roth, R., & Ferron, J. (2015). Development and initial validation of the Student Rating of Environmental Stressors Scale (StRESS): Stressors faced by students in accelerated high school curricula. *Journal of Psychoeducational Assessment, 33*(4), 339–356.

Suldo, S. M., & Fefer, S. A. (2013). Parent–child relationships and well-being. In C. Proctor & P. A. Linley (Eds.), *Research, applications and interventions for children and adolescents: A positive psychology perspective* (pp. 131–147). New York: Springer.

Suldo, S. M., Frank, M. J., Chappel, A. M., Albers, M. M., & Bateman, L. P. (2014). American high school students' perceptions of determinants of life satisfaction. *Social Indicators Research, 118*(2), 485–514.

Suldo, S. M., Friedrich, A. A., & Michalowski, J. (2010). Factors that limit and facilitate school psychologists' involvement in mental health services. *Psychology in the Schools, 47*(4), 354–373.

Suldo, S. M., Friedrich, A. A., White, T., Farmer, J., Minch, D., & Michalowski, J. (2009). Teacher support and adolescents' subjective well-being: A mixed-methods investigation. *School Psychology Review, 38*(1), 67–85.

Suldo, S. M., Gelley, C. D., Roth, R. A., & Bateman, L. P. (2015). Influence of peer social experiences on positive and negative indicators of mental health among high school students. *Psychology in the Schools, 52*(5), 431–446.

Suldo, S. M., Gormley, M., DuPaul, G., & Anderson-Butcher, D. (2014). The impact of school mental health on student and school-level academic outcomes: Current status of the research and future directions. *School Mental Health, 6*(2), 84–98.

Suldo, S. M., Hearon, B. V., Bander, B., McCullough, M., Garofano, J., Roth, R., et al. (2015). Increasing elementary school students' subjective well-being through a classwide positive psychology intervention: Results of a pilot study. *Contemporary School Psychology, 19*(4), 300–311.

Suldo, S. M., Hearon, B. V., Dickinson, S., Esposito, E., Wesley, K. L., Lynn, C., et al. (2015). Adapting positive psychology interventions for use with elementary school children. *NASP Communiqué, 43*(8), 4–8.

Suldo, S. M., & Huebner, E. S. (2004a). Does life satisfaction moderate the effects of stressful life events on psychopathological behavior during adolescence? *School Psychology Quarterly, 19*(2), 93–105.

Suldo, S. M., & Huebner, E. S. (2004b). The role of life satisfaction in the relationship between authoritative parenting dimensions and adolescent problem behavior. *Social Indicators Research, 66*(1–2), 165–195.

Suldo, S. M., & Huebner, E. S. (2006). Is extremely high life satisfaction during adolescence advantageous? *Social Indicators Research, 78*(2), 179–203.

Suldo, S. M., Minch, D. R., & Hearon, B. V. (2015). Adolescent life satisfaction and personality characteristics: Investigating relationships using a five factor model. *Journal of Happiness Studies, 16*(4), 965–983.

Suldo, S. M., Savage, J. A., & Mercer, S. (2014). Increasing middle school students' life satisfaction: Efficacy of a positive psychology group intervention. *Journal of Happiness Studies, 15*(1), 19–42.

Suldo, S. M., & Shaffer, E. J. (2008). Looking beyond psychopathology: The dual factor model of mental health in youth. *School Psychology Review, 37*(1), 52–68.

Suldo, S. M., Thalji, A., & Ferron, J. (2011). Longitudinal academic outcomes predicted by early adolescents' subjective well-being, psychopathology, and mental health status yielded from a dual factor model. *Journal of Positive Psychology, 6*(1), 17–30.

Suldo, S. M., Thalji-Raitano, A., Hasemeyer, M., Gelley, C. D., & Hoy, B. (2013). Understanding middle school students' life satisfaction: Does school climate matter? *Applied Research in Quality of Life, 8*(2), 169–182.

Suldo, S. M., Thalji-Raitano, A., Kiefer, S. M., & Ferron, J. (in press). Conceptualizing high school students' mental health through a dual-factor model. *School Psychology Review*.

Terry, J., Strait, G., McQuillin, S., & Smith, B. H. (2014). Dosage effects of motivational interviewing on middle-school students' academic performance: Randomized evaluation of one versus two sessions. *Advances in School Mental Health Promotion, 7*(1), 62–74.

Tilly, W. D. III. (2014). The evolution of school psychology to science-based practice: Problem solving and the three-tiered model. In P. L. Harrison & A. Thomas (Eds.), *Best practices in school psychology: Professional foundation* (pp. 17–36). Bethesda, MD: National Association of School Psychologists.

Thompson, E. R. (2007). Development and validation of an internationally reliable short-form of the Positive and Negative Affect Schedule (PANAS). *Journal of Cross-Cultural Psychology, 38*(2), 227–242.

Tkach, C., & Lyubomirsky, S. (2006). How do people pursue happiness?: Relating personality, happiness increasing strategies, and well-being. *Journal of Happiness Studies, 7*(2), 183–225.

Tolan, P. H., & Larsen, R. (2014). Trajectories of life satisfaction during middle school: Relations to developmental–ecological microsystems and student functioning. *Journal of Research on Adolescence, 24*(3), 497–511.

Tschannen-Moran, M., & Hoy, A. W. (2001). Teacher efficacy: Capturing an elusive construct. *Teaching and Teacher Education, 17*(7), 783–805.

van Horn, J. E., Taris, T. W., Schaufeli, W. B., & Schreurs, P. J. G. (2004). The structure of occupational well-being: A study among Dutch teachers. *Journal of Occupational and Organizational Psychology,* 77(3), 365–375.

Veronneau, M.-H., Koestner, R. F., & Abela, J. R. Z. (2005). Intrinsic need satisfaction and well-being in children and adolescents: An application of the self-determination theory. *Journal of Social and Clinical Psychology, 24*(2), 280–292

Walker, H. M., Horner, R. H., Sugai, G., Bullis, M., Sprague, J. R., Bricker, D., et al. (1996). Integrated approaches to preventing antisocial behavior patterns among school-age children and youth. *Journal of Emotional and Behavioral Disorders, 4*(4), 194–209.

Ware, J. E., Snow, K. K., Kosinski, M., & Gandek, B. (1993). *SF-36 Health Survey Manual and Interpretation Guide.* Boston: The Health Institute.

Warner, R. M., & Vroman, K. G. (2011). Happiness inducing behaviors in everyday life: An empirical assessment of "the how of happiness." *Journal of Happiness Studies, 12*(6), 1063–1082.

Watkins, C. L., & Slocum, T. A. (2003). The components of direct instruction. *Journal of Direct Instruction, 3*(2), 75–110.

Watson, D., Clark, L. A., & Tellegen, A. (1988). Development and validation of brief measures of positive and negative affect: The PANAS scales. *Journal of Personality and Social Psychology, 54*(6), 1063–1070.

Weist, M. D., Lever, N. A., Bradshaw, C. P., & Owens, J. S. (Eds.). (2014). *Handbook of school mental health: Research, training, practice, and policy* (2nd ed.). New York: Springer.

Weisz, J. R., & Kazdin, A. E. (2010). *Evidence-based psychotherapies for children and adolescents* (2nd ed.). New York: Guilford Press.

Weisz, J. R., Sandler, I. N., Durlak, J. A., & Anton, B. S. (2005). Promoting and protecting youth mental health through evidence-based prevention and treatment. *American Psychologist, 60*(6), 628–648.

Wentzel, K. R. (1993). Motivation and achievement in early adolescence: The role of multiple classroom goals. *Journal of Early Adolescence, 13*(1), 4–20.

West, A. E., Weinstein, S. M., Peters, A. T., Katz, A. C., Henry, D. B., Cruz, R. A., et al. (2014). Child- and family-focused cognitive-behavioral therapy for pediatric bipolar disorder: A randomized clinical trial. *Journal of the American Academy of Child and Adolescent Psychiatry, 53*(11), 1168–1178.

White, M. A., & Waters, L. E. (2015). A case study of "the good school": Examples of the use of Peterson's strengths-based approach with students. *Journal of Positive Psychology, 10*(1), 69–76.

Wilmes, J., & Andresen, S. (2015). What does "good childhood" in a comparative perspective mean?: An explorative comparison of child well-being in Nepal and Germany. *Child Indicators Research, 8*(1), 33–47.

World Health Organization. (1948). *Constitution of the World Health Organization.* Geneva, Switzerland: Author.

Yeager, D. S., & Walton, G. M. (2011). Social–psychological interventions in education: They're not magic. *Review of Educational Research, 81*(2), 267–301.

You, S., Dowdy, E., Furlong, M. J., Renshaw, T., Smith, D. C., & O'Malley, M. D. (2014). Further validation of the Social and Emotional Health Survey for high school students. *Applied Quality of Life Research, 9*(4), 997–1015.

You, S., Furlong, M. J., Felix, E., & O'Malley, M. D. (2015). Validation of the Social and Emotional Health Survey for five sociocultural groups: Multigroup invariance and latent mean analyses. *Psychology in the Schools, 52*(4), 349–362.

Index

Page numbers followed by *f* indicate figure, *t* indicate table